The Portable Ethicist for Mental Health Professionals

Other Books by the Authors

The Portable Guide to Testifying in Court for Mental Health Professionals: An A–Z Guide to Being an Effective Witness (2005), John Wiley & Sons, Inc.

The Portable Lawyer for Mental Health Professionals: An A–Z Guide to Protecting Your Clients, Your Practice, and Yourself, second edition (2004), John Wiley & Sons, Inc.

The Portable Ethicist for Mental Health Professionals
A Complete Guide to Responsible Practice

Second Edition

With HIPAA Update

Thomas L. Hartsell Jr., JD
and
Barton E. Bernstein, JD, LMSW

WILEY

JOHN WILEY & SONS, INC.

Library of Congress Cataloging-in-Publication Data:

Hartsell, Thomas L. (Thomas Lee), 1955-
  The portable ethicist for mental health professionals: a complete guide to responsible practice: with HIPAA update/by Thomas L. Hartsell Jr., Barton E. Bernstein.—2nd ed.
        p. ; cm.
  Bernstein's name appears first on the earlier ed.
  Includes bibliographical references and index.
  ISBN 978-0-470-14030-7 (pbk. : alk. paper)
  1. Mental health personnel–Professional ethics. 2. Psychiatric ethics. 3. United States. Health Insurance Portability and Accountability Act of 1996.
I. Bernstein, Barton E. II. Title.
  [DNLM: 1. United States. Health Insurance Portability and Accountability Act of 1996. 2. Psychiatry–ethics. 3. Codes of Ethics. 4. Confidentiality.
5. Professional-Patient Relations–ethics. WM 62 H335p 2008]
  RC455. 2.E8B476 2008
  174'.2–dc22

                                                    2007045712

Printed in the United States of America
SKY10082568_082124

To all of the mental health practitioners who struggle to ethically serve their clients.

Contents

PART I
CLIENT ISSUES

PART II

ETHICS CODES AND LICENSING

PART III

PRACTICE CONSIDERATIONS

PART IV

PROFESSIONAL ISSUES

PART V

SPECIAL THERAPY CONSIDERATIONS

Preface

Having been longtime observers of the mental health profession, we have come to know the value and benefits that its professionals offer to consumers of their services. Unfortunately, many of the consumers whom professionals take into therapy try to do them harm in return. With a proliferation of licensing boards and other regulatory authorities, consumers have easier and more numerous options to seek redress for perceived malevolent and negligent acts. With the advent of the Health Insurance Portability and Accountability Act (HIPAA) Privacy and Security Rules, mental health professional clients come to us for assistance with a state licensing board complaint while seeking our help with a duplicate complaint filed by the same client with the Office of Civil Rights or the Centers for Medicare and Medicaid. The same therapist may hold two or more state licenses and each board may pursue its own investigation, disciplinary action, and sanctioning. Add to this, membership in professional organizations and specialty certifications, and you can see just how many outlets a client wishing to do harm or mischief to a mental health professional has to choose from.

The world is not a kinder and gentler place for mental health professionals. Professional associations, licensing boards, the federal government, certifying authorities, media, and clients are quick to judge negatively and punish the conduct of mental health professionals. There are more technical rules in place for mental health professionals to be aware of and to comply with. Jurisprudence exams are a direct result of the complexities in ethical codes and legal statutes and the need for regulatory authorities to increase knowledge and compliance with all of these rules and requirements of practice. It is much easier and more probable now for an overworked, undercompensated, and unappreciated mental health professional to make a technical mistake that results in sanctioning even if the client has not been harmed or has even benefited from the therapy.

There has never been a more precarious time to practice one of the mental health disciplines. It is our goal to present ethical information and advice on how mental health professionals can practice with less risk of harm from clients. We want the book to be both a guide and a practice aid for practitioners as well as a teaching tool for instructors in mental health discipline educational programs. We weave in HIPAA rules where applicable as well as the ethical codes and canons of the major national professional associations. We devote entire chapters to identifying risky and dangerous clients.

Practitioners must remember, though, that they need to become knowledgeable about the specific state rules and statutes for the state and locations where they are providing services. It is not possible in a book of this length to be state specific, although the major ethical principles are applicable across the country.

Many years ago, the authors were asked to serve on a panel of experts; the topic was "Ethical Problems of Mental Health Professionals." The other two panel members were both providers in the field of mental health; one was a PhD psychologist employed by a fledgling managed care company and the other was a clergyman who, at about age 40, decided to earn a counseling degree and change professions from the ministry to counseling. Armed with his advanced degree, he was pursuing a career as a counselor in a group practice.

When we assembled to prepare for the presentation, both mental health professionals were ready to deal with global questions, such as counseling with children about abortion, dealing with "tough love," or the ethical consequences of needed treatment with limited funds. They wanted to discuss the big picture, ethical dilemmas that would make the participants think. These were problems that would evoke a thought process but would not necessarily provide concrete answers the participants could rely on and carry back to their offices. So the question arose: Did the attendees want to learn how to think or did they seek some practical suggestions about the ethical nuts and bolts of their profession?

When we suggested that ethics, in our opinion, concerned the published ethical canons or codes of their professions, we received only a blank stare. The psychologist allowed that she had taken an ethics course in graduate school about 10 years ago but remembered little about it; while the counselor admitted he had never taken a course specifically called "ethics," but he received annual copies of the licensing law that contained the ethical codes. And where were these codes now? Lying unread in the bottom of his desk drawer, available to be studied on a moment's notice should a complaint ever be filed against him with the state licensing board.

We were shocked and disappointed. As advocates and practicing attorneys who have represented mental health professionals before licensing boards, we assumed (incorrectly, apparently) that when the subject of ethics came up, we were referring to canons of ethics promulgated either by licensing boards or by national professional organizations. We were aware of the many individuals who had been disciplined by local boards or threatened with expulsion by national organizations. We faithfully read the publications of the various mental health disciplines that list by name and city the professionals disciplined for all manner of infractions or violations of ethical guidelines and list those who have been found guilty of misconduct. These individuals needed representation to protect their licenses, livelihood, and reputation. General postulates of ethical rights and wrongs are interesting topics to banter around in a profound conversation, but as attorneys educated in the adversary system, we felt that the target audience of mental health professionals would be more interested in ethical questions such as: How many ways are mental health professionals vulnerable? What does the state require regarding informed consent? Can you accept a referral fee for referring clients? What are some obvious and some subtle boundary violations or dual relationships? What kind of records can you keep and what kind of records must you keep? Guidance for all these problem areas is set forth in the published codes of ethics of the state board (and published in one form or another in the board rules of most sister states).

The argument was long and spirited without resolution. Since we couldn't agree on anything else, each of the four presenters spoke for about 10 minutes followed by a question period. And what were the questions? Just what we had anticipated. None of the participants were interested in global issues or clever hypothetical ethical dilemmas that taxed their intellect to find options or solutions. Instead, they wanted to know about records, preservation and documentation, prohibited client relationships, reporting obligations concerning another therapist who was acting inappropriately, and how to deal with managed care and remain ethical while earning a living.

Most of the participants, licensed people all, were concerned with self-preservation and making a living in peace. They wanted knowledgeable individuals to discuss the important parts of their specific ethical canons so they would recognize any ethical problem on the horizon and could conform their conduct to the requirements of their local board and national organizations. Perhaps they might be inspired to read the codes of conduct, but failing that, they would, at least, through seminars and workshops, understand the crucial points and most commonly violated rules of their profession. So the lawyers answered specific and general questions like these: How long does the professional have to keep and preserve records? What is therapeutic confidentiality? Is what is told to a therapist 100 percent confidential? What happens, ethically, if you know a colleague has had sex with a client or is impaired by drugs or alcohol?

What we discovered in our prepanel conversation with the counselor and the psychologist was frightening. Professionals who had graduated from universities only a few years ago might have been exposed to a course in ethics, while those who received their degrees more than 10 years ago viewed professional ethics in summary: "We know the difference between right and wrong, and we don't do what's wrong." Common sense will prevail. They were shocked when we told them that in a conflict between common sense and the licensing law, the licensing law prevails.

More recently, we learned that mental health professionals are still not truly familiar with the canons of ethics and rules that govern their delivery of mental health services. Many have been slow to educate themselves regarding the HIPAA Privacy and Security Rules and are still not compliant.

From the point of view of the federal government, a state licensing board, or the disciplinary committee of a national organization, these mental health professionals are dangerously naive. Many ethical violations are not intentional wrongs, consciously and maliciously performed, but are actions that in years past might have gone unnoticed and unpunished. Today they are understood by the consuming public and the board members appointed to represent the consumer of mental health services.

When the authors first started representing mental health professionals, there were few complaints to state boards. Today, litigious clients with a perceived wrong realize they can request a free investigation by federal authorities, a state agency, or national organization at no inconvenience and no expense. In fact, mental health professionals are required to inform clients how and to whom they can file complaints if they are dissatisfied with the services provided. Thereafter the only question is whether a rule or regulation has been violated. Heartache, expense, embarrassment, and notoriety await the professional who receives a letter from a licensing entity or regulatory authority suggesting that his or her future is on the line. An adverse ruling can ruin a professional career and deprive a person of a lifetime of positive community service.

Practitioners are anxious to know, understand, and honor the rules and regulations of their profession. Once they put these commandments in place, practitioners can relax, proceed with self-assurance, and serve the community with honor and distinction.

The mental health profession is in a constant and often anxiety-producing state of flux. Practices, procedures, and rules are changing with lightning speed. Earning a living is complex enough without worrying about a disciplinary committee breathing over your shoulder. And how can you avoid this? By knowing the rules in the same way that an athlete knows the rules, a lawyer knows courtroom procedures, or a musician knows the score.

This book can help avoid a tragedy. The tragedy is that a person completes undergraduate and perhaps graduate school. The graduate is then armed with advanced degrees and pursues either the advanced designations of his or her professional organization or applies for and receives a state license. The degree and the license are framed and proudly mounted on the wall of the clinical office, and then a complaint is filed. Some unhappy client writes to the state licensing board, the federal authorities, or the national organization and an investigation begins. Then, if the investigation uncovers an act that is unethical or can be construed to be unethical, the license, loaned to the licensee in the first place, is withdrawn. The licensee can no longer practice the profession for which he or she invested so much study, expense, dedication, and hard work. Fines and even imprisonment can be imposed for serious violations.

This tragedy can be avoided by practicing ethically. And how can you practice ethically? By knowing the ethical canons, codes, and guidelines and practicing within them. But first, you must learn what they are. That is why this book was written and has been revised.

Throughout this book, we have selectively used different codes and code summaries to illustrate problems being discussed. References to the HIPAA Privacy and Security Rules are included where appropriate. When a real problem occurs, practitioners should consult the most current version of the ethical canons in their jurisdiction, the HIPAA Privacy and Security Rules as well as the national standards of their discipline. Ignorance of any of these rules and regulations is not an excuse when a complaint is filed and some disciplinary board or the federal government is called on to act. Almost all codes and rules can be found on the Internet. Others may be obtained by a telephone call or a letter of inquiry to the publishing authority.

Today the codes are understood by the consuming public and the boards appointed to represent the customer of mental health services. You, the professional, must be as well-versed as the consumer and the boards appointed to represent them.

We encourage mental health professionals to get to know a local attorney who is either well versed in the rules and laws governing their discipline or who is inclined to learn and study them. The attorney-client privilege is much stronger than the patient-therapist privilege. It would be a rare circumstance whereby an attorney would have to report a therapist for an ethical mistake or violation. We have always made ourselves available for consultation when a mental health professional has a question. We would prefer to spend a few minutes helping someone avoid a problem than many hours and many dollars to assist that person when trouble comes calling.

The time to call a knowledgeable attorney is as soon as a potential ethical dilemma presents itself, before mistakes of commission or omission occur. The amount spent on legal services is usually far less when advising a client on how to avoid or prevent a problem. It is harder and more expensive to defend a mental health professional after the facts or events have occurred. Risk management means avoiding risk where possible and ameliorating problems when they arise.

We include study or research questions at the end of each chapter to encourage review and study of individual state ethical canons and statutes. We also include a jurisprudence exam in Appendix D, to test state-specific knowledge of ethical and legal rules and principles.

THOMAS L. HARTSELL JR.
BARTON E. BERNSTEIN

Acknowledgments

It is hard to believe that it has been a decade since Bart and I first worked on a project for John Wiley & Sons. The same folks I have thanked and credited for inspiration in the past are still there for me. For that fact and for all of the publishing professionals involved, I continue to be very appreciative. Working with Wiley has generated two careers as authors. I love you all.

My biggest shout out goes to Barbara, my wife, my best friend, companion, cheerleader, critic, nurse, and supporter. Lady, you mean the world to me.

Right behind her I have to express my deep affection and delight in my special four-legged pal, Dexter, my Jack Russell terrier. He is like a fine wine, getting better with age. I miss him almost as much as I miss Barbara when I am away.

Speaking of fine wine, my parents, Tom and Julie Hartsell, enjoying their 55th year of wedded bliss, continue to give me support and inspiration to be a better person. Bless you both.

I would like to congratulate my in-laws, Bill and Paula Edwards, who celebrated their 50th wedding anniversary last year. They, too, are an inspiration. The Colonel is a West Point graduate and retired army officer, and I would like publicly to thank him and Paula for their service and sacrifice for all of us. And for Barbara.

To my sons, Ryan and Jason, and stepsons, Glenn and Chandler, you have my thanks and Barbara's for becoming fine, productive young adults despite our flawed parenting. You are making us proud and happy.

To my program director and boss at Southern Methodist University (SMU), Dr. Tony Picchioni, thank you for allowing me to become a contributing faculty member in the two wonderful programs, Conflict Resolution and Counseling, that you were so instrumental in establishing. You have presented me with wonderful opportunities that have enriched my life. I hope I always warrant your trust and confidence.

Last but definitely not least, I want to thank my mentor, my good friend, and my collaborator, Bart Bernstein, for all that he has done and continues to do for me. Bart, I hope I am still as intellectually active, curious, and sound as you are when I get an equal number of years under my belt. Keep on being you.

T. L. H.

Thank you to my ever-loving, patient, brilliant, and supportive wife, Donna Jean Bernstein, with special thanks for her continuing enthusiasm and confirmation. She set the tone and provided the inspiration for this edition.

To my children, Alon Samuel Bernstein, merchant, and Talya Bernstein Galaganov, lawyer and mother of my grandchildren, Sima Galaganov and Haya Galaganov, and her husband, Misha Galaganov, professor of music, and to my stepdaughter, Amy Huck, with good wishes as she embarks on her life's accomplishments.

To my sisters, Rona Mae Solberg and Dr. Berna Gae Haberman, and her husband, Wolf (Bill) Haberman, and in loving memory of my brother-in law, Dr. Myron "Mike" Solberg, professor emeritus, Rutgers University. And in loving memory of my parents, Samuel and Suetelle Bernstein, who always thought Fall River, Massachusetts, was the Garden of Eden.

With special thanks to my colleague, friend, and distinguished attorney and lead author Tom Hartsell who has continued to inspire, invigorate, and motivate both of us to serve the legal and mental health communities, me as a grand old man of the law and Tom as a distinguished professor and lecturer in the fields of ethics, law, alternate dispute resolution, and peaceful decision making. With Tom, conflict resolution is always a pleasure.

B. E. B.

We again want to thank the staff at John Wiley & Sons, Inc. for realizing the importance of the connection between law and the mental health professions and for understanding the magnitude of the ethical component in any mental health practitioner's practice. We especially want to thank Isabel Pratt for giving us the opportunity to update this material with a second edition and for her support of this project.

We thank Nancy Marcus Land of Publications Development Company for her terrific job in editing our work.

In writing this book, the authors received invaluable support, encouragement, and inspiration from family members, friends, and colleagues. Encouragement came from many special friends. We want to mention especially Dr. Tony Picchioni, LPC, LMFT, program director of Conflict Resolution and Counseling, Southern Methodist University; Dr. Hal Barkley, LPC, LMFT, Director of Counseling, Southern Methodist University; Dr. Gay McAlister, LPC, RED, Associate Director: Supervision, Counseling, Southern Methodist University; Terry Towne, president, and Gayle Sutch, past president, of the Art Therapy Credentials Board; and all the mental health professionals we have had the pleasure of meeting and working with over the years.

T. L. H.
B. E. B.

Introduction

Professional ethics can be considered in terms of both a big picture and a little picture. The big picture consists of countless complex philosophical dilemmas that keep graduate students, ethicists, and philosophers in business, endlessly pondering and filling the literature with the "right" and "wrong" answers to unanswerable problems and esoteric, hypothetical, interpersonal ethical situations. The little picture consists of everyday situations that therapists have faced since the dawn of the mental health profession. Such situations, if perceived incorrectly, can cause a professional to be summarily expelled from his or her national organization or subjected to severe disciplinary action revoking his or her license to practice within the profession. The net effect is that the professional loses the means to earn a living in his or her chosen field.

The big picture is heady, deep, penetrating, and profound. However, in this era of credentials, initials, and licenses, the little picture is usually more important to the treating practitioner. These testimonials grant the professional the cloak of governmental authority, representing to the consumer the approval of the state authorizing the individual to practice a profession. In most jurisdictions, the psychologist, social worker, counselor, therapist, addictions specialist, or mental health provider of any description cannot practice without a license. Therefore, it is important for practicing professionals to protect their credentials from being compromised by charges of an ethical violation.

Definitions

A composite of dictionary definitions of ethics would include:

- The study of standards of conduct and moral judgment
- The system of morals of a particular person, religion, group, and so on

- Of or relating to ethics or morality, relating to or dealing with questions of right or wrong
- Involving or expressing approval or disapproval
- Being in accord with approved standards of behavior socially or in a professional code
- Conforming to professionally endorsed principles or practices
- Pertaining to or dealing with morals or the principles of morality: pertaining to right and wrong in conduct
- In accordance with rules or standards for right conduct or practice, especially the standards of a profession

Ethics has been defined in dictionaries, philosophical tomes, literary and religious works, countless theoretical treatises, and psychological and psychiatric texts. Definitions such as those listed are subject to different interpretations, and making a decision about what is or is not considered ethical is often relative to a particular situation.

Establishing a rule or guideline for individual conduct becomes even more difficult when one considers that each state has its own professional ethical standards, and national and state mental health organizations create, augment, and interpret published public ethical standards differently. The federal government now plays a greater role as a result of the Health Insurance Portability and Accountability Act (HIPAA) Privacy and Security Rules that are in force. In addition, each mental health professional has individual inclinations influenced by theoretical orientation, religious background, training, education, experience, and biology. An individual's total feelings of what is right and wrong affect decisions in any given situation. The result by any objective standard is a somewhat unworkable and amorphous set of guidelines that may offer little specific help to the practitioner who is trying to practice in an ethical manner and maintain a professional license at the same time.

Even the various mental health disciplines differ on fundamental issues. Consider the following questions and their underlying ethical concerns:

- Is it ever acceptable to date a client, and if so, when and under what circumstances?
- How long must records be maintained for adults? For children?
- How much information must be divulged to a parent after a child has requested confidentiality?
- Exactly what must a therapist do when he learns a colleague is seducing a client, has covertly entered into a business arrangement with a client, has traded (bought or sold) stocks based on insider information learned from a patient, cheated an insurance company by submitting fraudulent claims or overbilling, or otherwise has violated permissible boundaries and ethical norms?
- If a parent brings a child to the therapist for treatment, who is the client, the parent or the child? If it is the child, can the therapist date the parent? Or can the therapist date the uncle of the child?

Can one depend on a gut reaction or a broad definition of common sense to protect a license? The answer is a resounding "No"! When common sense and published rules conflict, the published rules should control the therapist's conduct. The professional against whom a complaint is filed cannot build a defense on the basis of a purely common-sense approach to an ethical problem.

Personal Ethics versus Professional Standards

General ethical principles might serve as a comprehensive guide for social or professional conduct, but if mental health professionals want to remain members in good standing of a local, state, or national organization, they must scrupulously adhere to the published standards of that organization. Likewise, mental health professionals who want to keep and maintain a professional license must unerringly honor the published rules, regulations, and mandates of the licensing board or whatever state agency publishes, enforces, and disseminates the board's rules. For those states that have no directly published standards, but incorporate by reference national published standards into state board rules, there is a double whammy. If a rule is violated, the individual is disciplined by both the national organization and the state licensing board.

Practice Implications

An awareness of your personal moral code in relation to knowledge of the professional standards and regulations of your state and national associations and licensing boards dictates that in the area of mental health ethics, common sense, gut reactions, individual morality training, and personal preference—*even actions which in the opinion of the clinician are in the best interest of the client*—take a back seat to the published guidelines of the profession. As noted, in most jurisdictions a professional license is required to practice. Thus, competence, experience, and compassion are of no value if the practitioner cannot share that expertise with the public (the consumer) because of a revoked license.

In a simpler age, the mental health professional's personal instincts and moral compass would usually provide a protective shield, shelter, or umbrella. A dependable feeling guided the conscience and thoughts of what was right and wrong. The pendulum could shift from one side to the other, depending on the individual therapist, the client, and the circumstances. Blatant forms of ethical violations could be avoided by old-fashioned common sense.

In today's litigious society, however, where the "someone has to pay" mentality pervades the minds of consumers, an ethical complaint often follows even when a malpractice case is not pursued. One reason, perhaps, is that filing a complaint and letting the board know of alleged inappropriate activity might be good therapy for that individual. Another reason seems to be that state tort reform measures have made it more difficult for consumers in some states to bring, maintain, and prevail in malpractice suits against health-care professionals. Filing a complaint against a mental health professional costs the client nothing but a little time in filling out and forwarding the complaint. State rules and HIPAA require mental health professionals to advise their clients on how and where to submit complaints they may have with the treatment provider.

"Getting even" for an actual or perceived wrong is as American as apple pie. What better way is there to get back at someone than having the federal government or the alleged offender's state licensing board or a national organization fight the battle for the allegedly wounded consumer? These entities serve as free compliance investigators, enforcers, and punishers through their complaint processes.

So what does this mean for the practitioner? It is simple. Read the provisions of the HIPAA Privacy and Security Rules as well as the canons of the professional organizations and state licensing boards. Understand them and don't violate them. Treat each regulation as a commandment or as gospel, and avoid compromising situations.

But what happens when the professional follows all the rules and is still confronted with an ethical dilemma?

How This Book Is Organized

This book covers common ethical problems encountered by providers, educators, supervisors, and consumers of mental health services. The goal is to avoid ethical confrontations and conflicts by recognizing what they are and how they come about; to attain and maintain an ethical and profitable practice, one must know the rules and regulations of the profession and be guided by them.

The book is divided into five parts: Client Issues, Ethical Codes and Licensing, Practice Considerations, Professional Issues, and Special Therapy Considerations. Each part is subdivided into chapters. Each chapter follows a similar format: first, a vignette or vignettes illustrate the basic ethical dilemma. Second, a big-picture explanation of the problem indicates how the situation in the vignette can be used to clarify other similar situations frequently confronting practitioners. Third, selected passages from the various federal, state, and national organization codes or canons of ethics portray the general concept and ethical guidelines that, if violated, can lead to a malpractice suit, loss of license, fine, imprisonment, or removal from membership in a national organization. The *Ethical Flash Points* serve as maxims for the practitioner throughout his or her professional career. Finally, we have

included suggested research projects and discussion questions at the
end of each chapter to encourage greater reflection and study into ethical issues presented in the chapter.

Using the Vignettes

The vignettes can be used for general discussion or assigned for analysis to individual members of the class. (Supervisors required to instruct
their supervisees in ethics could assign the text and use it in much the
same way as an educator or professor.) In general, the discussion questions might be as follows:

- What ethical problems are involved in the vignette?
- List or itemize the various options available to the therapist. (*Note:*
  Here, as throughout the text, the words therapist, provider, mental
  health professional, counselor, and social worker are used inter-
  changeably. Where ethics are concerned, the general guidelines of
  the so-called talking professions are remarkably similar.)
- Which option would you exercise?
- Why would you choose this particular option and why would you *not*
  choose another option?
- What are the risks involved in exercising this option?
- What are the potential rewards in exercising this option?

In many cases, the problem and the answer change completely by
altering the situation slightly; for example:

- If a person is male, change to female.
- If a person is a minor (under 18, unmarried, and unemancipated),
  change the age to 18 or older, married or unmarried.
- If the client and therapist went to a bar, make it a health food juice
  bar.
- If the client or therapist is married, change the status to single, or
  cohabiting.
- If the therapist is under the influence of medication, increase the
  dosage gradually to the point of intoxication. If the therapist is

under the influence of alcohol, make it only one drink at first, then two drinks, a "few" beers. As the consumption increases, notice how the attitude of the class changes.

- If the individuals are heterosexual, make them homosexual, but in the same "significant other" pairing.

Use your imagination and consider how the preceding questions might be discussed differently and answered differently as the situation changes.

When a lawyer first visits with a client, the client normally narrates the facts to the lawyer conveniently omitting any admissions that are contrary to the result the client desires. Only after serious, sometimes aggressive cross-examination do all the critical facts emerge. Often the details pulled reluctantly from the client determine the ultimate outcome of the case. In therapy, it is much the same. The therapy will take a different twist if the parties are heterosexual or homosexual, minors or have reached the age of majority, drunk or sober when abuse took place, male or female, normal or disabled or mentally impaired, and so forth. Each situation can be utilized for numerous discussions and will produce a different result in its ethical emphasis depending on the twist of the verbiage.

Using the Big-Picture Explanation

The big picture serves as the catalyst between the vignette and the various ethical codes. Keep in mind that the actual ethical problem faced will not be *exactly* the same as the scenarios provided in the book. Even slight variations can completely change the ethical risk to the provider and client. The text extrapolates from the facts a general proposition that illustrates an ethical problem. From this general presentation, rules are determined that the professional can apply to other situations. In one class, the dilemma of whether to date a client was presented. The answer was clear to everyone. Then a shaky hand went up: "How about a client's second cousin?" Although the codes are clear about direct family and friends, there has not been a second-cousin case. Our answer to the student: "It's a bad idea. Do you want to be the first second-cousin case?" That would be a dubious honor.

Using the Ethics Codes

Selected portions of the HIPAA Privacy and Security Rules as well as various national and some state ethical canons are included in the text. Many of these rules are so similar as to be almost identical in verbiage and theory. They are set out in the text for easy reference, so you can go directly to the source when an ethical dilemma comes up. HIPAA provisions and current codes for each of the national and state professional organizations are also available from the issuing organization and on the Internet. If the answer to a particular ethical question is not answered in the text, you may find the answer in the codes themselves. A call to the professional association, licensing board, or an Internet search may also produce the answer. Should a reading of the code reveal a conflict in wording or ambiguous interpretation, the organizations involved usually have staff available to answer questions. In addition, all malpractice carriers, ever anxious to avoid litigation, and knowing that ethical canons can be introduced into evidence to indicate minimum standards of conduct, will be happy to be of assistance. They often will make their risk management professionals available for consultation. Nevertheless, when conferring with any source of advice and interpretation, take copious notes and document the advice offered. These notations can be invaluable if a decision is ever challenged; also remember that ethical guidelines are updated on a regular basis. When a real problem arises, obtain the latest code available.

We have been shocked over the years by the large number of practitioners who have given little attention to their national and state ethics codes since graduate school. Some have updated their knowledge at lectures and seminars, especially in states that require ethics continuing education units to maintain a license. More often than not, however, practitioners receive copies of the ethical canons that remain unread until a complaint is filed.

We are concerned about the lack of detailed knowledge by mental health professionals of the HIPAA Privacy and Security Rules. Even more worrisome is the lack of compliance we are seeing on the part of many mental health professionals with respect to these rules. Although the rules are *scalable*, which means the smaller the entity (solo practitioner versus national hospital chain) the less the federal government will expect in terms of compliance, this does not mean that you do nothing.

Ethical codes and federal and state law are not stimulating reading. There is no plot, no character development, and good does not triumph over evil. Ethical codes and laws are only listings of potential evils with the admonition to avoid committing the "sins" set out in the rules and regulations of each discipline.

This text offers an introduction to the codes or canons of professional ethics in mental health. This introduction may, as a practical matter, be the only time the novice provider has to discuss and absorb the technical rules and regulations under which he or she operates. Such knowledge is not an academic exercise. It is essential to keeping a license, avoiding a malpractice lawsuit, and practicing within a profession.

Using the Ethical Flash Points

The Ethical Flash Points are maxims or sayings for risk-free practice. They are set out in list form for easy reference.

To the educator, they might serve:

- As subjects for discussion and debate.
- As a basis for essay questions that trace the root of the maxim or state the rationale for its existence.
- As a source of argument: Is this rule really necessary and does it serve the best interest of most of the clients most of the time, or some of the clients some of the time?
- As a basis for true-and-false or multiple-choice questions.
- As a test question: The Flash Point is the answer, but where is it found in the profession's code of ethics?
- As a handy reminder of ethical practice.

The provider, supervisor, consumer, and educator can use this book as a general guide to ethical practice. The text, vignettes, published codes, and Ethical Flash Points were designed for ease of presentation in the lecture format as well as for class discussion and case review. The Ethical Flash Points can also be used as a quick reference in avoiding an ethically questionable situation. It is our hope that long after receiving degrees and entering professions, practitioners will avert ethical problems because they recall these Ethical Flash Points and recognize that a path about to be taken with a client is dangerous and that a step backward, together with a sensitive review, is warranted and appropriate.

Using the Suggested Research Assignments and Discussion Questions

The suggested research assignments and discussion questions are intended to stimulate further discussion and research concerning the ethical problems presented in the chapter.

To the educator they will provide:

- Research and assignment possibilities for work by students outside the classroom
- An opportunity to focus students on the specific rules in jurisdictions in which they intend to practice or provide services
- The ability to familiarize students with the differences in rules between jurisdictions
- A basis for examination questions or problems
- Additional discussion opportunities for the students in or out of class or in practicum

One of the things that makes ethics so interesting and complex is that despite all the specific rules that exist to instruct and regulate the profession, there are always shades of gray and circumstances that can present uncertainty about the course of conduct to pursue. By encouraging more detailed investigation and consideration of the rules, we hope that students, educators, and mental health professionals will be better able to make correct choices when uncertainty about a rule or a course of conduct presents itself.

How to Use This Book

How can mental health services providers use this book? Each mental health services provider, whether psychologist, psychiatrist, marriage and family therapist, counselor, addictions professional, social worker, or pastoral counselor, faces ethical dilemmas daily. An ethical violation could lead to personal discipline and the end of a professional practice.

Some ethical problems are easily solved, such as rearranging office furniture to prevent prying eyes from peering over a receptionist's desk at a computer screen. Other problems are more difficult in that they involve matters of degree. Every ethical code states clearly that a therapist cannot offer treatment to a spouse. Such treatment would defy common sense as there would be no clinical objectivity. But what about a brother-in-law? Or the girlfriend of the brother-in-law? Or the husband of the sister of the brother-in-law? How far removed from the primary relationship must a person be for therapy to be proper and ethical? When you consider stepparents or godparents, the issue can become even cloudier. And who wants to take a chance? Who wants to have his or her name attached to the first test case?

Although this book cannot explicitly address all these situations, Chapter 9, "Prohibited Clients," highlights some of the problems involved in working with individuals with whom there is an external relationship and provides guidelines for deciding who is an inappropriate client. Mental health providers need to consider such relationships to avoid ethical complaints, as well as the appearance of committing an ethical violation. In psychotherapy, as in other professions, perception is important, and any act or activity that *appears* to be unethical, will, if supported by media exposure, rumor, gossip, and table conversation, become reality.

The Portable Ethicist for Mental Health Professionals: A Complete Guide to Responsible Practice tackles dozens of ethical questions in a straightforward manner. It uses the ethical codes of mental health professional associations and federal HIPAA law, where applicable, to respond to these questions and provides guidelines for avoiding ethically questionable behavior. You can review the Contents to find information on a particular area of ethical concern or use the extensive Index to find additional references to the topic elsewhere in the book.

Armed with this information, the practitioner can determine how best to avoid an ethical violation or how to best handle the situation if a complaint has been filed. The material in this book may not always provide a definitive answer to the ethical dilemma, but mental health professionals who use this book will be in a better position to make an informed decision or judgment about the appropriate action to take. No book can answer all ethical questions with absolute authority. The point to remember is that whatever action is taken, the rationale should be clearly stated and the steps fully documented. The best interest of the client should be the therapist's primary concern.

The best advice may be that if after considering all aspects of the ethical dilemma, you still feel uneasy, don't do it. If you have already done it, call your lawyer first, before saying or doing anything else. Remember that in most cases, an attorney will not be obligated to report a therapist's unethical conduct, but a colleague would be.

How can the consumer of mental health services use this book?

Dorothy is a consumer of mental health services. She is the client of Dr. Silverstone, whom she has been seeing for two years. Occasionally, as small talk at the beginning of a session, they visit and share ideas about music.

Sitting in Dorothy's garage is an unused organ that has been in her family for as long as she can remember. Dorothy assigns a value of $2,000 to the organ and offers to trade it to Dr. Silverstone in exchange for 25 sessions. She feels this is a good bargain since Dr. Silverstone's normal charge is $100 per session. He accepts the offer, has the organ removed from her garage, and sends it to a restoration facility. After it is repaired, Dr. Silverstone displays it in his music room where he enjoys its elegance and sound.

Meanwhile, Dorothy feels remorse about trading the favorite family organ. She hears through the friend of a friend of Dr. Silverstone that the now mint-condition organ has a beautiful tone, looks like new as a restored valuable antique, and is worth a "fortune." She feels resentful, but is not sure whether the trade was inappropriate or unethical. She ponders the circumstance.

How can Dorothy determine if she has been taken advantage of by this mental health professional?

The Portable Ethicist provides a pathway to the answer in its discussion of bartering. Although ethical codes and standards of professional associations and licensing boards are augmented and amended from time to time, the basic principles generally remain the same. But there are differences. For example, certain ethical codes absolutely prohibit bartering with a client. Cash and cash only is the rule. Some codes allow bartering under limited circumstances. Should bartering occur, and should the client complain later, the burden is on the provider to show that the arrangement was fair. If the provider can do so, the practice may be considered ethical in that location.

This text also provides insight to the consumer for a laundry list of other ethical issues. Consider this sampling of situations in which a client might be involved:

- The client responded to an ad in a newspaper, a magazine, or a telephone book that was false or misleading. "Give up smoking/drinking/drugs for good in 10 convenient sessions."
- The client consented to therapy but failed to understand the goals, techniques, purposes, or methods of therapy.
- The client was unaware of the limitations on the authorized methods of treatment, the risks of treatment, or alternative treatments available.
- The client found out that her therapist was paying her physician a fee for the referral.
- The therapist suggested that the client attend her church, take a class offered by her at the university, or have coffee with her after a session.
- The therapist made no record of visits or payments and did not maintain clinical notes or progress notes of treatment.

- The client was gay and the therapist seemed (to the client) uncomfortable around him and uncomfortable when the subject of a gay lifestyle arose.
- The therapist offered treatment by fax and e-mail without ever interviewing the client.
- The client felt that although the therapist never made any overt advances toward her, he seemed to her to be preoccupied with her sexual history over and above what she considered appropriate under the circumstances.
- The client wanted assurances that whatever was said in the clinical setting was *absolutely confidential* and the therapist would not offer such assurances; instead the therapist initiated a dialogue concerning the numerous exceptions to confidentiality.
- The therapist asked the client to sign a consent form that obligated the client to pay the therapist for all time in court on any client-related case, which the client was reluctant to sign.
- The client knew little about client rights and therapist obligations and wanted an in-depth explanation of these rights and obligations.
- The client's repeated requests for copies of his records were ignored and the records were not provided.

In these and many other areas, consumers of mental health services need objective and educational information.

To many clients, especially those who are relatively unsophisticated about the mental health field, therapy of any type is somewhat of a mystery. The consumer/client not only is unschooled in the treatment methods being used but, more to the point, does not know the mental health professional's ethical obligations. This book can be a resource for such information because it uses clear examples, explanations, and Ethical Flash Points, along with excerpts from the ethical canons of major mental health professional associations to illustrate both ethical and unethical behavior. The client who feels uneasy with the therapy or the therapist should consult this text to determine if the uneasiness stems from unethical and improper actions of the provider as a consumer of health services:

- You have a right to know the therapist's credentials, licensing, educational background, and experience.
- You have a right to be informed of the nature of the treatment being offered, the fees for treatment, and the amount of copayments expected as well as third-party payments. You should be informed of the provider's no-show and cancellation policy and whether the provider is or will be available should you for any reason be involved in litigation.
- You have a right to know whether what is said in therapy will be confidential and when confidentiality may be legally breached, such as if the therapist is subpoenaed to testify in court. The HIPAA Privacy Rule dictates how your health-care information may be disclosed. All the exceptions to confidentiality are important, and you should understand them fully before beginning therapy.
- You have a right to know what to do should the provider prove to be incompetent, dishonest, or unethical in any way, including the right to sue, or to report the provider to the state board, national organization, or district attorney, if appropriate. You may choose not to pursue these options; however, you should be aware of your rights.
- You have a right to rely on claims made by and about the therapist, and if the claims seem grandiose, to seek verification.
- You have a right to discuss the treatment plan, the diagnosis, and the prognosis. The more you participate in the treatment process, the greater the opportunity for treatment to succeed.
- Informed consent includes the right to know the alternative treatments available, the ability to refuse the treatment or any part of the treatment, a full explanation of the risks of treatment (e.g., one risk of marital therapy is that the parties might get a divorce), and the risks of forgoing treatment.
- You have the right not to be exploited by the therapist, who has a duty to refrain from blurring professional boundaries, to respect professional distances, and to refrain from any act that suggests or implies a dual relationship of any type: social, business, intellectual, personal, sexual, or artistic. Remember, your therapist is your therapist only, not your friend, and any attempt to create any other relationship is unfair, unwise, and unethical. Therapists should not

attend a client's family events, religious ceremonies, or parties. Nor should they participate in any other function that might in any way affect clinical objectivity, even remotely. Therapists should not accept gifts, tickets, or invitations. Your therapist should not have personal or business relationships with your family members and friends. The therapist's relationship with you should be limited to the therapeutic treatment.

- You have a right to a copy of your file, but keep in mind that reading a clinical record is not always a good idea, especially if you do not understand clinical jargon and technical terms and concepts. A freshman course in psychology is typically not adequate preparation when trying to understand a professional file. One basic purpose of the clinical file is to communicate information to a subsequent or collaborating treatment provider or to serve as a basis for consultation between mental health professionals.

- Honor the rights of teenagers or children if they are seeing a therapist. Once a child realizes a parent or guardian is viewing a clinical record, trust evaporates. Most children want to tell the therapist what they do not tell their parents, and if the therapist is a snitch, frank and honest communication comes to an abrupt halt.

- If you have time, and if the method of therapy has a label, read some of the literature on the subject. Clinicians often are using a kind of therapy that a layperson can understand in general terms. Read an article or book or watch a movie that illustrates the type of problem you are facing. Sometimes the therapy moves faster if you know the direction and method in advance. Therapists like to deal with educated clients.

- You have a right to limited confidentiality in one-on-one therapy. In a group, you can count on the facilitator to respect what is said, but signed statements of confidentiality, oral pledges, and announcements that "what is said here, remains here" are no guarantee that another group participant will not gossip. Group therapy can be economical and helpful. However, there is a downside risk of breached confidentiality.

- You have a right not to be discriminated against because of race, color, creed, religion, nationality, or disability. However, if the therapist is unable to understand parts of your ethnic or cultural background, a referral may be made or a consultant engaged. Therapists are aware that some cultural diversities are difficult to understand and even more difficult to treat. No therapist is knowledgeable in all religions, ethnic varieties, and national customs to the extent that he or she can understand the impact of that background and put it into perspective. If you feel the therapist does not understand your background, explain as best you can and then discuss the problem with the therapist. An agreeable solution can usually be reached. The same is helpful if a clinician does not fully comprehend the full physical or emotional impact of a disability.

- You have the right to terminate therapy at any time, unless it is court ordered. Your therapist has a duty to terminate therapy when progress is not being achieved or all goals have been reached. If further mental health care is necessary, you have a right to be advised of the kind of care needed and to be provided with referral sources for such care.
- You have the right to be better informed about the ethical standards of the mental health profession by reading the rest of this book.

If a mental health consumer decides that the therapist has acted unethically, he or she may take the following actions:

- Call a lawyer and discuss the problem.
- Confront the therapist, explain the ethical perception, and resolve the matter between the two parties.
- Call the therapist's licensing board for an opinion.
- File a complaint with the licensing board. (*Note:* Once a complaint is filed with a licensing board, there is no turning back. The complaint is a serious matter and is taken seriously. The complainant must realize that filing a complaint means getting involved in an administrative process that concerns a governmental agency, a licensing board and board members, perhaps a state attorney and investigators, and a permanent state record. Filing a complaint is not something to do lightly or in haste.)

- File a complaint with federal authorities, Office of Civil Rights, for HIPAA Privacy Rule violations and the Centers for Medicare and Medicaid if a HIPAA Security Rule violation is suspected.
- Terminate the therapy and ask the therapist to make a referral or independently seek treatment from another provider.

Mental health consumers should carefully consider all the options before taking any action. There are times when a violated client whose mental health provider has acted unethically should take immediate affirmative action to redress the wrong, seeking the maximum punishment available from a disciplinary body. There are also times when a violated client's personal mental health would benefit from talking the violation through with a compassionate professional and letting it drop, perhaps with a telephone call or a note. It is appropriate for each client to personally make the final decision about how to handle such situations . . . as long as the decision is informed.

Ethical Flash Points

- Become sensitive, be aware. Learn to recognize potential ethical dilemmas.

- If you anticipate a complaint is coming, prepare a response plan and gather supporting materials.

- Develop a network of professional colleagues and discuss possible scenarios for ethical violations and how to resolve them. Ensure all scenarios are hypothetical or theoretical, so that the problem can be discussed without anyone feeling uncomfortable.

- Read the ethical guidelines for your professional organizations and licensing boards carefully. Learn what the HIPAA Privacy and Security Rules require of your practice. When a complaint is filed, the reviewing authority must prove a published rule or regulation was violated. To avoid violations, practitioners must be aware of the existence, content, and interpretation of the guideline rules. Even a letter of reprimand from a licensing authority has serious repercussions when seeking malpractice insurance, applying for hospital privileges or for managed care, seeking employment, and renewing a license.

- When there is a gray area, or if a legitimate question arises concerning whether a particular act or action might be a shade unethical, don't do it. If it tweaks your conscience or smells bad, don't do it ever!

- If an ethical question arises, talk with a lawyer.

- Even if a particular act may appear to be moral, ethical, appropriate, or in the best interest of the client in the big picture, if it violates a published ethical canon, rule, or regulation in the little picture, the big picture does not count. Violating an ethical rule in the little picture means the license is in peril. And a license is a terrible asset to lose.

PART I

CLIENT ISSUES

1

Alternative Treatment Methods

In the past, clients arrived for their appointments, took off their shoes, relaxed on the clinical couch, and in a soft and unemotional voice discussed the day's problems. They were encouraged to ramble in the hope that they would reveal significant information enabling the therapist to garner insight into the client's emotional issues. The clinician, meanwhile, sat in a comfortable chair jotting down occasional phrases, intermittently making a suggestion or two to keep the conversation focused. At the end of 50 minutes of practically uninterrupted monologue, the parties shook hands, the client paid cash, and left. The therapist closed that client's file and then picked up the file of the next client. "Thank you, Dr. Freud," the client thought.

Today, Dr. Freud III has a busy schedule and is happy to talk to clients over the phone in an emergency. He makes his fees clear on his intake form, which states that phone calls under 6 minutes (0.1 hour) are free, but calls over 6 minutes are charged at his usual hourly rate computed in 10-minute segments. He has a timer on his telephone, and each call is coded and transferred electronically to the client file. One day, Dr. Freud receives an emergency call from a prospective client. The potential client *was properly referred to Dr. Freud, but they had not yet met. Should he offer emergency treatment over the phone without first seeing the client, or should he refuse to offer any consultation without first insisting on an office interview? If he chooses the latter, may he continue telephone therapy after the initial consultation using his electronic billing method? Is telephone therapy an accepted method of treatment? Would it make a difference if each phone had a picture monitor so the client could be seen on the screen? How much of therapy is voice transmission and how much is body language, facial expression, or other visual hints of a person's attitude, demeanor, and meaning? And what about the ethical requirements in some licensing acts and numerous jurisdictions that require certain clarifications prior to the commencement of treatment, such as indicating the exceptions to confidentiality or charges in the event litigation becomes relevant?*

Dr. Freud III was tired of practicing the same old "talk therapy" he'd been using for years. True, his dad and granddad made history by listening to clients' problems, recording their findings, and publishing the results, but he was a modern therapist of the electronic age, and he sought to offer modern treatment. Many ethics guidelines provide that primary therapy should be offered in person and imply that other communication methods such as e-mail, telephone, fax, or other electronic transmission should be selectively used on an emergency basis or, perhaps, only as a supplement to established face-to-face therapy methods. One day, a thought flashed in his mind: He would create a web page; advertise his credentials, experience, writings, publications, and interests; and offer (with a certain amount of built-in name recognition) e-mail therapy. He searched his profession's ethics codes. The codes did not contain an absolute ethical prohibition against e-mail therapy. He would insist that prospective clients use a credit card to open an account with him before beginning therapy, and then he would respond to their e-mail inquiries and bill their credit card for his time. He would no longer suffer through face-to-face confrontations with clients who started talking and then, being on a roll, refused to leave. Could this be the dawn of a new era—treating and receiving payments from clients without ever seeing them?

A Plethora of Treatment Options

Years ago—and not so long ago—most therapy followed the model in the first example, one-on-one individual interpersonal therapy. Today, there is much more to do before therapy can even begin. First, clients must sign a carefully worded *consent-to-treatment form* (see *The Portable Lawyer for Mental Health Professionals*, Bernstein and Hartsell 2004, p. 50) that is often drafted and reviewed by a knowledgeable lawyer, with therapist protection in mind. Next, clients complete an *intake form*, listing all the mental health details of their lives so the therapist can never be accused of failing to discover some important fact or circumstance about a client's past life that might be critical to continuing therapy. No investigative stone is left unturned before treatment begins. Ethics guidelines dictate what therapists must explain to clients prior to beginning therapy to secure "informed consent" to treatment. And, whereas talk therapy was the most favored treatment in the past, therapists now use a plethora of techniques to effect behavioral change in their clients.

Distance Therapy

Is it ethical to offer distance therapy? Many ethics guidelines provide that primary therapy should be offered in person and imply that other communication methods such as e-mail, telephone, fax, or other electronic transmission should be used selectively on an emergency basis or, perhaps, only as a supplement to face-to-face therapy. Ethics codes provide some direction for distance therapy, and the Health Insurance Portability and Accountability Act (HIPAA) Security Rule provides specific instructions for preserving and protecting electronically transmitted health- care information. It will likely take legal proceedings to set precedents for these treatment options. Once a court or a regulatory authority disciplines a practitioner for committing an ethical infraction when inappropriately practicing therapy using the telephone or computer, we will have a better idea how to caution therapists about practicing distance therapy.

E-Mail

Today, many therapists offer e-mail counseling either as a primary form of therapy or as an adjunct to regular therapy sessions. E-mail therapy began as a matter of convenience for many practitioners: a way to schedule appointments or answer a quick question between sessions. Others strategically added computer-based education, counseling, or therapy sessions to build a varied menu of private pay services. Many licensed clinicians now offer therapy services ranging from a single interaction, to ongoing sessions, to hypnotherapy by electronic mail (see *Practice Strategies: A Business Guide for Behavioral Healthcare Providers*, March 1999, p. 1, American Association for Marriage and Family Therapists, for an early article on this subject). There are several problems with this approach. Therapists cannot observe a client's physical disability using only electronic communication. Likewise, if clients do not complete a mental health intake form or if they complete it untruthfully, therapists may be unaware of all existing conditions (e.g., the client may be a pedophile with a criminal record). They may also be unaware of existing sources of support (e.g., a client who asks about moderate drinking may be a member of Alcoholics Anonymous). Using electronic communication, therapists usually cannot see their clients' physical appearance, which often gives clues to their mental health state. Might a face-to-face therapeutic interface yield different results from one across a screen?

Other difficulties exist with online therapy. First, fees for different types of e-mail therapy may vary, and collecting fees for e-mail services is difficult unless prearranged credit card charges are approved. Second, it is hard to identify clients because the therapist is not meeting them face-to-face. Is the e-mail client a sincere client or someone having a good time at the therapist's expense? Third, how confidential can e-mail therapy be? How can a therapist ensure that an e-mail client will complete and sign an informed consent form and complete the intake form, which includes information required by state licensing laws? Fourth, if an e-mail communication crosses state lines, does the provider need to be licensed to practice in the recipient's state? Can the provider ethically process third-party payments in another state? How (or will) e-mail communications be stored? And in states where client files must be preserved and maintained for a specific number of years, must the clinician always ensure that the particular method of preservation is available in the future? Do you have to save every disk, every hard drive, every obsolete computer, and a hard copy of everything? One way to avoid ethical problems is to label any e-mail or online communication between therapist and client *educational* rather than *therapeutic*. If therapists take this route, the rules change. For example, if the advice is considered education rather than therapy, informed consent is not necessary, nor is a detailed intake form required. The therapist is not entirely free of responsibility by using this option. Even if the therapist has stated numerous times that the communication is only educational, there can be a problem if online clients interpret the advice as therapy. In such cases, there is a good chance that a court or licensing board will side with the complaining or damaged client.

Distance therapy has its proper place in the therapist's toolbox. It is easy to see how it can be of great benefit and assistance to clients in rural communities who live hundreds of miles from the nearest mental health practitioner or treatment facility. In large metropolitan communities, people with disabilities may have difficulty getting out and traveling even a few miles to a therapist's office. Distance therapy can be appropriate for certain clients; handicapped, disabled, and mentally impaired clients are as entitled to treatment as unimpaired individuals.

Even if it was established that distance therapy's risks significantly outweighed its usefulness, there does not appear to be any effective and viable means of preventing it. Policing voice and Internet communications has proven to be no easy matter. To stop distance therapy would deprive people of their privacy rights. For this reason and because it does have appropriate applications, regulatory authorities have not made any serious attempts to ban distance therapy. Eventually, regulation will catch up with our advanced telecommunications. Until licensing boards publish definitive rulings or legal cases and precedents determine the limits to be placed on the practice, mental health professionals who augment their practice with online

One way to avoid ethical problems is to call any e-mail or online communication between therapist and client educational rather than therapeutic. The best option is to consult the ethics codes, the licensing boards, and the malpractice carrier before beginning any online communications with clients.

education or distance therapy could be vulnerable to sanctions. For now, therapists should exercise caution when exploring their options to practice over the Internet or use other means of distance therapy. If advice is sought from a licensing board or an attorney, document the advice, print a hard copy, and insert it in a file. Many well-intentioned mental health practitioners received oral advice on the phone, acted in accordance with the advice, and then, when challenged, the advisor was no longer available to back up the therapist.

Agreed-on therapy in an office is clearly therapy. The boundaries begin to blur when clinicians use e-mail or answer therapeutic questions in "Ask Dr." columns in the newspaper, on television, or on the radio. Self-help books and newspaper and magazine articles purport to offer educational information but often provide therapeutic instructions. To date, few consumers have complained about the errors in self-help books or "feel good" articles. However, the electronic age, coupled with the enthusiastic enforcement of licensing and disciplinary boards throughout the country, opens a new avenue of ethical concerns. The best option is to consult the ethics codes, the licensing boards, and your malpractice carrier before beginning any online communications with clients. Find out if the malpractice policy covers new or novel treatment approaches before being sued or brought before the licensing board for an ethical complaint. Lawyers, liability insurance carriers, and licensing boards would rather avoid a problem than have to face an uncomfortable precedent. Be cautious and document everything.

Before providing any therapy, a mental health practitioner must advise potential clients about the limits of confidentiality. This is a requirement of the ethics canons. In addition, there must be a discussion of the risks and potential benefits of the treatment being offered. With distance therapies, there needs to be a greater emphasis on informing potential clients of the risks regarding disclosure of information and the limitations of this kind of treatment option.

Voice and e-mail communications are subject to capture and review by unauthorized persons. A person with the right kind of listening device or equipment can overhear a conversation with a client on a wireless or cell phone. We have all heard and read about the ease with which skilled computer hackers gain access to electronic information. The information garnered by the hacker is often unknown to the individuals involved in the conversation. It is the surreptitious gathering of confidential information that creates the anxiety and discomfort. Information once communicated through wireless communication can no longer be assumed to be absolutely confidential and private.

The inability to view body language or to hear voice inflection, pitch, or volume can certainly inhibit a therapist's insight about a client or the client's level of functioning. So if voice and video transmission of client contact and communication are not part of the distance therapy, there is a risk that some important clue or piece of information will be missed. The observable will not be observed. Most electronic communications between a client and therapist are typewritten and therefore pose what could be a significant risk of the therapy being ineffective or not as effective as it should or might be.

At a minimum, mental health practitioners need to advise their potential distance clients of inherent risks and limitations to this kind of therapy as indicated by the following ethical provisions:

National Guidelines for Providing Services via Electronic Communication

American Counseling Association (ACA) Code of Ethics (2005)

A.12. Technology Applications

A.12.a. Benefits and Limitations

Counselors inform clients of the benefits and limitations of using information technology applications in the counseling process and in business/billing procedures. Such technologies include but are not limited to computer hardware and software, telephones, the World Wide Web, the

(continued)

(*Continued*)

Internet, online assessment instruments, and other communication devices.

American Psychological Association (APA) Ethical Principles of Psychologists and Code of Conduct (2002)

4.02 Discussing the Limits of Confidentiality

(c) Psychologists who offer services, products, or information via electronic transmission inform clients/patients of the risks to privacy and limits of confidentiality.

National Association of Social Workers (NASW) Code of Ethics (1999)

1.03 Informed Consent

(e) Social workers who provide services via electronic media (such as computer, telephone, radio, and television) should inform recipients of the limitations and risks associated with such services.

The ACA *Code of Ethics* provides the most detail on what it charac-
terizes as "Technology Assisted Therapy." Under Section A.12, subsections (b) through (g) offer some specific guidance to counselors
who wish to practice distance therapy. The Code provides:

- When distance counseling is inappropriate, counselors should consider delivering face-to-face therapy.
- Before providing distance counseling, the counselor must ensure it
  does not violate any local, state, national, or international law.
- Counselors should provide themselves and clients reasonable access
  to computer applications.
- Counselors should get business, legal, and technical assistance, especially when applications will cross state or international boundaries.

- As part of the informed consent process, counselors should:
  - Address the difficulty of maintaining confidentiality of electronic communications.
  - Inform clients of all persons, including computer technicians, who might have access, authorized or unauthorized, to electronic transmissions.
  - Urge clients to be aware of all persons, authorized or unauthorized, who could access information on their end (i.e., the family or work computer).
  - Inform clients of any applicable rights and limitations governing the practice of a profession over state lines or international boundaries.
  - Use encryption software when possible.
  - When encryption software use is not possible, counselors should notify clients of this fact and limit electronic communications to general (educational) information that is not client specific.
  - Inform clients if and for how long the electronic information will be stored and maintained.
  - Discuss the possibility of electronic failure and alternative methods of delivering services.
  - Inform clients of emergency contact options (i.e., calling 911 or hotline numbers), if the counselor is unavailable.
  - Discuss time zone differences, local customs, and cultural or language differences that impact the therapy.
  - Inform clients when distance therapy will not be covered by insurance.

These provisions certainly offer sound ideas for ensuring informed consent and offering distance therapy to a client. But are they enough? No! Not even close.

Once a mental health practitioner ventures into the world of electronic transmission of health-care information to provide distance therapy, he or she becomes a "covered entity" and must comply with the HIPAA Security Rule. HIPAA's security standards apply to all protected health information (PHI) that is being stored or transmitted by a covered entity. The Security Rule does not cover health information that is on paper or communicated orally. The Security Rule, for example, would not cover doing phone therapy. Old-fashioned mail communication also would not be covered. Using a computer and the Internet to receive or send messages to a client would be covered.

The Security Rule deals with internal and external threats, risks, and weaknesses of all aspects of electronic transmission or storage of health-care information. These include outside threats (hackers, service interruptions, theft) and inside threats (unauthorized employees, fire or other casualty risks, environmental hazards, computer crashes). The Security Rule does not require specific technologies or practices, but it is intended to set a minimum level of security. Practitioners may choose to implement safeguards that exceed the minimum requirements.

To be compliant, a mental health practitioner who is a covered entity must:

- Ensure the confidentiality, integrity, and availability of all electronic PHI that is created, stored, maintained, or transmitted.
- Provide protection from any reasonably anticipated threats or hazards to the security or integrity of all electronic PHI.
- Provide protection from any reasonably anticipated uses or disclosures of electronic information not required or permitted by the Privacy Rule.
- Ensure all employees comply with the Security Rule.
- Have on hand a business associate contract pursuant to which any repairperson or technician guarantees the confidentiality of all information acquired as a result of working on or repairing equipment.
- Ensure employees and temporary help are trained and conversant with all security measures and that only persons with a need to access protected health information can do so.
- Ensure that those accessing client files only access the minimum information necessary for their job duties.

The therapist practicing distance therapy that involves the transmission or storage of electronic information pertaining to the client must develop and document internal and external administrative policies and procedures to prevent, detect, contain, and correct security violations. The Security Rule provides administrative safeguards that are scalable. This means they are designed to give covered entities the latitude to employ policies and procedures that make sense for their particular operation and size.

Administrative safeguards required by the Security Rule include:

- Security management process
- Assigned security responsibility
- Workforce security
- Information access management
- Security awareness and training
- Security incident procedures
- Contingency plan
- Evaluation
- Business associate contract or other arrangements

Before sitting down at a computer for an electronic "chat" with a client, the therapist must have documented safeguards in place that address each of these issues in a manner that is appropriate for his or her practice. It is not enough to know what the canons of ethics of the licensing board or professional organization have to say on the subject (see Chapter 18, "Centers for Medicare and Medicaid Services," this book, for a discussion of enforcement of the Security Rule; and *The Portable Lawyer for Mental Health Professionals,* Bernstein and Hartsell 2004, Chapter 46, "HIPAA Security Rule," for a more in-depth discussion of the Security Rule.).

Even the seemingly specific provisions of the ACA *Code of Ethics* and the HIPAA Security Rule do not provide the definitive and complete guidance that a mental health practitioner needs to safely and ethically practice distance therapy. Other state, federal, and international laws and state, national, and international regulatory and policing authorities could all determine how or if distance therapy is practiced. Mental health practitioners are required to be educated, informed, and current on all aspects of practice.

New and Novel Treatment Approaches

The Texas state licensing statute for professional counselors lists authorized counseling methods and practices, including individual counseling, group counseling, marriage counseling, family counseling, chemical dependency counseling, rehabilitation counseling, education counseling, career development counseling, sexual issues counseling, referral counseling, psychotherapy, play therapy, hypnotherapy, expressive therapies, biofeedback, assessing and appraising, and consulting. In all these fields, there is a constantly emerging body of literature with which the practicing professional is ethically obligated to be current, up-to-date, and informed. Moreover, many subspecialties have published ethical guidelines that bind their members.

Without question, more and different kinds of therapies can be listed (e.g., sand, art, music, psychodrama, equestrian) and over time, new and additional novel therapies will be advanced. A therapist who wants to use one must research the subject and take the time to become competent in offering the therapy and must advise the potential client of its potential risks and limitations. Without doing so, there could not be informed consent concerning the delivery of subsequent services.

National Guidelines for New and Novel Treatment Approaches

American Association for Marriage and Family Therapy (AAMFT) Code of Ethics (2001)

Principle III: Professional Competence and Integrity

3.7 While developing new skills in specialty areas, marriage and family therapists take steps to ensure the competence of their work and to protect clients from possible harm. Marriage and family therapists practice in specialty areas new to them only after appropriate education, training, or supervised experience.

American Counseling Association (ACA) Code of Ethics (2005)

Section C Professional Responsibility

C.2. Professional Competence

C.2.b. New Specialty Areas of Practice

Counselors practice in specialty areas new to them only after appropriate education, training, and supervised experience. While developing skills in new specialty areas, counselors take steps to ensure the competence of their work and to protect others from possible harm.

***National Association of Social Workers (NASW) Code of Ethics* (1999)**

4.01 Competence

(b) Social workers should strive to become and remain proficient in professional practice and the performance of professional functions. Social workers should critically examine and *keep current with emerging knowledge relevant to social work.* Social workers should routinely *review the professional literature* and participate in continuing education relevant to social work practice and social work ethics.

Obligations for Ethical Practice

The following guidelines are suggested:

- Professionals must keep current with the literature in their field. They must be conversant with the majority literature as well as that of a learned minority.
- Professionals must be knowledgeable in all areas in which they claim special expertise (e.g., couples therapy, school counseling).

- As various mental health disciplines develop new counseling or therapeutic theories or techniques, providers in those disciplines must become familiar with these emerging developments.
- New, novel, electronic, and computer-oriented methods are being used and developed every day. Mental health professionals have a responsibility to offer these developing options to their clients, who have a right to receive and may benefit from the latest proven treatment available.
- Nevertheless, when practitioners make use of a new or novel approach, they must be thoroughly knowledgeable about it, and ensure the new approach is appropriate to the particular client in treatment.
- Using new and novel approaches can be an ethical risk for providers because a substantiated body of empirical, scientific, or historic literature often does not support them. Thus, providers must provide excellent documentation to support all new therapeutic approaches to therapy, especially if they deviate from commonly accepted norms.
- Every ethical treatment modality must be generally accepted by a majority of practitioners or a learned minority. When challenged, the provider has the burden of proving that the modality used was appropriate to this problem and this client.

Ethical Flash Points

- Modern electronic communications such as e-mail do not have a long and professionally accepted therapeutic and academic history.

- Read all the published literature concerning electronic or other distance treatment before incorporating it into your practice.

- When using electronic communications, faxes, e-mail, chat rooms, or web sites, remember that the recipient may not be the person you envision. The provider is responsible for providing ethical treatment to specific, identifiable clients, from the time therapy begins to the time it ends and records are no longer preserved. All communications become part of the clinical record if they influence the diagnosis, treatment plan, or prognosis (see Chapter 13, "Terminating Therapy," Chapter 21, "Establishing a Practice," and Chapter 22,"Closing or Interrupting a Practice").

- Potential distance clients are entitled to the same disclosures and information as regular clients and to additional information of risks and limitations unique to distance therapy.

- Distance clients have the same rights as any other clients.

- Licenses apply to the state of issuance only, leading to ethical questions if the distance therapy client resides in another jurisdiction. Does therapy originate from the provider's workstation or the client's computer? Which location has jurisdiction over the therapeutic consultation? Should a problem occur, who has the enforcement obligation: the state of transmission, receipt, where the harm was done where the parties reside, or some other location?

- Each state and discipline as well as subspecialties within each discipline may have its own directive concerning distance therapy. Each must be consulted.

- Don't take unnecessary risks in implementing modern technology in therapy, but don't ignore such methods either.

- Additional information is required to ensure informed consent from potential clients when distance therapy is utilized.

- Ethical codes do not provide guidance on local, state, national, and international law that may apply to distance therapy. Ethical codes are not uniform. What is allowable under one code may be prohibited under another. The scribes of ethical canons or codes of professional responsibility do not necessarily coordinate their efforts or products. There may be conspicuous inconsistencies (e.g., how long you are mandated to keep, preserve, and maintain records).

- Knowledge and compliance of the HIPAA Security Rule is required if the distance therapy will involve the electronic transmission and retention of health information.

- Computer knowledge is required to determine how long computer records last and how and when they might begin to become garbled and compromise the information contained on the computer disk, tape, or drive.

Summary

Ethics codes have begun to incorporate guidelines for using modern communication methods in therapy, but practitioners should consider what the canons say as well as what they don't say before embarking on a new treatment plan or using a diagnostic tool that depends in whole or in part on electronic or computer-generated methods. Being trendy or ahead of the pack is wonderful as long as one's professional reputation or license is not placed at risk.

Technological developments are occurring rapidly and any comments made today might be totally obsolete tomorrow, as emerging technology changes the rationale behind the ethical guidelines. An old legal maxim states, "When the reason for the rule fails, the rule itself should fail." With advancing technology, today's rationale can be tomorrow's failing. Thus practitioners should consider new technological treatment options but use caution when employing them. Contact your board, national association, malpractice carrier, and lawyer before using a new technology or plunging headlong into a new therapeutic theory. If a new technology is employed, be sure to document its efficacy.

Suggested Research Assignments

1. Locate and discuss any rules promulgated by licensing boards in your state that deal with distance therapy.
2. Locate and discuss any national, state, or local laws or statutes that affect the delivery of distance therapy services.
3. Compare and contrast these state licensing board rules and state or local laws with the ethical rules found in the *ACA Code of Ethics* for technology-assisted therapy.
4. Contact the national, state, and local organizations and request their latest publications on the subject.
5. Create security safeguards and guidelines to ensure compliance with the HIPAA Security Rule and ethical canons for your present or future practice. Do you need to amend or modify your intake form?

6. Identify another novel therapeutic approach other than distance therapy, research its literature, and create a plan to implement its use in a practice in a manner that reduces risk to the practitioner from ethical or legal claims.

7. Identify resources or persons you would consult to safely and ethically implement distance therapy.

8. Interview mental health practitioners and attorneys in your area about their experiences with distance therapy.

9. Research the decisions of your state licensing boards and state and national professional association ethics committees for distance therapy violation sanctions.

10. Research civil case decisions of your state involving distance therapy. What damages, if any, were awarded?

Discussion Questions

1. What kinds of distance therapy technology do you use or plan to use in your practice? What risks do you see with distance therapy? What are its benefits?

2. What type of clients would you consider targeting for distance therapy? How would you go about reaching this targeted patient population?

3. Would you insist on at least one face-to-face session with a client before or during distance therapy? State your reasoning for or against this practice.

4. Would price determine or affect distance therapy differently from traditional face-to-face therapy? If so, why? And if not, why not?

5. What are other emerging novel or new therapies, and what risks do they present to mental health professionals implementing them in their practices?

2

Boundary Violations

During a recent therapy session, a client (Sue) asks Carol, a licensed professional counselor, to attend a marriage commitment ceremony she and her husband are scheduling for their 25th wedding anniversary, which will take place in 2 weeks. The client says her marriage could not have survived except for the therapy Carol provided and the results it achieved in the client's life. Should Carol accept the invitation?

One day at the beauty shop, Dr. Good talks with her beautician. As soon as the beautician realizes Dr. Good is a therapist, she starts talking about her son, a poor student, who has taken up with a bad crowd and who, she thinks, has a drinking problem. Dr. Good handles just this sort of problem in her therapeutic practice and thinks she could help this child. After the appointment, the beautician asks if she can talk to Dr. Good in private. She admits her son does have a proven alcohol problem and wants help, but she is low on funds. She suggests a trade, in which Dr. Good would treat her son in exchange for beauty services. She already has a similar arrangement with her lawyer, dentist, and physician. On its face, the offer seems like a win, win, win (Dr. Good, child, mother) situation. Should Dr. Good accept her offer?

Dr. Moore consults with a team of professionals to manage his practice. He retains a lawyer, a stockbroker, and a financial planner, as well as an accountant, a banker, and an insurance agent. At church, he is a friend of the minister, the choir director, the janitor, and the church secretary. All of them (along with his family members) know that Dr. Moore is a therapist and often share their problems on a "by the way" basis when they see him. Should Dr. Moore offer to treat any of these individuals as in-office clients or accept them for treatment if they approach him first? Is there a potential danger if Dr. Moore engages in a conversation that he considers small talk but the other person considers an insightful exchange of therapeutic perceptiveness, that is, a sort of informal treatment session?

A therapy client of Dr. Megabucks is a venture capitalist–stockbroker. The client shares a hot tip with her that could make her an instant millionaire once the stock comes on the market. Is it ethical for Dr. Megabucks to surreptitiously subscribe to this new issue by opening an account with her client? What if she chose a different broker? Would therapeutic objectivity be compromised if the stock she purchased decreased in value or if it were later discovered that the new issue was the result of hype and fraud?

Identifying Boundary Violations

Encounters with more or less subtle overtones might seem harmless at first glance but nonetheless represent an ethical violation that can haunt the mental health service provider.

Boundary violations sometimes sneak up on the mental health professional when least expected. In the case of sexual or very close social or intimate contacts, the inappropriateness of the encounter is obvious. Chapter 12, "Sexual Misconduct," carefully sets out how a sexual need, activity, or satisfaction can bring disastrous consequences to the helping professional. When we discuss personal needs and activities in this chapter, we are referring to a less obvious type of relationship that would appear to be innocent, customary, and acceptable for most professionals, but when applied to mental health providers is unethical or has the appearance of unethical conduct. Encounters with more or less subtle overtones might seem harmless at first glance but nonetheless represent an ethical violation that could haunt the mental health service provider.

Most ethics codes have both general and specific statements concerning therapists meeting personal needs and promoting personal activities at their clients' expense. In fact, such activities need not be at a client's expense to be considered unethical. These activities would also be inappropriate if engaging in them would compromise the therapist's objectivity toward the client or even have a tendency to compromise it.

National Guidelines for Identifying Potential Boundary Violations

American Association for Marriage and Family Therapy (AAMFT) Code of Ethics (2001)

Principle 1: Responsibility to Clients

1.3 Marriage and family therapists are aware of their influential positions with respect to clients, and they avoid exploiting the trust and dependency of such persons. Therapists, therefore, make every effort to avoid conditions and multiple relationships with clients that could impair professional judgment or increase the risk of exploitation. Such relationships include, but are not limited to, business or close personal relationships with a client or the client's immediate family. When the risk of impairment or exploitation exists due to conditions or multiple roles, therapists take appropriate precautions.

American Psychological Association (APA) Ethical Principles of Psychologists and Code of Conduct (2002)

Ethical Standards

3. Human Relations

3.05 Multiple Relationships

(a) A multiple relationship occurs when a psychologist is in a professional role with a person and (1) at the same time is in

(continued)

(*Continued*)

another role with the same person, (2) at the same time is in a relationship with a person closely associated with or related to the person with whom the psychologist has the professional relationship, or (3) promises to enter into another relationship in the future with the person or a person closely associated with or related to the person.

A psychologist refrains from entering into a multiple relationship if the multiple relationship could reasonably be expected to impair the psychologist's objectivity, competence, or effectiveness in performing his or her functions as a psychologist, or otherwise risks exploitation or harm to the person with whom the professional relationship exists.

Multiple relationships that would not reasonably be expected to cause impairment or risk exploitation or harm are not unethical.

National Association of Social Workers (NASW) Code of Ethics (1999)

1.06 Conflicts of Interest

(c) Social workers should not engage in dual or multiple relationships with clients or former clients in whom there is a risk of exploitation or potential harm to the client. In instances when dual or multiple relationships are unavoidable, social workers should take steps to protect clients and are responsible for setting clear, appropriate, and culturally sensitive boundaries. (Dual or multiple relationships occur when social workers relate to clients in more than one relationship, whether professional, social, or business. Dual or multiple relationships can occur simultaneously or consecutively.)

Anticipating Potential Boundary Violations

There is no way to predict all the circumstances under which a client or prospective client might approach or seek the services of a therapist. Therapists do not treat family, friends, business associates, or individuals with whom they have an existing relationship that might impair their objectivity or affect their clinical judgment. The following 12 situations describe some not-so-obvious conflicting relationships:

1. After several sessions, a therapist discovers that two clients in therapy for help in choosing a mate are actually talking about each other. To avoid any possible conflict, therapists should terminate treatment when they discover a previously unrecognized relationship between two clients.

2. Therapists cannot control whom a relative marries. If a client marries into the family, the therapist should refer that person to another provider.

3. Resist the temptation to offer informal therapeutic services to friends and family. Most will respect the boundaries a therapist firmly establishes. Remember, therapists cannot control whether an individual will consider their comments to be casual conversation or therapeutic advice. Develop a stock response that clearly and firmly sets the boundaries. Once set, be careful to enforce the boundaries. No exceptions.

4. Avoid cocktail chatter that has therapeutic or counseling overtones. It is unusual to meet a mental health professional who has never been tapped for free consultations at a social gathering. Not only is such talk unethical but it compromises the whole concept of obtaining informed consent and taking a mental health history. Therapy should be conducted in the proper forum after all preliminary steps have been completed, including an informed consent to treatment agreement and a clinical history.

5. A shift in boundaries is usually gradual, not abrupt. A lawyer drafts a therapist's will and then casually asks about omitting his rebellious daughter from his own will. An insurance salesperson, after reviewing a therapist's policy, wants to talk about his

Therapy should be conducted in the proper forum after all preliminary steps have been completed, including an informed consent to treatment agreement and a clinical history.

feelings concerning the allocation of his own insurance proceeds between the children of his first marriage and his current wife. A therapist's banker, always a supportive father, feels guilty when he does not want to endorse and guarantee his son's note so his son can go into business. All mental health professionals have to be sensitive to the gradual shifts that blur boundaries and compromise objectivity. Therapists can engage a lawyer, a banker, or insurance professional but cannot then offer professional consultations to any of them. Helping professionals want to help. But there can be no dual relationships. Therapists, in this area, have to resist the temptation to offer help to prohibited clients. If there is any doubt, resolve the doubt in favor of maintaining a strict boundary demarcation.

Do not buy from or sell anything to clients, or accept any service from them.

6. Avoid accepting proffered tickets to sporting events, cultural performances, or journeys to exotic places using clients' frequent flyer miles. Do not buy from or sell anything to a client, nor accept any service from them.

7. In a small city or town where contact is inevitable, make sure that clients recognize the limits and guidelines imposed by the therapeutic relationship and insert a carefully drawn clause into your intake form that sets out the nature of unavoidable contacts and the manner in which such contacts are being handled in your community. Repeat guidelines as needed. Don't assume that once said and heard, they will be remembered forever.

8. Your client has a mint condition 1957 Chevrolet that you would love. It cannot be traded for a lifetime of therapy.

9. You treat a client who is a locally recognized painter, now selling paintings with a fair market value of $200 each, retail. Can you take a painting and credit $200 to the account? Suppose the painting increases in value to $20,000 and the client feels you took advantage of her?

10. Painters, plumbers, mechanics, and roofers may have personal problems or problem children. But you should not trade or barter for their services. Would your clinical objectivity be compromised if you traded services with your hairdresser and a day after having your hair treated it turned green? Also ask the question: What are

you bartering for? Is it a certain number of clinical hours, a cure, perpetual consultations as long as the client needs help or thinks help is needed, or is it result oriented? And if there is an additional need in the remote future? Is the provider obligated to provide services into the foreseeable future or so long as there is a treatable diagnosis? When the contract is for dollars per contact hour, the limits are more certain. When barter is involved, the financial boundaries become hazy and subject to interpretation, as each person interprets the contract according to his or her own purposes and subjective thoughts.

11. Do not invite a client to sing tenor in your barbershop quartet or participate in other groups to which you belong.

12. Your lawyer calls you at night in a panic. He claims an emergency with his child, and only you can help. Should you offer assistance? Probably yes, but document the nature of the emergency, the reason for seeing the lawyer's child in this particular emergency, and then make a referral as soon as is practicable. Make sure the lawyer understands this is a response to an "emergency" situation.

Potentially Beneficial Interactions

All ethics codes for the mental health disciplines advocate the avoidance of nonprofessional relationships with clients, former clients, and those in close relationships with a client. Some codes provide exceptions for interactions that are potentially beneficial to the client. Consider the following provisions from the *ACA Code of Ethics* (2005):

A.5.c. Nonprofessional Interactions or Relationships (Other Than Sexual or Romantic Interactions or Relationships)

Counselor-client nonprofessional relationships with clients, former clients, their romantic partners, or their family members should be avoided, except when the interaction is potentially beneficial to the client.

A.5.d. Potentially Beneficial Interactions

When a counselor-client nonprofessional interaction with a client or former client may be potentially beneficial to the client or former client, the counselor must document in case records, prior to the interaction (when feasible), the rationale for such an interaction, the potential benefit, and anticipated consequences for the client or former client and other individuals significantly involved with the client or former client. Such interactions should be initiated with appropriate client consent. Where unintentional harm occurs to the client or former client, or to an individual significantly involved with the client or former client, due to the nonprofessional interaction, the counselor must show evidence of an attempt to remedy such harm. Examples of potentially beneficial interactions include, but are not limited to, attending a formal ceremony (e.g., a wedding/commitment ceremony or graduation); purchasing a service or product provided by a client or former client (excepting unrestricted bartering); hospital visits to an ill family member; mutual membership in a professional association, organization, or community.

In the opening scenario, a grateful client (Sue) invited Carol to a marriage commitment ceremony. Pursuant to the ACA rule cited, if Carol concluded that her attendance would be beneficial to the client, she could attend. However, if something went wrong, Carol would have a duty to attempt to remedy the harm. What could go wrong? What if a stranger comes up to Carol and asks, "Are you Sue's therapist?" How does she answer the question? Can she indicate she is a friend of Sue's? What if no matter what Carol says, the inquiring guest proceeds to introduce her to everyone as Sue's therapist, which badly embarrasses Sue. It will be a rare case where the benefit realized by the client will exceed the potential risk of harm. Once these conversations are initiated by strangers or third parties, they are hard to limit or control. Whenever a therapist speaks with a talkative and gossipy individual, there is a risk that the entire conversation, with embellishments, will be repeated, often with striking inaccuracies and creative exaggerations. Our recommendation: the fewer out-of-therapy contacts, the better.

What if Sue decides to take the relationship up a notch and invites Carol to have lunch with her? Once boundary walls are chipped away or taken down, it is sometimes impossible to put them back in place without hurt feelings that can discourage future relationships and potential referrals. Carol could be inclined or forced to terminate effective therapy before the work is completed. Although the ACA rules give the therapist some latitude in making the decision about nonprofessional relationships, the better course to follow is to instruct clients at the outset that there can be no relationship other than the therapeutic one and then to stick to that declaration.

Because most relationships have gray areas of tolerance, clients often cannot understand the absolute need for therapeutic objectivity, single-focused relationships, or strict boundaries. Clients have no ethical problems in encouraging interpersonal dealings and associations. The mental health professional, however, has codes, ethical canons, rules, and traditions that mandate a wall between the provider and the client. Woe to the therapist who breaches the wall and allows the client to enter the professional's private space. The whole wall can crumble once a single brick is removed.

Ethical Flash Points

- There is no absolute guide or therapist-related written commandment concerning boundary violations that indicates a provider is meeting personal needs or promoting personal activities at a client's expense. Rather, therapists must be aware that the wall of professionalism between the therapist and the client is high and should be impenetrable. A therapist who feels any urge to compromise an ethical boundary should immediately raise and reinforce that wall.

- Therapists, like other workers, need to earn a living. This concept of "need" (as in meeting personal needs) only comes into question when clients use something other than dollars to pay for treatment. Only dollars have a fixed, recognized value that cannot be questioned later. Dollars provide, "This note is legal tender for all debts. Public and private." The fixed value is determined. In bartering, the many possible variations on both sides of the relationship make mutual understanding difficult. If at all possible, use the coin of the realm.

- For the dedicated mental health professional, saying no to a client is difficult, but saying no is easier than defending a claim for unethical conduct. And, financially and emotionally, it is less expensive in the long run.

- Although a code of ethics may allow for a nonprofessional relationship with a client if it is beneficial to the client, the risk of harm is too great to pursue or allow such contact with a client or former client.

Summary

Before embarking on a questionable relationship, call your lawyer for suggestions concerning worst-case scenarios.

In each situation described at the beginning of this chapter, what started out as an innocent supportive venture or gesture could turn into an ethical nightmare if the client or a colleague becomes unhappy. Before embarking on a questionable relationship, call your lawyer for suggestions concerning worst-case scenarios. Think through all the "what if" possibilities and then check those scenarios against your professional association's or licensing board's published guidelines and the disciplinary actions taken under those guidelines. A lawyer with extensive education, training, and experience in dealing with the risks faced by mental health professionals usually can create a worst-case situation. If there is none, and the therapist feels comfortable with the evolving situation, it is probably ethical and within the appropriate professional boundaries. If possible, obtain the opinion of the expert in writing. If a written memorandum is not possible, at least take copious notes of the conversation and insert the notes in the clinical file.

Suggested Research Assignments

1. Locate and discuss any rules promulgated by licensing boards in your state that deal with dual relationships.
2. Locate and discuss any state and national professional association ethical guidelines that deal with dual or multiple relationships. In reviewing ethical guidelines, do you notice any glaring inconsistencies?
3. Compare and contrast these state licensing board rules with the ethical rules promulgated by the state professional associations.
4. Compare and contrast state licensing board and professional association guidelines with the guidelines of national professional associations.
5. Identify resources and persons you would consult with to safely and ethically make a decision about a potential dual relationship.
6. Call the chairman of the ethics committee of the state board. Determine how available the chairman or the board members are when professionals need guidance in subtle or tricky ethical problems.

Is the office staff any more helpful? And, if you are fortunate enough to obtain a ruling, can you count on it should a real problem occur in the future and no one remembers your conversation?

7. Research the decisions of your state licensing boards and state and national professional association ethics committees for dual relationship violation sanctions.

8. Research civil case decisions of your state involving dual relationships. What damages, if any, were awarded?

Discussion Questions

1. What would you tell a client about boundaries and dual relationships prior to initiating treatment?

2. What would you tell another mental health practitioner, who is a close friend of yours, who has agreed to attend the bar mitzvah of a child she is treating? Would it make a difference if therapy had concluded? Does it make a difference if your friend is or is not Jewish?

3. What steps would you take if a client persistently tried to draw you into a dual relationship? How do you document this?

4. Would there be a problem with entering into a lucrative business relationship with a wealthy former client if 5 years have elapsed since you last saw the client?

5. Can you develop a response that will eliminate the problem of blurring boundaries without offending the client?

6. How would you respond to a person who knows you are a therapist and comes up to you in the grocery store checkout line and asks, "You are a therapist. Would you mind my asking a simple question?" Is "Buzz off" an appropriate response?

3

Confidentiality

Anita was a patient in the local hospital when she was seen by the hospital social worker. Anita's adult daughter was also present and asked the social worker many questions about her mother's health care. The social worker on rounds grew impatient, but she answered the questions and finally left the room in what might be called a controlled "huff." About an hour later when the daughter was meandering through the halls taking a break from sitting with her mother, she overheard the social worker in the nursing station talking with the nurses about the "hysterical daughter in 504 who asks silly and irrelevant questions." The target of the invective could be identified since 504 was a room on the floor and the daughter was the only person, in addition to the patient, who was in the room. Is this a breach of the patient's right of privacy? Is this an example of unethical behavior or simply unprofessional behavior? Does this turn a professional conversation into inappropriate gossip?

Dr. Knight counsels clients with sexual dysfunction. One day, a client entered the office for his weekly therapy session and told Dr. Knight about his remarkable recovery from impotence after using Viagra. Dr. Knight dutifully recorded the information and then altered his treatment plan to indicate that the client's sexual functions had improved with this specific medication and that future treatment would shift to handling the client's other interpersonal problems. Later, while sitting in a booth in the office building cafeteria, he shared with another therapist the information that the client who came in at 10:00 AM was helped by Viagra and now is facing the world with renewed potency. Both twitter a little, as men sometimes do, as they discuss this subject. Unknown to either therapist, the client's "significant other" is sitting in the next booth. She overhears the entire conversation. No names were ever used; however, she knows exactly whom they are talking about because she can recognize the other details of the conversation, and their amusement is extremely distressing to her.

Dr. Green is active on the lecture circuit in addition to her busy clinical practice. She uses many case illustrations to illustrate the points she wants to emphasize in her seminars but always changes the names, the location, and any descriptive or identifying data. If possible, she does not use an example in a city where the situation might have gained some notoriety. In one complex case study, she has made what she thinks is a complete deidentifying transition. Nothing is the same and no stranger, or perhaps even a friend, could identify the client. Unbeknownst to her, the client to whom she is referring in the case study has become a licensed therapist during the past 3 years and is sitting in the audience. Although all names and personal information have been changed, Dr. Green's former client is able to identify herself as the source for the case study. Certain phrases in the dialogue are unmistakably identifiable. As a result, she feels that the entire mental health community (or at least all those in the audience) now knows her problems. As with many individuals in therapy, she has shared her problems with some of her friends, many of them classmates in the counseling curriculum, and knows that, if they think about it, they could gather the evidence, compare their conversations with her to Dr. Green's example, and conclude correctly that she is the client being described. The example used was not an assemblage of different cases and clients but an accurate description of her personal, intimate, and former therapeutic situation, including her diagnosis, treatment plan, and the outcome of her therapy. Has the client's confidentiality been breached? Will the client exacerbate the problem if she makes further disclosures to friends and colleagues?

Dr. Strange, a professor of clinical psychology, has retired after 30 years with the university. During all those years, he maintained a log of bizarre cases, and in retirement, he intends to disguise all the cases and write a book about the clinical practice he maintained while he was teaching and consulting. Word has leaked out around the campus about Dr. Strange's book, although it is only rumor and gossip. One of Dr. Strange's former clients is now involved in litigation in which the client's mental health is an issue. The attorney for the defendant (the person the client/plaintiff is suing) hears about the future manuscript and the bizarre cases file and, on a whim, issues a subpoena to compel Dr. Strange to bring the client's file as well as the manuscript to a deposition where it will be examined. Then Dr. Strange will be asked questions about both. Is Dr. Strange's manuscript considered a clinical record? Must Dr. Strange bring this manuscript, which refers to actual cases, but is not a part of a particular client's clinical file, to the deposition? And how about the other cases referenced in the manuscript that are not connected with the defendant or the plaintiff? Should Dr. Strange be required to discuss their particulars or surrender these underlying case files as well?

When Dr. Pepper retired, she took all her files home and stored them in a locked room constructed in the corner of her garage. Finally, after 10 years, at age 75, she needed the space, so she disposed of them by carting off one cardboard box at a time, one each week, and putting it in a dumpster behind the Dairy Queen. Imagine her surprise when a group of children, playing in the dumpster, found a box, opened it up, and took out selected files . . . the ones that concerned the preacher, schoolteachers, and neighbors. Surprise was only the beginning of her troubles.

Dr. Smiley started practicing as a clinician about 45 years ago, when therapy began with a handshake and a one-sentence consent form. She has preserved all her clinical files in locked cabinets, even though the new licensing law only requires her to keep and maintain them for 7 years. Jackie, a client treated by Dr. Smiley 15 years ago, becomes involved in litigation concerning custody of a teenage daughter. The angry husband/plaintiff issues a subpoena to Dr. Smiley to appear in court with the 15-year-old record. Jackie is furious. She was never informed that her old clinical files could be subpoenaed and further tells Dr. Smiley that she would never have been so honest, revealing, and loquacious if she knew her words would come back to haunt her. There is nothing in the file to indicate an understanding of this particular exception to confidentiality. Indeed, 15 years ago, few therapists were concerned about the technical exceptions. What can Dr. Smiley do now?

Confidentiality and Therapy

The words *confidentiality* and *trust* are inextricably tied together in the lexicon of therapy. Few clients would consent to therapy if they thought that what they said in a therapy session would become part of the public domain or community gossip. Clients have a right to expect confidentiality. That is why under normal circumstances what is said in therapy is absolutely confidential and will *never ever* be repeated. Absolute confidentiality is the general rule, however, and is subject to many exceptions, especially when the client or the therapist is involved in legal proceedings. Absolute confidentiality, while discussed as a maxim, cannot be guaranteed.

The rules of confidentiality state that what is said to the therapist in therapy is confidential and cannot be voluntarily repeated, but under the direction of a judge or other magistrate, or when directed under other rules of law, the therapist may be compelled to testify concerning the client, the client's records, or the

In litigation, the rules of evidence in that jurisdiction prevail, and the question of confidentiality becomes one of privilege. Privilege issues are decided by judicial authority; the judge determines what is or is not subject to revelation in court. In such cases, the rules of confidentiality state that what is said to the therapist in therapy is confidential and cannot be voluntarily repeated, but under the direction of a judge or other magistrate, or when directed under other rules of law, the therapist may be compelled to testify concerning the client, the client's records, or the client's history as contained in the therapist's notes and intake data. The questions we must answer are: What are examples of confidentiality and privilege, and how do they differ?

Masking Identity of Clients and Cases in Conversation

Some elements of confidentiality are clear, especially when reduced to simple terms and in simple situations. Therapists do not gossip about identifiable clients. Identifiable does not just mean using a name but also providing enough information so that anyone knowing the person and the facts could make the connection. In conversation, the names, circumstances, places, ages, number of children, and professions must be eliminated, along with other details that might lead to self-identification or allow one individual to identify another. Using composite examples is helpful, but even then all principal facts must be so distorted that identification is impossible.

Informed Consent

A client can waive confidentiality in writing, as in a "Consent to Therapist-to-Therapist Disclosure of Client Records/Information," "Consent for Release of Information upon Insurance Assignment," or "Authorization for the Use and Disclosure of Protected Health Information" form (examples of these forms can be found in *The Portable Lawyer for Mental Health Professionals*, Bernstein and Hartsell 2004). In that case, information about the client can be shared freely but consistent with the terms and limitations of the written authorization. When providers solicit the written authorization from the client, they must be careful if the information is to be made public or semipublic. The rule of unintended consequences confines client consent to the waiver of confidentiality regarding predictable consequences. If the consequences prove to be terribly harmful to the client in an unintended, unpredictable, or unanticipated manner, the client could complain that the waiver was overreaching and that the release of information was not appropriately consented to by the client. Put another way, the client may consent to the release of information, but it must be an informed consent, that is, informed of all the foreseeable consequences of the release.

client's history as contained in the therapist's notes and intake data. Identifiable does not just mean using a name but also providing enough information so that anyone knowing the person and the facts could make the connection.

The client may consent to the release of information, but it must be an informed consent.

Confidentiality versus Privilege

Confidentiality is both an ethical precept and a traditional rule when offering therapy. Privilege, on the other hand, is a rule of law. Without a statute, there is no privilege. Bernstein and Hartsell (2004), *The Portable Lawyer for Mental Health Professionals*, indicated:

Privilege . . . belongs to the client. If the client tells the therapist to make the record public, then the therapist must do so. (The client's request should be written, signed, and dated. In some states, it may have to be notarized. HIPAA's Privacy Rule also requires specific language to be included in a client's authorization including a specific consent or request to release psychotherapy notes. (45 C.F.R. §164.508 (3)) If a therapist feels, as a matter of professional judgment, that the file should not be made public, he or she may file a motion with the appropriate court to restrict publication of the file. This motion will lead to a hearing and a judicial determination. The therapist does not possess the right to refuse to disclose the file if the client and court determine it should be made public. The burden of proof is on the therapist. The court must be shown that revealing the file to the client would be harmful to the client and that the best interest of the client would be served by keeping the file confidential, even from the client. (pp. 5–6)

Privilege is granted by statute, applies to the judicial or court system only, and must be claimed by the client.

Many states allow a therapist to block a client's access to their confidential information without court intervention if he or she, in the exercise of professional judgment, believes disclosure of the information will be harmful to the client. Usually the client must be notified in writing of the therapist's decision. The client then will have the option of having a second mental health professional review the information and make an independent analysis on disclosure or may file a court action and seek judicial review and determination. The Health Insurance Portability and Accountability Act (HIPAA) Privacy Rule has similar provisions and includes an additional requirement of advising the client how a complaint can be filed with the therapist or the therapist's employer's designated Privacy Officer and the Department of Health and Human Services (45 C.F.R. §164.524 (3) (i)).

Privilege is granted by statute, applies to the judicial or court system only, and must be claimed by the client. If, in the context of litigation, a third party requests client information or records and the client does not consent to the release of information or the therapist believes therapeutically that a disclosure would harm the client, the therapist must file a motion for a protective order or motion to quash and assert privilege. Privilege, if granted, allows that certain information, although possessed by a therapist, is protected by law from disclosure in a court proceeding. Some examples of privilege include the priest-penitent, lawyer-client, or husband-wife relationships, among others. Although some statutes grant a privilege for mental health information, many of them are so diluted by the statutory exceptions that they have little effect. If a privilege is to be claimed, the client and the therapist must consult a lawyer and then assert the appropriate specific privilege in court by motion before a judge. The judge will rule if the privilege applies and will either grant the privilege and block testimony or overrule it and compel testimony or disclosure of records, in which case the therapist as a witness must either testify or risk being held in contempt for failure to testify and possibly be fined or incarcerated.

There are many exceptions to privilege. When the question arises in any jurisdiction, the therapist should consult an attorney in that jurisdiction to determine the verbiage of the local privilege statute, the limits indicated by case law, the exceptions, and the client-related public relations aspects. Sometimes it is better for the therapist to raise the privilege question loudly and clearly before the court just so the client understands that the therapist has made every effort to protect a file if ordered to testify or reveal a record. The therapist, however, does not have to object so enthusiastically that the judge holds the therapist in contempt and orders the therapist to be incarcerated. When ordered by the court, the therapist must be sworn in by the bailiff, take the witness stand, answer questions, and give testimony in the traditional manner. Whenever a therapist is ordered to testify by a judge or magistrate, it would be wise to have the therapist state the objection to testifying into the record, and to later request a copy of the transcript from the court reporter. In this way, the therapist's efforts to refrain from testifying are part of the record of the case and available to the therapist if the client should later complain that confidentiality was breached. It is evidence that the testimony was proffered under the direct order of the court.

The HIPAA Privacy Rule

This body of law provides the first comprehensive federal protection for the privacy of health information. It establishes a foundation of federal protections for the privacy of protected health information. It does not, however, replace or supersede other federal or state laws that grant clients greater privacy protection. Covered entities (which include mental health professionals who transmit protected health information electronically) are free to implement measures allowed by state law that are more protective. It allows the mental health professional the flexibility to create privacy procedures that fit his or her size and need (the requirements are scalable).

The HIPAA Privacy Rule grants to individuals specific privacy rights governing the use and disclosure of their protected health information. It provides a general rule that use or disclosure of protected health information for purposes other than treatment, payment, or health-care operations is permitted only with the client's written authorization (45 C.F.R. §164.508 (a) (1)).

However, the HIPAA Privacy Rule backs in the kinds of exceptions that mental health professionals have become familiar with under state law and the professional association canons of ethics. Examples include reporting statutes for child abuse and neglect and, in some states, domestic violence, judicial and administrative proceedings, and billing for services.

National Guidelines for Protecting Confidentiality

American Association for Marriage and Family Therapy (AAMFT) Code of Ethics (2001)

Principle II: Confidentiality

Marriage and family therapists have unique confidentiality concerns because the client in a therapeutic relationship may be more than one person. Therapists respect and guard the confidences of each individual client.

2.1 Marriage and family therapists disclose to clients and other interested parties, as early as feasible in their professional contacts, the nature of confidentiality and possible limitations of the clients' right to confidentiality. Therapists review with clients the circumstances where confidential information may be requested and where disclosure of confidential information may be legally required. Circumstances may necessitate repeated disclosures.

2.2 Marriage and family therapists do not disclose client confidences except by written authorization or waiver, or where mandated or permitted by law. Verbal authorization will not be sufficient except in emergency situations, unless prohibited by law. When providing couple, family or group treatment, the therapist does not disclose information outside the treatment context without a written authorization from each individual competent to execute a waiver. In the context of couple, family or group treatment, the therapist may not reveal any individual's confidences to others in the client unit without the prior written permission of that individual.

2.3 Marriage and family therapists use client and/or clinical materials in teaching, writing, consulting, research, and public presentations only if a written waiver has been obtained in accordance with Subprinciple 2.2, or when appropriate steps have been taken to protect client identity and confidentiality.

2.4 Marriage and family therapists store, safeguard, and dispose of client records in ways that maintain confidentiality and in accord with applicable laws and professional standards.

2.5 Subsequent to the therapist moving from the area, closing the practice, or upon the death of the therapist, a marriage and family therapist arranges for the storage, transfer, or disposal of client records in ways that maintain confidentiality and safeguard the welfare of clients.

2.6 Marriage and family therapists, when consulting with colleagues or referral sources, do not share confidential information that could reasonably lead to the identification of a client, research participant, supervisee, or other person with whom they have a confidential relationship unless they have obtained the prior written consent of the client, research

(continued)

(Continued)

participant, supervisee, or other person with whom they have a confidential relationship. Information may be shared only to the extent necessary to achieve the purposes of the consultation.

American Counseling Association (ACA) Code of Ethics (2005)

Section B: Confidentiality, Privileged Communication, and Privacy

Introduction

Counselors recognize that trust is a cornerstone of the counseling relationship. Counselors aspire to earn the trust of clients by creating an ongoing partnership, establishing and upholding appropriate boundaries, and maintaining confidentiality. Counselors communicate the parameters of confidentiality in a culturally competent manner.

B.1. Respecting Client Rights

B.1.a. Multicultural/Diversity Considerations . . .

B.1.b. Respect for Privacy

Counselors respect client rights to privacy. Counselors solicit private information from clients only when it is beneficial to the counseling process.

B.1.c. Respect for Confidentiality

Counselors do not share confidential information without client consent or without sound legal or ethical justification.

B.1.d. Explanation of Limitations

At initiation and throughout the counseling process, counselors inform clients of the limitations of confidentiality and seek to identify foreseeable situations in which confidentiality must be breached.

B.2. Exceptions

B.2.a. Danger and Legal Requirements

The general requirement that counselors keep information confidential does not apply when disclosure is required to protect clients or identified others from serious and foreseeable harm* or when legal requirements demand that confidential information must be revealed. Counselors consult with other professionals when in doubt as to the validity of an exception. Additional considerations apply when addressing end-of-life issues.

B.2.b. Contagious, Life-Threatening Diseases

When clients disclose that they have a disease commonly known to be both communicable and life threatening, counselors may be justified in disclosing information to identifiable third parties, if they are known to be at demonstrable and high risk of contracting the disease. Prior to making a disclosure, counselors confirm that there is such a diagnosis and assess the intent of clients to inform the third parties about their disease or to engage in any behaviors that may be harmful to an identifiable third party.

B.2.c. Court-Ordered Disclosure

When subpoenaed to release confidential or privileged information without a client's permission, counselors obtain written, informed consent from the client or take steps to prohibit the disclosure or have it limited as narrowly as possible due to potential harm to the client or counseling relationship.

(*continued*)

---

*Such disclosure, called the "duty to warn" concept, is controlled by statute in some jurisdictions and by case law in others. The HIPAA Privacy Rule provides for this exception as well (45 C.F.R. §512 (j) (1)) (see Chapter 27, "Duty to Warn"). When the problem arises, contact the state board for your profession, your malpractice insurance carrier, your lawyer, and your national organization. This is an area of law where states differ (see Chapter 27, "Duty to Warn").

(Continued)

B.2.d. Minimal Disclosure

To the extent possible, clients are informed before confidential information is disclosed and are involved in the disclosure decision-making process. When circumstances require the disclosure of confidential information, only essential information is revealed.

B.3. Information Shared with Others

B.3.a. Subordinates

Counselors make every effort to ensure that privacy and confidentiality of clients are maintained by subordinates, including employees, supervisees, students, clerical assistants, and volunteers.

B.3.b. Treatment Teams

When client treatment involves a continued review or participation by a treatment team, the client will be informed of the team's existence and composition, information being shared, and the purposes of sharing such information.

B.3.c. Confidential Settings

Counselors discuss confidential information only in settings in which they can reasonably ensure client privacy.

American Psychological Association (APA) Ethical Principles of Psychologists and Code of Conduct **(2002)**

4. Privacy and Confidentiality

4.01 Maintaining Confidentiality

Psychologists have a primary obligation and take reasonable precautions to protect confidential information obtained through or stored in any medium, recognizing that the extent and limits of confidentiality may be regulated by law or established by institutional rules or professional or scientific relationship.

4.02 Discussing the Limits of Confidentiality

(a) Psychologists discuss with persons (including, to the extent feasible, persons who are legally incapable of giving informed consent and their legal representatives) and organizations with whom they establish a scientific or professional relationship (1) the relevant limits of confidentiality and (2) the foreseeable uses of the information generated through their psychological activities.

(b) Unless it is not feasible or is contraindicated, the discussion of confidentiality occurs at the outset of the relationship and thereafter as new circumstances may warrant.

(c) Psychologists who offer services, products, or information via electronic transmission inform clients/patients of the risks to privacy and limits of confidentiality.

4.03 Recording . . .

4.04 Minimizing Intrusions on Privacy

(a) Psychologists include in written and oral reports and consultations, only information germane to the purpose for which the communication is made.

(b) Psychologists discuss confidential information obtained in their work only for appropriate scientific or professional purposes and only with persons clearly concerned with such matters.

4.05 Disclosures

(a) Psychologists may disclose confidential information with the appropriate consent of the organizational client, the individual client/patient, or another legally authorized person on behalf of the client/patient unless prohibited by law.

(b) Psychologists disclose confidential information without the consent of the individual only as mandated by law, or where permitted by law for a valid purpose such as to (1) provide needed professional services; (2) obtain appropriate

(*continued*)

(*Continued*)

professional consultations; (3) protect the client/patient, psychologist, or others from harm; or (4) obtain payment for services from a client/patient, in which instance disclosure is limited to the minimum that is necessary to achieve the purpose. (See also Standard 6.04e, Fees and Financial Arrangements.)

4.06 Consultations

When consulting with colleagues, (1) psychologists do not disclose confidential information that reasonably could lead to the identification of a client/patient, research participant, or other person or organization with whom they have a confidential relationship unless they have obtained the prior consent of the person or organization or the disclosure cannot be avoided, and (2) they disclose information only to the extent necessary to achieve the purposes of the consultation. (See also Standard 4.01, Maintaining Confidentiality.)

4.07 Use of Confidential Information for Didactic or Other Purposes

Psychologists do not disclose in their writings, lectures, or other public media, confidential, personally identifiable information concerning their clients/patients, students, research participants, organizational clients, or other recipients of their services that they obtained during the course of their work, unless (1) they take reasonable steps to disguise the person or organization, (2) the person or organization has consented in writing, or (3) there is legal authorization for doing so.

National Association of Social Workers (NASW) Code of Ethics (1999)

1.07 Privacy and Confidentiality

(a) Social workers should respect clients' right to privacy. Social workers should not solicit private information from

clients unless it is essential to providing services or conducting social work evaluation or research. Once private information is shared, standards of confidentiality apply. . . .

(f) When social workers provide counseling services to
families, couples, or groups, social workers should seek
agreement among the parties involved concerning each
individual's right to confidentiality and obligation to preserve
the confidentiality of information shared by others. Social
workers should inform participants in family, couple, or
group counseling that social workers cannot guarantee that
all participants will honor such agreements. . . .

(k) Social workers should protect the confidentiality of clients
when responding to requests from members of the media. . . .

(o) Social workers should take reasonable precautions to
protect client confidentiality in the event of the social worker's termination of practice, incapacitation, or death. . . .

(p) Social workers should protect the confidentiality of deceased clients consistent with the preceding standards.

Common Threads among Ethics Codes

- Clients are entitled to confidentiality as that word is commonly
  understood by laypersons.
- Therapists have to resist the temptation to gossip, tell war stories,
  or use thinly disguised examples of clients in social conversations.
  A client should never be identified.
- Clients have the right to be informed, before services are provided,
  of the exceptions to confidentiality, such as child abuse; elder abuse;
  duty to warn, where it applies; exceptions when there is involvement in the judicial system; custody cases; and other situations
  that, when they become part of litigation, are not protected by
  confidentiality.
- The HIPAA Privacy Rule requires that clients be informed in writing of all permitted uses and disclosure of their protected health

Therapists have to resist the temptation to gossip, tell war stories, or use thinly disguised examples of clients in social conversations. A client should never be identified.

information. A "Notice of Privacy Practices" must be given to each potential client.

- The limits to absolute confidentiality should be stated on the informed consent form and clearly discussed before therapy begins.
- Records have to be both maintained and preserved according to professional guidelines or state statute.
- Clients have a right to waive confidentiality in writing.
- Client confidentiality continues after the death of the therapist or the client.
- Preparations have to be made to accommodate the death of the client or the death or incapacity of the therapist. Every person, including professionals, should have a valid and current will. The will must conform to the ethical canons so that in the event the professional dies, the administrator or executor of the estate may probate the will in conformity with the ethical guidelines of the profession. The client file is handled with more delicacy than personal property or real estate, because rules of confidentiality govern the disposition of the clinical file and protect its contents.
- The final word has not been established concerning contagious diseases, especially AIDS. The HIPAA Privacy Rule provides that if a public health authority (Center for Disease Control) is authorized by law to collect or receive information for public health purposes, entities may disclose protected health information without client authorization. Other protective statutes dealing with HIV come into play. There is some confusion between the various disciplines and the law at local, state, and federal levels.
- Where confidences have to be disclosed, the least information possible or necessary should be disclosed ("minimum necessary standard").
- Confidentiality binds employees, subordinates, agents, and servants, as well as temporary help, technicians, repair people, copy personnel, individuals, and others who retrieve and scan faxes. All have to be educated and trained concerning the applicability of confidentiality rules that apply to the therapist and understand that these rules apply directly to them. Each person in the office should sign or initial a lawyer-drafted confidentiality memorandum. HIPAA Privacy and Security Rules require documentation of such training.

- Clients being treated by a treatment team have a right to know who is on the team and why.
- Information received and shared should be on a need-to-know basis.
- Families, couples, and groups need special sensitivity. The individual rights of each person in the system must be protected.
- Beware of the media. Clever reporters can put words in a therapist's mouth that may be embarrassing, misleading, and downright dangerous to the therapist and the client, especially when taken out of context. In pursuit of a good story, many reporters will have no hesitancy disclosing confidential information.
- HIPAA Privacy Rule requires a written record be kept of many disclosures of a client's protected health information.

Ethical Flash Points

- Punishment for violating confidentiality can be meted out by licensing boards, federal authorities, and national organizations. Punishment can also lead to a malpractice suit.

- The client must be informed, prior to the commencement of therapy, of all the limits to confidentiality. This includes the special situations that can arise if there is involvement in the judicial system. The clinician should talk with the client about the possibility of litigation during the initial interview and explain the therapeutic pitfalls. Often litigation and the threat of litigation create their own mental health problems.

- Confidentiality continues to be an issue after the death of either the client or the therapist. A protocol has to be established by every mental health provider or agency to take care of the client, the clinical file, and the continuation of therapy if needed. The intake and consent form is the place to provide for disposition of the file on the death of either.

- Check the local legal rules when a client threatens to commit suicide or threatens to injure or kill another readily identifiable person. The instinct is to warn the potential victim. It may not be ethical. Check your state law. Check it now. The therapist may not have time when the actual threat occurs, especially if the threat occurs at night or over a weekend.

- Store records so as to protect them from curious eyes. They should be locked and safe from fire and natural disasters.

(*continued*)

(Continued)

- If using case examples in lectures or otherwise, explain that the case represents a composite problem, not a real person, and then deidentify the case as much as possible. No one should be able to discern the identity of any case illustration.

- With proper information, a client can always waive confidentiality.

- The therapist, with motion and order before the proper court, can object to waiving confidentiality if the therapist feels it would be a danger to the client or others. This would include letting the client see his or her own file. The law in many states and the HIPAA Privacy Rule allow for the withholding of information from a client if it is perceived to be harmful to the client. Follow your state-specific requirements including notice requirements when deciding not to provide a client with information about his or her treatment.

- Protecting confidentiality includes training agents, employees, servants, receptionists, transcription services, answering services, and others who learn about therapists' files, to recognize that from their point of view *everything is confidential*. The provider alone issues the order to share information.

- Train all temporary help and new employees regarding issues of confidentiality.

- When information is shared, it should be the minimum necessary to do the job (the least necessary amount of information to convey what needs to be known by the other person).

- Where there are multiple members of a group, keep a separate file for each member, including children. This will lead to more paperwork, but less confusion if an individual file must be examined.

- When in doubt, call your lawyer and your malpractice insurance carrier.

Summary

Communications between a provider and client and a client's records, however created or stored, are confidential.

HIPAA and all ethics canons or codes of the mental health professions and most of its subgroups provide that communications between a provider and client and a client's records, however created or stored, are confidential. Further, the codes charge that the therapist shall not disclose any communication, record, or identity of a client except when required under rules of law or statute. Improper breaches of confidentiality are unethical and can lead to regulatory authority disciplinary actions and malpractice suits. Thus, although records are mandated under the mental health codes, these records are represented to the client as being confidential and not available to the curious eyes of others. They are, in a sense, sacrosanct and untouchable. But there are exceptions to confidentiality, and under HIPAA and the ethics canons, the client has a right to be fully informed of the exceptions to confidentiality before treatment begins.

One concept is clear: Although reporting statutes provide for reporting such offenses as child abuse, the therapist is vulnerable if he or she recklessly disregards the confidentiality of the clients who have placed their trust in a professional relationship. There is zero tolerance for the gossipy provider, the chatty clinician, or the talkative therapist who reveals too much confidential information to the wrong person or people. The exceptions often apply to the judicial system. They do not ever give license to the clinician to reveal confidences in an inappropriate context or setting. Such is grounds for disciplinary action. The disciplinary actions of the various licensing boards are replete with actions taken against therapists who shared information when it was inappropriate to do so. Table talk with friends or even one's spouse should not include the repetition of anything learned in a therapy session. Therapeutic information is to be used for the benefit of the client only, not as social small talk.

The professional cannot gossip, identify a client in a verbal conversation, or use an identifiable client in a lecture to illustrate a point, or in a written work or electronic presentation. When disclosure is mandated, the wall surrounding confidentiality seems to crumble. Confidentiality may be compromised in cases of child abuse or elder abuse, in response to a lawfully issued subpoena, when mental health is a concern in litigation, when the client sues a therapist, when a judge orders a therapist to testify under penalty of contempt of court, or when a therapist sues a client (ill-advised) for an unpaid bill. Confidentiality may also be compromised when a therapist is called to testify in court.

Although state and federal rules differ, a therapist cannot represent to a client that the record is absolutely sacred and sacrosanct and the contents of a record or the therapeutic session that created the record or produced the record will never be disclosed. Ethically, then, what is confidentiality and what are the limitations? The broad concepts are set out in the various guidelines. The exceptions usually arise when the therapist is involved in a judicial system that is seeking the truth. This quest sometimes affects the therapist's ability to protect the client from disclosure. However, the therapist in many jurisdictions has the right and obligation to seek the protection of the court for testimony that may be intrusive, irrelevant, or requested mainly for the purpose of intimidation or harassment. Such protection would be sought after a motion, hearing, and ruling of the court. If the court does not grant the protection, then the therapist must comply with the order of the court.

A review of the HIPAA Privacy Rule and the ethical standards of the mental health organizations indicates that the federal government and each organization seeks to protect clients from the disclosure of their personal remarks, thoughts, histories, and inner feelings as well as the records made of all these therapeutic moments. The codes differ in verbiage but are nearly identical in their philosophy of client protection. Some are more comprehensive than others, but all are remarkably consistent. In a general sense, the client has a right to know what might have to be disclosed to a third party and when.

Suggested Research Assignments

1. Locate and discuss any rules promulgated by licensing boards in your state that deal with confidentiality and its exceptions.
2. Locate and discuss any state and national professional association ethical guidelines that deal with confidentiality and its exceptions. In reviewing ethical guidelines, do you notice any glaring inconsistencies?
3. Compare and contrast these state licensing board rules with the ethical rules promulgated by the state professional associations.
4. Compare and contrast state licensing board and professional association guidelines with the guidelines of national professional associations.

5. Locate and discuss the HIPAA Privacy Rule provisions regarding confidentiality and its exceptions. What similarities or differences are there between these federal rules and the state and professional organization rules and state licensing board rules that you examined?

6. Identify resources/persons you would consult with to safely and ethically make a decision regarding confidentiality and its exceptions.

7. Consult with mental health professionals in your area and find out what are the most common issues regarding confidentiality they are confronted with in their practices.

8. Research the decisions of your state licensing boards and state and national professional association ethics committees for confidentiality-related violation sanctions.

9. Research the civil and criminal case decisions of your state for confidentiality-related violations. What penalties or damages were assessed and awarded?

10. Research the decisions of the Office of Civil Rights for privacy violations. What penalties or sanctions were assessed?

11. Apply the ethical canons of the state licensing board for your discipline to the scenarios at the beginning of this chapter and answer the questions that are posed.

Discussion Questions

1. What would you tell a client about confidentiality and its limitations prior to initiating treatment?

2. How do you document Question 1?

3. What would you tell another mental health professional who wants to discuss a case with you before going any further with the conversation?

4. What steps would you take to ensure confidentiality of group therapy?

5. If you were approached by a publisher with a serious offer to write a book detailing your most interesting and successful cases, could you

say yes? What support would you give for your decision to say yes
or no?

6. What would you tell a lawyer for a client who called to discuss the
   client's treatment?

7. Are you required to answer questions about treatment posed to you
   by the parent of a 16-year-old client?

8. How would you respond to a client who comes up to you in a bookstore and starts telling you how bad, sad, and depressed he is feeling
   that day?

9. Do you have a rehearsed technique for rejecting inappropriate clinical conversations, generated by inappropriate potential clients in
   inappropriate locations? Is "Buzz off" an acceptable response to the
   aggressive individual who assaults you with therapeutic questions
   in unprofessional places? Is there a better method?

4

Dangerous Clients

Sharon has a hair-trigger temper. In the past, she committed several physical assaults, most of which were papered over, except one that ended with a conviction and a 6-month stay in the county jail. The girl she assaulted with an ax handle suffered several facial fractures and a concussion. Sharon's friends are a residual small group of high school classmates who just "hang out" and get by begging money from family members and working occasional minimum-wage jobs. In this group, physical assaults and threatening confrontations are the rule rather than the exception. Sharon has now managed to get an associate degree from the local community college and knows that a second assault conviction will result in serious penitentiary time. She is contemplating making an appointment to see a counselor at the suggestion of a college advisor.

John was a tough high school athlete who has used physical force or the threat of it in every conflict. His mother died when he was 3, and he was raised by an abusive and alcoholic father. He has a record for spousal abuse, and misdemeanor assault and battery, and has been a person of serious interest to the police in two investigations, one for an arson in which a person was seriously burned and the other for a homicide in which the victim was

*bludgeoned to death. During divorce proceedings involving his second
spouse, the judge ordered John into counseling as a condition of future access
to his 4-year-old daughter.*

Some clients are risky. You can't practice in the field of mental
health without an occasional risk. The clients served by mental health
providers are inherently more problematic than the average person.
These clients bring their problems to the clinician for help in solving
them.

In Chapter 10, "Risky Clients," we list characteristics of clients
who, because of their educational background, learning or therapeutic
experiences, personal instability, or psychological diagnosis pose a
complaint or practice risk to the therapist. Treating these clients can
be a source of intense personal aggravation and tension.

These risky clients should not be accepted into therapy without in-
depth inquiry and should often be refused or referred. Treating them
can certainly upset the mental health professional's peaceful practice.
Other potential clients, however, are downright dangerous from a
physical safety perspective and should be declined by all but the most
experienced and skilled mental health professionals. Prudence in these
instances is the better part of valor. A merely *risky* client deserves second thoughts, and as such might present a challenge, but a truly *dangerous* client is to be avoided unless some compelling reason mandates
accepting the presenting dangerous client into a therapeutic relationship. A protective antenna should go up as soon as the provider clinically determines that the presenting client has a diagnosable
propensity to do real harm.

The dangerous client may have many obvious characteristics and
may be a danger to themselves (the suicidal client), a danger to others
(the homicidal client), a danger to the community (a potential mass
murderer), or a danger to themselves and the community (such as the
mass murderer who commits suicide by shooting at a police officer
knowing the officer will shoot back). These potential clients are dangerous as well to the mental health provider and must be identified
and appropriately treated by skilled therapists before real damage is
done. When you cannot filter the dangerous from the harmless with

any degree of certainty, caution is the best policy. If there is any doubt, the policy of avoidance should be followed.

A therapist who treats a client who does serious harm to himself or others may be closely scrutinized by law enforcement, victims, the victims' families and their attorneys, and ultimately by judges, juries, and licensing boards. Just imagine the intense focus on a treating counselor that would occur if a youthful client enters his school and kills several students and teachers.

Clients can become dangerous in numerous ways, often unpredictably, but usually following events that trigger the temper or violent tendency of the client. Some examples of situations that have resulted in violent outbursts by clients of mental health professionals are:

- A serious fee dispute over the amount charged for a particular service that, whether real or feigned, is considered to be unjust, unwarranted, unfair, or that did not produce the effect expected or anticipated by the client.
- Courtroom testimony of a therapist on behalf of a client or another that does not, in the client's mind, appear to be supported by the therapy or that, though truthful and objective, results in a litigation result unfavorable to a client.
- Clients have been known to become violent when supportive therapy is not backed up by helpful testimony in court. And in this situation, "helpful" means that in the eyes of the client the testimony did not produce the desired result. Any client who loses a case will have a tendency to criticize his lawyer and his witnesses. Clients who lose are often unwilling to accept personal blame for the result but will review all collateral reasons they lost, aiming their venom at their lawyer, their mental health professional, or "lying" neighbors, antagonistic jurors, or prejudiced judges.
- Failing to take prescription medication or using inappropriate medication. Or, taking medication with substances that produce an undesired effect. Certain medications should not be taken with alcohol, and others should be taken with water or food. While most nonmedical professionals do not prescribe medications, they must be aware of the misuse of medications. Misuse or nonuse can be equally

dangerous and produce unexpected clinically observable behavioral patterns. One prerequisite for effective therapy consists of determining if prescription medications have been suggested or prescribed and if these medications are being ingested in the proper dosage and at the proper times. Although only physicians prescribe medications, the therapist must be aware of the client's attitude while in the office. The question? Is the person being treated the true person without medication, or is the demeanor of the person in the office so medicated or so affected by a mental illness requiring medication that the client's conduct is adversely or profoundly affected either by medication or lack of medication? A client who overdoses on medications, either prescription or nonprescription, can show behavioral signs that alert the provider to signs of dangerousness. An immediate inquiry should be made concerning medication. This inquiry, with permission of the client, should be made to the treating physician. You can anticipate that a client who is not following directions for medications will lie or exaggerate when challenged.

- Contact with a former spouse or lover.
- Loss of a job or employment-related discipline.
- Confrontations with spouse's or lover's paramour. Attacks on the "other" man or woman occur with frequency. The typical lovers' triangle is a most dangerous social situation.
- Threats by the therapist to terminate if the client does not become compliant.

These are just a handful of the possible stressors or triggers that can result in violent and harmful outbursts. Think about the challenges of taking on Sharon or John, the potential clients in the opening scenarios. Is it hard to imagine a client like these getting angry with their therapist who is firm and unapproving when the client refuses to follow sound therapeutic advice?

Avoiding Dangerous Clients

The mental health professionals we are mainly speaking to here are those who are not trained and experienced in treating clients with anger management issues or who exhibit sociopathic, or worse, behavior. Most therapists lack this kind of expertise and inclination. To avoid treating dangerous clients, it is imperative to identify who they are prior to commencement of the therapeutic relationship. Insisting on and conducting an evaluative session or interview before a decision is made to initiate therapy is the best approach. Just as with risky clients (see Chapter 10, "Risky Clients"), a mental health professional may wish to add questions to an intake form that solicit information about problems with anger, relationships, arrests, lawsuits, and criminal convictions. Be sure to review any written intake form carefully and follow up with questions posed to the potential client. If the client indicates he was arrested for spousal abuse, spend some time getting a clear history of what has occurred. If the potential client is evasive or seemingly dishonest, refer him or her to a therapist in the area with expertise in treating persons with anger management or sociopathic tendencies. Turn the client away even if the presenting problem the client wishes to work on is something that the mental health professional feels competent treating.

Remember, it is ethical to decline to treat clients you do not feel competent to treat.

National Guidelines for Competency

American Association for Marriage and Family Therapy (AAMFT) Code of Ethics (2001)

Principle III: Professional Competence and Integrity

Marriage and family therapists maintain high standards of professional competence and integrity.

3.1 Marriage and family therapists pursue knowledge of new developments and maintain competence in marriage and family therapy through education, training, or supervised experience.

(continued)

(Continued)

American Counseling Association (ACA) Code of Ethics (2005)

Section C: Professional Responsibility

C.2. Professional Competence

C.2.a. Boundaries of Competence

Counselors practice only within the boundaries of their competence, based on their education, training, supervised experience, state and national professional credentials, and appropriate professional experience. Counselors gain knowledge, personal awareness, sensitivity, and skills pertinent to working with a diverse client population.

American Psychological Association (APA) Ethical Principles of Psychologists and Code of Conduct (2002)

2.01 Boundaries of Competence

(a) Psychologists provide services, teach, and conduct research with populations and in areas only within the boundaries of their competence, based on their education, training, supervised experience, consultation, study, or professional experience.

National Association of Social Workers (NASW) Code of Ethics (1999)

Ethical Principle: *Social workers practice within their areas of competence and develop and enhance their professional expertise . . .*

1.04 Competence

(a) Social workers should provide services and represent themselves as competent only within the boundaries of their education, training, license, certification, consultation received, supervised experience, or other relevant professional experience.

When a Potentially Dangerous Client Becomes a Risk

There are clients who exhibit and cause danger to themselves and others. Former and present clients have been known to murder their parents, siblings, and others, while unstable clients have been known to commit suicide or murder students or coworkers in their workplaces. Violent behavior often becomes a media event, or sometimes a media circus. Then an investigation commences by prosecutors, investigators, curious interlopers, and members of the ever-inquisitive press. The inquiry may begin when family members, unable or unwilling to accept any responsibility for a client's (their sibling, parent, or friend) unhappy life, seek an avenue to obtain redress from the person who last or recently visited with the deceased or accused. This is often the mental health professional, who is vulnerable to accusations by the family of the deceased that he or she could have or should have prevented the untimely death or violent act of the loved one. What can the professional do when informed that a present or former client has committed a violent act or has injured or killed himself or another person? Many prescribed steps should be undertaken. Protecting yourself is a key interest when the death of a client occurs or when the client has killed or maimed others. What does the provider do? Here are some suggestions; however, they are not necessarily done in this order:

- Review and correct all progress or case notes. Make sure they are current, fulfill and accommodate all professional and ethical requirements, and determine that such clinical records do not contain mistakes. If so, follow the published rules of the location or licenses to correct, augment, change, or alter clinical records whether written, printed, or computer generated.
- Consult with your personal lawyer and make sure the lawyer has more than a casual acquaintance with mental health law. When a death occurs, consult a recognized expert. Determine your exposure to liability and possible defenses to anticipated litigation. Determine the civil, criminal, and licensing board ramifications. Begin to prepare a defense or at least conceptualize the defense with your lawyer.

- Call your malpractice or professional liability carrier. Discuss the case with the carrier's lawyer and risk management experts. Develop a defensive plan with them. Gather self-protecting information with this professional team and preserve it with the advice and consent of the insurance carrier, the lawyers, and such advisors as they recommend. Then arrange your defense and wait. If a case develops, you are prepared. If no case is ever processed, file the information away and give thanks. No harm was done in excessive preparation.

- Do a little research. The best professional defense is that the treatment plan is a plan accepted by the majority of therapists in your discipline or a plan accepted by a learned and accepted minority of professionals. Be prepared to show that your diagnosis, prognosis, and treatment plan are professionally acceptable. If available, find a local expert who will review the file and agree with you, in general. Since therapy is really a combination of art form and science, no two therapists will ever treat a client exactly the same way, and so a general agreement is all that is required. Did you do what other professionals would have done in the case? Remember, it is not essential that every client recover 100 percent, only that you did what a professional and licensed person would do for this specific client under these presenting circumstances (the treatment was professionally acceptable).

- Have either the liability carrier or your attorney hire another therapist to review your file as part of your defensive work so this expert's reports and opinions cannot be subpoenaed by another party. If there were flaws in your diagnosis, prognosis, or treatment plan, create a sensible rationale for what you did. If necessary, show that while your client did not get better, at least the client did not get worse; or if the client deteriorated, it was at a slower pace than might have happened without your effective treatment.

Do not discuss the case with anyone other than your lawyer, your hired experts, or the risk management supervisors of your insurance carrier. Loose talk among colleagues can return to haunt you. And do not talk to media people of any type, especially investigative reporters without your personal attorney present. Do not be seduced by the media or the promise of media exposure. Remember TV reporters want to sell TV time, and print reporters want to sell papers. Both will put words into your mouth if given the opportunity.

The Transition

Every client who seeks the help of a mental health professional enters the relationship with great hope. Sometimes he or she is seeking a cure. Sometimes the hope is the relief of anxiety, and on occasion the treatment is for the purpose of just having someone to talk to who will listen and reflect, respond, and reinforce. At the beginning of therapy, both the client and the provider feel that the relationship will be mutually rewarding and hopeful. As time passes, the relationship may change, and when and if the client becomes upset and dangerous, there is a transition. The client suddenly becomes adversarial and combative. The client may be revealing these negative characteristics for the first time. The dangerous client must be handled differently from the time of the confrontation to the time the confrontation is resolved. While helping and serving the client is still the goal, the subtle transition indicates that the client is slowly becoming part of the problem and must be sensitively treated to avoid changing from a client-serving experience to one where serving the client is secondary to the treatment provider protecting himself or herself. Defensive therapy at this point suggests that all contact with the client be faithfully documented, and any conduct that might result in action on behalf of the client be scrupulously reviewed. If there is any antagonism on the horizon, with the permission of the client, there should either be a referral or a consultation that supports the current treatment plan or offers another that is more acceptable to both the client and the provider.

As soon as the therapist has an uneasy feeling with a client, the therapist should seek the advice of a learned colleague. Without identifying the client (which would require client permission), the therapist should seek a consultation concerning the client. Explain the transition from satisfied client to belligerent antagonist and trace the changing relationship. Discuss a change in therapeutic modality that might relieve the antagonism and resistance. Then proceed with augmented or modified therapy. The client must know that the modification is for the purpose of serving the client, and that some tensions will be ameliorated if the current treatment plan is adjusted and a new treatment plan is adopted. At this point, continued documentation should indicate that the modified plan is client serving and resistance is being overcome. If the client continues to be antagonistic, and the provider feels that this antagonism could become more violent, then termination and a referral would be merited.

It is not unethical to terminate under these circumstances (see Chapter 13, "Terminating Therapy").

The initial intake and consent form by which the client consents to treatment must contain a clause that authorizes the provider to terminate treatment when the therapist does not feel the client is progressing or when the therapist feels, in his or her professional judgment, that the client can best be served by another helping professional. An appropriate referral, and the reasons for the referral, should be carefully documented, and, if possible, consent for the referral should be signed by the client and inserted in the file.

Can the Mental Health Professional Call the Police?

What can the mental health professional do when the client turns on the therapist and threatens the therapist or begins stalking the therapist? Is it unethical or a breach of confidentiality to contact the police or hire a lawyer to obtain a restraining order? Under such circumstances, it would not be unethical for a therapist to take protective action such as contacting the police or pursuing legal action. Every ethical code allows the mental health professional to take some action to prevent clients from harming themselves or a third party (which would include the treating mental health professional).

Even states that do not follow the holding in *Tarasoff v. Regents of University of California*, 17 Cal. 3d 425, 551 P.2d 334, allow a mental health professional to contact law enforcement if he or she has cause to believe a third party is in danger from a client (see Chapter 27, "Duty to Warn").

Additional authority is found in HIPAA Privacy Rule §164.512 (f) (5):

> Permitted disclosure: Crime on premises. A covered entity may disclose to a law enforcement official protected health information that the covered entity believes in good faith constitutes evidence of criminal conduct that occurred on the premises of the covered entity.

If the client while on the therapist's premises strikes (battery) or threatens to strike (assault) the therapist or becomes a stalker, the police should immediately be called. If a crime has been committed, prosecution should be pursued. If the police do not believe enough evidence exists for a criminal prosecution, consult a lawyer about civil action including a restraining order. The mental health professional has the right to seek protection and to be safe as he or she goes about everyday and professional life.

Ethical Flash Points

- Develop intake forms that seek to ascertain a potential client's propensity for violence.

- Be extremely sensitive to clients who exhibit words or actions that indicate a propensity toward dangerousness, either to self, others, or the community in general.

- As soon as this possibility occurs, do a little extra research and call a learned colleague and your risk management or liability insurance carrier. Take advice and proceed defensively from this point on.

- If the risk of dangerousness is too severe and it is beyond your level of competence to treat, terminate and make an appropriate referral. Keep detailed notes and maintain a defensive record from that point on. Maintain a balance between self-protective clinical notes and an accurate record of the treatment.

- Discuss all possibilities and alternatives with your personal mental health lawyer. Orchestrate your next movements with the knowledgeable attorney, documenting the advice given and pursued. The mental health provider makes the final decision, but to do so, legal and therapeutic input is required.

(continued)

(*Continued*)

- Review the canons of ethics or the published ethical principles in your state. See which clauses cover dangerous or risky clients. Be aware, there is an ethical and an unethical way to terminate treatment or make an appropriate referral. In this situation, make sure you have followed all the required standards and documented the fulfillment of each and every obligation.

- Some therapists use a "no suicide" or "no homicide" contract. If this is utilized, remember that even a signed memorandum of the client's agreement not to commit suicide or homicide is not a contract in the legal sense of the word. Rather, it is a therapeutic tool. If a client signs a no suicide contract and then commits suicide, the client's estate cannot be sued for breach of contract.

- Before determining whether to treat a client or continue treating a client, do a risk assessment. Mental health professionals are vulnerable civilly if they are negligent, criminally if they break the law, and professionally if they violate their licensing acts. A professional license is a terrible thing to lose.

- If the client crosses the line into criminal and dangerous conduct directed at a third party, including the therapist, the police should be contacted and criminal or civil legal action should be pursued.

Summary

Dangerous clients do not usually present themselves initially as being dangerous. Rarely, if ever, will a client present to a therapist that the overarching requested diagnosis is or should be "dangerousness." It is imperative therefore for therapists to ask intelligent and probing questions on intake to ferret out a propensity for violence.

Perhaps in anger management therapy or classes, or court-ordered cases, dangerousness is an obvious observation, but sometimes an occurrence in someone's life triggers dangerous and threatening acting-out that places the client, the therapist, or some other third person or the community in danger. When these signs appear, the treating clinician must pause and take note. If the client does, in fact, commit homicide or suicide, or hurt others, the treating provider is surely going to be called on to explain the circumstances: how the dangerous propensities developed, and how and why the diagnosis, treatment plan, and prognosis can be defended as the appropriate treatment for this client. With 20/20 hindsight, the ultimate question is, why wasn't the danger prevented? To substantiate that the plan was appropriate, some research may be required, and in addition, conventional wisdom would indicate that confidential input from colleagues would be helpful. Signs of dangerousness may be subtle or blatant, sudden or developed over an extensive period. In either case, the dangerous client represents a difficult challenge to the mental health professional.

Handle with care!

Suggested Research Assignments

1. What words, if used by a client, would indicate dangerousness?
2. What kind of past behavior would indicate a propensity toward violence?
3. What techniques can be used to handle an upset client?
4. Talk to mental health professionals in your area to learn how they screen for dangerous clients and how they treat dangerous clients that they accept.
5. Identify professional colleagues or resources that you could consult with when a client becomes hostile toward you or another person.
6. Develop a detailed client history form to help you identify dangerous or potentially dangerous clients.

Discussion Questions

1. You are visiting with a friend at the local McDonald's when a distraught client walks in. She slips into a booth next to you and tells you how unhappy she is because you were not able to "fix" her husband and she is now a single mom with all the attending financial problems. "If only," she says, you had been a more directive therapist, she "would be happily married and fully supported." Her misery is all your fault, and she will get even. What should you do? Her husband had mentioned to you that she carries a handgun in her purse and that she is expert at using it.

2. You keep getting late-night calls at home from a client who says she got your home phone number from your office staff, which you know is not true. She gets increasingly belligerent each time you tell her it is not appropriate to call you at home. What should you do? What do you document?

3. A potential new patient appears in your office for the initial evaluation and tells you that he terminated with his previous therapist when he filed a complaint against her with the state licensing board after they got into a physical altercation. What should you do? What do you document?

4. A mother calls and wants to schedule an appointment for you to see her daughter, of whom she is fearful. The mother advises you that the daughter is a martial arts instructor and her temper outbursts are becoming more frequent and explosive. What would you say? What do you document?

5

Discrimination

Katherine is a right-to-life supporter, both politically and religiously. She belongs to a church that regularly pickets abortion clinics and has participated in many of these protests. She does not condone violence against physicians or abortion clinic employees, but she supports her constitutional right to exercise free speech. Her views did not change when she attended graduate school or when she received her graduate degree in social work. She is now employed at an agency that offers general counseling to any woman who walks in the door. All women are entitled to a reduced fee scale in what is considered to be a clinically objective atmosphere. One day a woman (who is 4 weeks pregnant) comes in for abortion counseling. Her mind is not made up. She wants to consider the ramifications of all her options rather than feel pressured to select any particular alternative. Katherine is not married. The client is not married. Can Katherine have a definite point of view and still be clinically objective? Katherine and the woman like each other and enjoy the therapy session. All the options are presented. A few days later, the woman seeks additional counseling at the local abortion clinic. Katherine is outside with a picket sign. They exchange glances, but do not speak. After seeing Katherine picketing at the abortion clinic, will her client ever feel the abortion options were presented objectively?

Dr. Stevens is a heterosexual therapist in private practice. Her practice has been limited to couples contemplating divorce, and she has a fine community reputation for reconciling couples in troubled marriages. On the third visit, John, a married client, asks whether he can bring in a friend. Dr. Stevens reluctantly says yes, and John appears for the next session with Billy Bob, his significant other. Dr. Stevens has had no experience with gay clients and is very uncomfortable as the two men sit in her office holding hands. However, she is convinced John needs therapy to help with his marriage, his sexual identity, and other problems. As the session continues, her discomfort grows. What should Dr. Stevens do next?

Martha works for an agency where she deals with adults and teens. A change of administration indicates she must now handle preadolescent children. She is a single woman, does not like being around young children, and underwent sterilization to avoid the risk of ever having a child. At first, she makes deals with other therapists to handle her child caseload. Finally she faces the facts. Much to her chagrin, her new job description mandates that she must work with children. Considering her attitude toward children, can she handle her growing caseload of 5- to 10-year-olds? Will she discriminate without intending to be prejudicial? How will her antichild bias affect her clinical objectivity?

Judy is a card-carrying Oklahoma Republican and a strong supporter of the Republican president. Her client Bill is an enthusiastic Democrat, but that does not seem to make any difference to either of them and conversations rarely develop about their political preferences. The therapy Judy offers is effective and competent. Her client Bill surmises Judy's political leanings by seeing her picture with the president on the wall in her office. One day after a session, Judy observes Bill walk slowly by her car and stop for a moment, placing a flyer on her windshield. When she heads to the parking lot at the end of the day, there is the flyer: "HILLARY RODHAM CLINTON FOR PRESIDENT, THE PEOPLE'S CHOICE." How should Judy react during the next session? Or should she react at all? Can Judy continue to treat this client although he is a Democrat?

Melissa comes from a dysfunctional family where her father and mother were alcoholics. She hates liquor and married a man who never touches alcohol. The thought, sight, or smell of any liquor makes her ill. When she enrolled in graduate school, she resolved to take any other type case, but not addictions of any classification, including drugs, smoking, or drinking. Recently, her husband, an engineer, was transferred to a new community. The only therapy position available is with a substance abuse clinic. She and her husband need a second income. Should Melissa apply for the job?

Overt versus Subtle Discrimination

Whether old or young, in robust health or infirm, a client is entitled to competent therapy. Every client, whether a man or woman, gay or straight, is entitled to therapeutic objectivity. Color, race, nationality, religion, ethnicity, or country of origin should not in any way affect the availability of competent therapy. Physically and emotionally challenged individuals are also entitled to mental health counseling and treatment. All types of politically affiliated and unaffiliated individuals are entitled to treatment regardless of the label they carry. Age, race, gender, color, national origin, religion, disability, sexual orientation, or political affiliation should never influence the availability or quality of therapy. The right to such treatment is codified in the canons of ethics, and practitioners are subject to disciplinary action if they ignore their profession's ethical canons and exhibit discrimination in any form.

> *Age, race, gender, color, national origin, religion, disability, sexual orientation, or political affiliation should never influence the availability or quality of therapy.*

> *Discrimination in any form is unethical.*

The guidelines are clear. Discrimination in any form is unethical. Yet calling someone a "racist" either directly or implicitly seems to be common when a disagreement rises to the surface. This is especially true when differences arise in political or church-related disputes where race and religion are the subjects of the conflict. Discrimination is a subtle problem because *although discrimination exists in the mind of the person who feels discriminated against, it does not necessarily exist in the mind of the person accused.* Therapists must strive for objectivity and fairness with all clients and be particularly sensitive to issues of discrimination to avoid problems. Not all discrimination problems can be solved by a therapist, but they must all be recognized for therapy to be effective.

National Guidelines Regarding Discrimination

American Association for Marriage and Family Therapy (AAMFT) Code of Ethics (2001)

Marriage and family therapists provide professional assistance to persons without discrimination on the basis of race, age, ethnicity, socioeconomic status, disability, gender, health status, religion, national origin, or sexual orientation.

American Counseling Association (ACA) Code of Ethics (2005)

A.4.b. Personal Values

Counselors are aware of their own values, attitudes, beliefs, and behaviors and avoid imposing values that are inconsistent with counseling goals. Counselors respect the diversity of clients, trainees, and research participants.

C.5. Nondiscrimination

Counselors do not condone or engage in discrimination based on age, culture, disability, ethnicity, race, religion/spirituality, gender, gender identity, sexual orientation, marital status/partnership, language preference, socioeconomic status, or any basis proscribed by law. Counselors do not discriminate against clients, students, employees, supervisees, or research participants in a manner that has a negative impact on these persons.

C.6. Public Responsibility

6.a. Sexual Harassment

Counselors do not engage in or condone sexual harassment. Sexual harassment is defined as sexual solicitation, physical advances, or verbal or nonverbal conduct that is sexual in nature, that occurs in connection with professional activities or roles, and that either:

1. Is unwelcome, is offensive, or creates a hostile workplace or learning environment, and counselors know or are told this; or

2. Is sufficiently severe or intense to be perceived as harassment to a reasonable person in the context in which the behavior occurred.

Sexual harassment can consist of a single intense or severe act or multiple persistent or pervasive acts.

American Psychological Association (APA) Ethical Principles of Psychologists and Code of Conduct (2002)

Principle E: Respect for People's Rights and Dignity

Psychologists respect the dignity and worth of all people, and the rights of individuals to privacy, confidentiality, and self-determination. Psychologists are aware that special safeguards may be necessary to protect the rights and welfare of persons or communities whose vulnerabilities impair autonomous decision-making. Psychologists are aware of and respect cultural, individual, and role differences, including those based on age, gender, gender identity, race, ethnicity, culture, national origin, religion, sexual orientation, disability, language, and socioeconomic status and consider these factors when working with members of such groups. Psychologists try to eliminate the effect on their work of biases based on those factors, and they do not knowingly participate in or condone activities of others based upon such prejudices.

3. Human Relations

3.01 Unfair Discrimination

In their work-related activities, psychologists do not engage in unfair discrimination based on age, gender, gender identity,

(continued)

(*Continued*)

race, ethnicity, culture, national origin, religion, sexual orientation, disability, socioeconomic status, or any basis proscribed by law.

3.02 Sexual Harassment

Psychologists do not engage in sexual harassment. Sexual harassment is sexual solicitation, physical advances, or verbal or nonverbal conduct that is sexual in nature, that occurs in connection with the psychologist's activities or roles as a psychologist, and that either (1) is unwelcome, is offensive, or creates a hostile workplace or educational environment, and the psychologist knows or is told this or (2) is sufficiently severe or intense to be abusive to a reasonable person in the context. Sexual harassment can consist of a single intense or severe act or of multiple persistent or pervasive acts. (See also Standard 1.08, Unfair Discrimination Against Complainants and Respondents.)

3.03 Other Harassment

Psychologists do not knowingly engage in behavior that is harassing or demeaning to persons with whom they interact in their work based on factors such as those persons' age, gender, gender identity, race, ethnicity, culture, national origin, religion, sexual orientation, disability, language, or socioeconomic status.

American School Counselor Association (ASCA) Ethical Standards for School Counselors (2004)

E.2. Diversity

The professional school counselor:

a. Affirms the diversity of students, staff, and families.

b. Expands and develops awareness of his or her own attitudes and beliefs affecting cultural values and biases and strives to attain cultural competence.

c. Possesses knowledge and understanding about how oppression, racism, discrimination and stereotyping affects her/him personally and professionally.

d. Acquires educational, consultation, and training experiences to improve awareness, knowledge, skills and effectiveness in working with diverse populations: ethnic/racial status, age, economic status, special needs, ESL or ELL, immigration status, sexual orientation, gender, gender identity/expression, family type, religious/spiritual identity, and appearance.

National Association of Social Workers (NASW) Code of Ethics (1999)

4.02 Discrimination

Social workers should not practice, condone, facilitate, or collaborate with any form of discrimination on the basis of race, ethnicity, national origin, color, sex, sexual orientation, age, marital status, political belief, religion, or mental or physical disability.

4.03 Private Conduct

Social workers should not permit their private conduct to interfere with their ability to fulfill their professional responsibilities.

General Guidelines for Avoiding Discrimination

All mental health professions have guidelines for avoiding discrimination. People who seek help from clinicians are entitled to assistance regardless of their background, and they are entitled to competent treatment free from prejudice. The consuming public must obtain the services needed with clinical objectivity free from discrimination. The public is also sensitive to discrimination—more sensitive, perhaps, than the provider—because in many cases the recipient has lived with discrimination for years and has an antenna that picks up bigotry, intolerance, or narrow-mindedness of any type including strong preconceived opinions. The client is a reactive victim. Therapists therefore must be sensitive to their own feelings as well as their clients' feelings. A chance remark, mildly inappropriate under other circumstances, can produce a tornado of reaction among sensitive clients. Whenever a hint of discrimination appears, overt or subtle, internal or external, it must be eliminated at once. The therapist might require therapy or sensitivity training. If a bias is acted on, and if it interferes with any part of the therapy, it violates the ethical codes of the state licensing regulations as well as the antidiscrimination clauses of national organizations. Therapeutic objectivity as well as common sense precludes discrimination of any type. It is not necessarily important in therapy that providers agree with their clients. It is, however, important that the provider offer competent and objective services.

Therapeutic objectivity as well as common sense precludes discrimination of any type.

When Discrimination Interferes with Responsible Practice

Sometimes providers are concerned about treating clients who have a religious or cultural orientation completely foreign to them. The professional might believe that the client may misunderstand or misinterpret aspects of treatment, or the professional might feel incapable of understanding the client's background or point of view adequately enough to provide helpful therapy. Should the therapist provide therapy anyway or make a referral to another provider? Suppose the provider's political or religious orientation cannot be reconciled with the client's position and conduct regarding abortion, birth control, homosexuality, alcoholic beverages, or political leanings. The list of possible biases and prejudices is too numerous to be all-inclusive. Can the provider offer therapeutically appropriate services? Each provider, within his or her own frame of reference, must make this decision and document the rationale for the determination.

There is a delicate balance between discrimination and exceeding one's level of competence and objectivity. The friction must be recognized, considered, pondered, and then handled in an ethical manner. Treating a client from a background completely unknown to the therapist is difficult. If the therapist cannot understand the client's particular orientation, it would not be discriminatory to make a referral to a provider who can. Nevertheless, it is important to document all aspects of the decision to refer the client elsewhere. Recognizing your limitations concerning objectivity is not unethical, but it must be handled appropriately within the guidelines of the profession. In some situations, the position of the client, either emotionally or physically, is so contrary to that of the provider that offering therapy would present too many conflicts. When this occurs, it is unwise as well as inappropriate to work so hard to overcome these biases that concentration on the problem becomes impossible. Refer, but document. This is often a case where finesse and sophistication will prevent an accusation of abandonment.

If the therapist cannot understand the client's particular orientation, it would not be discriminatory to make a referral to a provider who can.

Recognizing your limitations concerning objectivity is not unethical, but it must be handled appropriately within the guidelines of the profession.

Ethical Flash Points

- Discrimination of any type is a violation of all ethical canons and codes.

- Discrimination comes in many forms. The clinician must be sensitive to his or her own feelings and instincts and work to eliminate any feelings that are negative to any specific person or class.

- Equal services are to be provided to all consumers of mental health services.

- If there is ever a hint, an accusation, or an intimation of discrimination, the problem is to be handled at once. The reaction and steps to handle must be documented.

- Discrimination complaints have a habit of becoming media events, political footballs, and public affairs. When the suggestion appears, the situation must immediately be sensitively handled.

- A mental health professional assigned to a geographic area, or to an agency that deals with the public at large, cannot insist on serving only a limited population in that area because of bias or prejudice.

(continued)

(*Continued*)

- Sometimes we have to look in the emotional mirror and see where our feelings take root. Then we have to control any feelings that hinder an open mind or clinical abilities.

- Do not ever disregard or minimize a discrimination complaint. It can be the professional's undoing. Keep in mind that discrimination in the thinking of a client is felt rather than objectively provable. The stronger the feeling, the more important it is to react to any intimation of bias, chauvinism, or prejudice. Offer a free session to ameliorate feelings of discrimination.

Summary

A mental health services provider must not refuse to perform any act or service for which the person is licensed or qualified solely on the basis of a client's age, gender, race, color, religion, national origin, ethnicity, disability, sexual orientation, or political affiliation. To refuse to provide effective treatment or services to any of these, or perhaps other, identifiable groups is unethical. And remember, each of the group members is sensitive and aware of his or her right to treatment and to the various laws, codes, rules, and regulations that protect them. If they are not aware today, they become aware quickly when a problem arises. Lawyers, ethicists, other clinicians, the boards, the literature, and other friends within a common interest group will educate unhappy clients quickly.

A complication arises when the client has a religious or national orientation that is completely foreign or unknown to the provider, and the professional feels that if services are granted, the client or the provider will be misunderstood. Or suppose the historic and religious orientation of the provider has irreconcilable differences with the client in the area of abortion, birth control, homosexuality, liquor or alcoholic beverages of any type, or even political orientation, and so on. Can the provider offer therapeutically appropriate services? Each provider, within his or her own frame of reference, must make this decision and document the rationale for the determination.

There is a delicate balance between exceeding your level of competence and objectivity, and discrimination. The friction must be recognized, considered, pondered, and then handled in an ethical manner. Treating a client whose orientation is so esoteric as to be misunderstood is difficult. Some backgrounds are hard to clinically fathom and are beyond the capacity of the therapist to understand. Making a referral in a case such as this would not be discrimination. It would be good sense and to the client's benefit, if properly documented.

Suggested Research Assignments

1. Locate and discuss any rules promulgated by licensing boards in your state that deal with discrimination and diversity issues.
2. Locate and discuss any state and national professional association's ethical guidelines that deal with discrimination and diversity issues. Do you note any differences?
3. Compare and contrast these state licensing board rules with the ethical rules promulgated by the state professional associations.
4. Compare and contrast state licensing and professional association guidelines with the guidelines of national professional associations.
5. Identify resources/persons you would consult to safely and ethically make a decision regarding discrimination and diversity issues.
6. You have received a quiet hint of an ethical complaint because of discrimination. What do you do in the form of risk management and damage control?
7. Consider and determine whether there are diversity issues or differences that a client might present that would impact your ability to provide objective and competent therapy. If so, develop a plan of action for confronting them including the possibility of referral.
8. Research the decisions of your state licensing boards and state and national professional association's ethics committees for discrimination-related violation sanctions.
9. Research the civil and criminal case decisions of your state with respect to discrimination. What penalties or damages were assessed and awarded?

10. Apply the ethical canons of the state licensing board for your discipline to the scenarios at the beginning of this chapter and answer the questions that are posed.

Discussion Questions

1. What would you tell a client who prior to consenting to therapy asks you what your position is with respect to same-sex marriages? Must you respond, and if so, what is the best response?

2. Is it ethical for you to attend a commitment ceremony between two people of the same sex?

3. What would you say to a colleague who consults with you about her difficulty in treating a client she finds increasingly morally reprehensible?

4. How would you respond to a client who accuses you of being insensitive to his sexual orientation?

5. How would you handle a client who during therapy continuously places blame for her failures on racial prejudice when you truly believe this is not true and therapeutic progress cannot be made until the client acknowledges that she is responsible, at least in part, for her difficulties?

6. How would you explain to a client your need to refer the client to another therapist when the client's lifestyle or behavior is precluding you from being objective in treating the client?

6

False and Misleading Statements

Sam's first love was engineering, and he pursued and received a PhD at the Colorado School of Mines. After 20 years in the field, he lost his job due to downsizing and later obtained a master's degree in counseling. He is now in private practice. His counseling business card and other office promotional materials do not indicate his PhD because he knows that would be conspicuously misleading and prohibited, but one evening while being introduced at a church forum to talk about "blended families," he was praised as "Dr. Sam Johnson, the eminent local counselor," with a profound expertise regarding second marriages. Is Sam obligated to explain that the degree that entitles him to be called "Doctor" was in engineering?

One day, while walking down the street with a friend and colleague, Susan, a social worker, was approached by an effusive former client. This client enthusiastically blurted out with hardly a pause to inhale, how, following therapy with Susan, her life had changed, her health had improved, and how Susan was the most marvelous therapist in the world. Susan sought some moderation in the monologue, but the praise continued until the former client rushed away to an appointment. Is Susan obliged to "set the record straight" with her friend and colleague, and can she do so without revealing confidential information about the client?

On his resume, used for introductions at lectures, Dr. Smith indicates he teaches at the state university. That is true. He teaches one course each year (3 hours) for one semester. At a recent seminar, the person introducing him referred to him as a practitioner in private practice and as a "professor at the state university." Does such an introduction mandate clarification? Would this be a false and misleading statement? Is it misleading without being unethical? Suppose an adjunct professor is introduced as "professor," or an assistant professor is introduced as "professor." At what point does a harmless error or an exaggeration become an ethical disaster? Remember that any jealous colleague sitting in the audience can file a complaint, and some boards accept anonymous complaints. In fact, fellow clinicians file many complaints concerning therapists, often anonymously.

National Guidelines for Responding to Exaggerated Claims

American Association for Marriage and Family Therapy (AAMFT) Code of Ethics (2001)

Principle VIII: Advertising

8.1 Marriage and family therapists accurately represent their competencies, education, training, and experience relevant to their practice of marriage and family therapy.

8.5 In representing their educational qualifications, marriage and family therapists list and claim as evidence only those earned degrees: (a) from institutions accredited by regional accreditation sources recognized by the United States Department of Education, (b) from institutions recognized by states or provinces that license or certify marriage and family therapists, or (c) from equivalent foreign institutions.

8.6 Marriage and family therapists correct, wherever possible, false, misleading, or inaccurate information and representations made by others concerning the therapist's qualifications, services, or products.

8.8 Marriage and family therapists do not represent themselves as providing specialized services unless they have the appropriate education, training, or supervised experience.

American Counseling Association (ACA) Code of Ethics (2005)

C.3.C. Statements by Others

Counselors make reasonable efforts to ensure that statements made by others about them or the profession of counseling are accurate.

American Psychological Association (APA) Ethical Principles of Psychologists and Code of Conduct (2002)

5.01 Avoidance of False or Deceptive Statements

(b) Psychologists do not make false, deceptive, or fraudulent statements concerning (1) their training, experience, or competence; (2) their academic degrees; (3) their credentials; (4) their institutional or association affiliations; (5) their services; (6) the scientific or clinical basis for, or results or degree of success of, their services; (7) their fees; or (8) their publications or research findings.

(c) Psychologists claim degrees as credentials for their health services only if those degrees (1) were earned from a regionally accredited educational institution or (2) were the basis for psychology licensure by the state in which they practice.

National Association of Social Workers (NASW) Code of Ethics (1999)

4.06 Misrepresentation

(c) Social workers should ensure that their representations to clients, agencies, and the public of professional qualifications,

(continued)

(Continued)

credentials, education, competence, affiliations, services provided, or results to be achieved are accurate. Social workers should claim only those relevant professional credentials they actually possess and take steps to correct any inaccuracies or misrepresentations of their credentials by others.

Therapists should not make any false, misleading, fraudulent, or exaggerated claims or statements and should discourage clients from holding overstated or inaccurate ideas about their professional services. There is a tendency for the satisfied client to speak well of the therapist, and such endorsements are appropriate and professional. In fact, private practices depend on the good words of satisfied clients.

There is always a tendency for the satisfied client to speak well of the therapist, and such endorsements are appropriate and professional.

Occasionally, the practitioner will hear through the grapevine or from a new client that a former client has made statements about the competence, credentials, experience, or even success of the therapist that the therapist knows to be untrue or so exaggerated as to be misleading. In such cases, the therapist is obligated to review what was said and put it in a correct perspective. People who introduce speakers and program directors, especially, may exaggerate credentials and depart from the prepared introduction material. When this occurs, don't make too much of a fuss, but do set the record straight. If you have furnished your introduction material, keep a copy in your file so that you are not responsible if the enthusiastic introducer departs from the prepared text. (Remember, there is a difference between an assistant professor, associate professor, and full professor, just as there is a difference between a lieutenant, a lieutenant colonel, and a lieutenant general.)

The therapist is obligated to review what was said and put it in a correct perspective.

Three social workers, two professional counselors, and three psychologists formed a group to market and practice together because they realized the benefits of size; that praising another was easier than self-praise; and that sharing experience, expertise, and expenses would be valuable. They also realized the importance of hiring a professional marketer. A week later, when the marketer presented the preliminary plan, they found it completely unacceptable. Each of the eight professionals had forgotten the same thing. They had neglected to give the marketer all the applicable advertising and promotional rules and regulations relating to each profession, with the admonition that any plan advanced would have to comply with every applicable state and national guideline and standard of the discipline of each and every participant. Once the guidelines were assembled, a workable marketing plan was easily generated.

A therapist took a lawyer to lunch and casually asked the lawyer to look over her most recent promotional literature from the advertising agency. It contained the following phrases: "guaranteed results" and "if you visit me, we will establish a relationship, and I will always be here for you if needed." The lawyer was appalled. No therapist can guarantee results and should not claim to be able to do so in promotional literature. Likewise, no therapist can represent to a client that he or she will "always" be there for the client. Consider what would happen if the therapist had to relocate when her husband's promotion took him to a new city.

National Guidelines for Advertising

American Association for Marriage and Family Therapy (AAMFT) Code of Ethics (2001)

Principle VIII: Advertising

8.2 Marriage and family therapists ensure that advertisements and publications in any media (such as directories, announcements, business cards, newspapers, radio, television, Internet, and facsimiles) convey information that is necessary

(continued)

(Continued)

for the public to make an appropriate selection of professional services. Information could include: (a) office information, such as name, address, telephone number, credit card acceptability, fees, languages spoken, and office hours; (b) qualifying clinical degree (see subprinciple 8.5); (c) other earned degrees (see subprinciple 8.5) and state or provincial licensures and/or certifications; (d) AAMFT clinical member status; and (e) description of practice.

American Counseling Association (ACA) Code of Ethics (2005)

C.3. Advertising and Soliciting Clients

C.3.a. Accurate Advertising

When advertising or otherwise representing their services to the public, counselors identify their credentials in an accurate manner that is not false, misleading, deceptive, or fraudulent.

American Psychological Association (APA) Ethical Principles of Psychologists and Code of Conduct (2002)

5. Advertising and Other Public Statements

5.01 Avoidance of False or Deceptive Statements

(a) Public statements include but are not limited to paid or unpaid advertising, product endorsements, grant applications, licensing applications, other credentialing applications, brochures, printed matter, directory listings, personal resumes or curricula vitae, or comments for use in media such as print or electronic transmission, statements in legal proceedings, lectures and public oral presentations, and published materials. Psychologists do not knowingly make public statements that are false, deceptive, or fraudulent concerning their research, practice, or other work activities or those of persons or organizations with which they are affiliated.

In general, providers may advertise as long as they "accurately represent their competence, education, training, and experience relevant to their practice." Also, they must assure that advertisements and publications in any media (such as directories, announcements, business cards, newspapers, radio, television, and facsimiles) convey information that is necessary for the public to make an appropriate selection of professional services.

In this competitive era, the mental health professional may seek professional help when preparing a logo, letterhead, brochures, and other advertising materials. The advertising agency may be familiar with the products the provider desires, but may not be aware of the ethical issues surrounding responsible and technically appropriate advertising of mental health services. An ad agency may be tempted to market the provider as a product, using inappropriate adjectives, solicited testimonials, or success stories that may be perfectly acceptable when selling cars, boats, or breakfast cereals but unacceptable when marketing mental health services. Keep in mind that the person punished for false advertising is the professional, not the advertising executive.

The advertising agency may be familiar with the products the provider desires, but may not be aware of the ethical issues surrounding responsible advertising of mental health services.

When hiring an outside agency for advertising or public relations services, mental health agencies should provide:

- A copy of the state standards or board rules concerning advertising.
- A copy of the standards concerning advertising of every state and national organization to which the provider belongs.
- An understanding that the provider may face serious consequences if advertising and promotional enthusiasm exceed acceptable standards.

As soon as any ethical violation is discovered, a correction or redaction should be issued. Keep the relevant agency informed of all corrections, and try to inform the appropriate enforcement group prior to any complaint being filed. Indicate the discovery of the error and the efforts made to correct any infractions.

The state of Texas Licensing Act for professional counselors publishes helpful guidelines concerning advertising and announcements to guide the ethical professional in developing sound promotional material (Title 22, Texas Administrative Code §681.49. Advertising and Announcements). The highlights include:

- Can't be false, inaccurate, misleading, incomplete, out of context, deceptive, or not readily verifiable.
- Can't create unjustified expectations about the results of a health-care service or procedure.
- Can't cause confusion or misunderstanding as to the credentials, education, or licensure of a health-care professional.
- Must be careful about the waiving of insurance deductibles.
- Can't make a representation that is designed to take advantage of the fears or emotions of a particularly susceptible patient.
- Can't cause confusion or misunderstanding as to credentials, education, or licensure.
- A licensee who retains or hires others to advertise or promote the licensee's practice remains responsible for the statements and representations made.

It is up to each advertising mental health professional to carefully review all material that is disseminated to the public to ensure compliance with these guidelines. A client who relies on false, deceptive, or misleading information about the therapist would be in a strong position to assert there was not informed consent given to the treatment. This could be the basis of a licensing board complaint, malpractice suit, or a suit to recover fees paid for the treatment. A wise move might be to seek the advice of a learned colleague for advance approval of all printed matter. A small exaggeration in an introduction or a promotional brochure could have disastrous consequences if discovered by a hostile professional or unhappy client.

Selecting a Name

Advertising may not include a statement or claim that

There are limits when using a business name that could mislead the public. Advertising may not include a statement or claim that is false, fraudulent, misleading, or deceptive. In addition, therapists must correct, wherever possible, false, misleading, or inaccurate information and representations made by others concerning the therapist's qualifications, services, or products. All mental health professionals must conform to their recognized and accepted standards for accurate representation of their practice and credentials.

is false, fraudulent, misleading, or deceptive.

National Guidelines for Selecting a Name

American Association for Marriage and Family Therapy (AAMFT) Code of Ethics (2001)

8.3 Marriage and family therapists do not use names that could mislead the public concerning the identity, responsibility, source, and status of those practicing under that name, and do not hold themselves out as being partners or associates of a firm if they are not.

For example, it would be improper for a licensed counselor to do business under an assumed name "ABC Psychological Services, Inc." This could cause consumers to assume the counselor was in fact a psychologist. It would be equally improper for a solo practitioner to conduct business under the name "Susan Jones, LMFT & Associates" when there are no other mental health professionals in the practice.

The authors represented a licensed master's level social worker who picked up the nickname "Dr. Smiley" while working with children for a state social services agency. When he started a private practice, his former colleagues with the state agency routinely referred clients to "Dr. Smiley." The private practice went well until the mother of an adolescent client became dissatisfied with advice she was given and began to examine "Dr. Smiley's" credentials. When she learned he did not have a PhD, she filed a complaint with the state licensing board that initially recommended a one-year probated suspension with a weekly supervision requirement. On appeal, the social worker ultimately received a letter of instruction (not a public sanction) to discourage people from referring to him as Dr. Smiley and to post a disclaimer on his web site that, although he has been known by a nickname in the past of "Dr. Smiley," he does not have a PhD or an MD and he does not encourage people to refer to him by that nickname.

Mental health professionals should describe themselves in an honest and forthright manner. Names should accurately portray the mental health professional in a manner that precludes misunderstanding. It is better to understate yourself than to exaggerate or mislead.

The Media

Dr. Smith, a clinical psychologist, was between patients when a call came in from a local newsperson. The reporter asked him about his time in practice, credentials, education, and publications and then asked a seemingly innocent question about the "mess" (the reporter's word) in the housing of mental health patients. Taken off-guard but somewhat flattered by press attention, Dr. Smith uttered a few innocuous (in his opinion) remarks and in a short time ended the interview. A few days later, his entire biography was published in an interview that implied that Dr. Smith agreed there was a "mess" in the housing of mental health patients. Indirectly, the published interview implied that Dr. Smith used the word "mess."

As long as the information concerning biographical information given to the reporter is factual and not misleading, there is no inherent problem in dealing with reporters or the press in general. Mental health professionals who are contacted by the media need to keep in mind that the reason for the interview is to get information that will sell newspapers or magazines. Once information is shared with the press, control over its use is in the hands of the reporter and the editor. Mental health professionals are permitted and even encouraged to speak with the press. But an interview can be cast in a context that is misleading and, in some cases, downright false.

Before granting an interview, seek and obtain information concerning its

Before granting an interview, seek and obtain information concerning its purpose. Then speak gingerly. Being quoted out of context may cause irreparable harm. If the reporter writes a flowery, but exaggerated and possibly misleading, description of you and your services, at the minimum call and inform the reporter of the facts and make a note of the call in case some person reading the article accuses you of inappropriate self-promotion.

purpose. Then speak gingerly.

Testimonials

Client testimonials have long been viewed with disfavor because of the concerns for the exploitation of vulnerable clients and the possible disclosure of confidential information. If the testimonial does not bear the client's name or signature, the issue becomes one of verifiability and of client consent. If it does contain a client's signature, there may have been a breach of confidentiality (disclosure of client's name), and this creates the potential for clients to come back after the fact and allege the therapist took advantage of them and that they didn't understand just what the therapist was going to do with the testimonial (exploitation).

The authors have been contacted by numerous providers who received favorable plaudits from clients, only to be devastated when they fell out of favor. The transition from hero worship to vilification would constitute one indication of a person suffering from borderline personality disorder (*DSM-IV;* American Psychiatric Association, 1994). The final results of therapy may not be what the client expected (e.g., the client's spouse files for divorce instead of reconciling with the client, or a chemically addicted child relapses). High esteem can be fleeting.

National Guidelines for Testimonials

American Counseling Association (ACA) Code of Ethics (2005)

C.3.b. Testimonials

Counselors who use testimonials do not solicit them from current clients nor former clients nor any other persons who may be vulnerable to undue influence.

(continued)

(Continued)

American Psychological Association (APA) Ethical Principles of Psychologists and Code of Conduct (2002)

5.05 Testimonials

Psychologists do not solicit testimonials from current therapy clients/patients or other persons who because of their particular circumstances are vulnerable to undue influence.

Despite their attractiveness from an advertising perspective, testimonials should be avoided. If clients, no matter the true reason, accuse the mental health professional of taking advantage of them after the testimonials become prominently featured in an ad, a brochure, or a web site, the mental health professional could have considerable difficulty in defending against the claims. After all, what benefit does a client derive from a testimonial? What competent and right-minded person wants the whole world to know about a problem for which he or she needed the services of a mental health professional?

Ethical Flash Points

- You can have a legitimate credential, but if it cannot be applied to the practice of mental health, it cannot be used.

- Therapists have an affirmative duty to correct false and misleading statements made about them.

- When determining guidelines for advertising and promotion, the practitioner is bound by the licensing law (more than one if there is more than one license) and the advertising ethical canons of every organization to which the professional belongs.

- If using a professional marketer, furnish the marketer with all applicable guidelines. See to it that they are understood and followed.

- Be careful that resumes are accurate.

- When creating an assumed name for business purposes, make sure it is not false or deceptive.
- Guidelines are constantly changing; keep your information up to date.
- When two or more professionals of different disciplines join in a professional venture, the codes of all must be respected.
- Avoid the temptation to include testimonials of clients in promotional materials.
- Remember—the buck stops with the professional.

Summary

The canons of ethics control advertisements, introductions, what we say, and what is said about us. It is the obligation of the professional, whether the situation concerns advertising, a simple introduction, or a public announcement, to guarantee that the announcement is true and correct, not false, deceptive, or misleading. When we hire another person to promote us, we face the same obligation. The professional has the ultimate obligation to see that the final promotional product conforms to all ethical standards. Begin with the standards in this book, then continue with your personal affiliations and determine the allowable, permissible, and prohibited. Use only ethically approved promotional materials. If possible, have an ethically aware colleague review all written materials.

It is the obligation of the professional whether the situation concerns advertising, a simple introduction, or a public announcement to guarantee that the announcement is true and correct, not false and misleading.

When speaking in public, prepare a card with your introductory material on it. Then hand this card to any person introducing you. Introducers appreciate this gesture because it saves reading a long vita and selecting the relevant material. Also it creates written proof of what you wanted the introducer to say.

Suggested Research Assignments

1. Locate and discuss any rules promulgated by licensing boards in your state that deal with advertising and promotion.

2. Locate and discuss any state and national professional association ethical guidelines that deal with advertising and promotion. Do you note any differences?

3. Prepare ethical guidelines for an advertising agency that is not familiar with mental health ethical rules.

4. Compare and contrast these state licensing board rules with the ethical rules promulgated by the state professional associations.

5. Compare and contrast state licensing and professional association guidelines with the guidelines of national professional associations.

6. Identify resources and persons you would consult with to safely and ethically make a decision regarding advertising and promotion.

7. Research the decisions of your state licensing boards and state and national professional association ethics committees for advertising- or promotion-related violation sanctions.

8. Research the civil and criminal case decisions of your state with respect to advertising or promotion. What penalties or damages were assessed and awarded?

9. Apply the ethical canons of the state licensing board for your discipline to the scenarios at the beginning of this chapter and answer the questions that are posed.

10. Create a set of guidelines for advertising and promotion that you will implement to ethically disseminate information about yourself and the services you provide or intend to provide in the future.

Discussion Questions

1. What would you tell a client who volunteers to give you a testimonial to include on your web site?

2. What do you tell the executive director of the counseling center that employs you when he asks you to solicit testimonials from clients or former clients to include in the new promotional materials the center is developing?

3. Is there anything improper about using the descriptive words "competent" and "quality" to describe the services you provide in your practice?

4. How do you respond to a grateful client who sings your praises every chance she gets, proclaiming you to be a "miracle worker"?

5. What steps would you take to ensure that your new web site is ethically compliant?

6. You have just been informed that one of your church organizations has published an unauthorized biography in a bulletin used for mutual networking purposes. Some statements are inappropriate. What steps do you take to institute damage control? How do you document the efforts you have made to correct the record?

7

Informed Consent

Dr. Kindheart, a licensed professional counselor, greets a potential new client, Harold, in his office late Friday afternoon at the end of a very slow week. Harold, in the midst of an affair, is concerned about confidentiality. When he asks Dr. Kindheart if their therapy sessions will be kept confidential, Dr. Kindheart responds, "Absolutely." Three months later, Harold is walking out of Dr. Kindheart's office when he is served with divorce papers. At the same time, Dr. Kindheart is served with a subpoena to appear at a temporary hearing to testify and produce Harold's records. Does Harold have anything to be concerned about? How about Dr. Kindheart? Is confidentiality ever absolute?

Carol, under the influence of alcohol and amphetamines, comes in for therapy at a local counseling center. A nonlicensed staff worker conducts the intake session and has Carol sign the center's standard consent for therapy form. She then ushers Carol into the office of one of the center's five therapists. After talking with the therapist for 2 hours, Carol leaves the center without paying for services. On receiving a bill from the counseling center, Carol tells them she is not going to pay. Can the counseling center confidently pursue collection action for payment? What happens when Carol *argues that she was too upset and did not have the capacity to consent at the time she presented herself at the counseling center?*

A concerned, noncustodial father, during an extended visitation period, takes his daughter to see a psychologist experienced in sexual abuse cases after the girl complains about her stepfather giving her baths when her mother is not at home. He completes the psychologist's intake forms and gives consent for evaluation and treatment if necessary. When the girl's mother finds out that her daughter is seeing a therapist, she angrily contacts the psychologist and faxes a copy of the relevant pages from the divorce decree giving her the exclusive right to consent to mental health care and treatment for the child absent an emergency. An emergency is defined as a serious and immediate threat to the health, safety, or welfare of the child. She asserts that the psychologist wrongfully provided mental health services and threatens to file an ethical complaint with the state licensing board and to sue for malpractice if her daughter is emotionally harmed by the sessions with the psychologist. In this case, what is considered appropriate informed consent? Can the noncustodial parent legally consent to treatment of a minor child during visitation periods?

Why Informed Consent Is Important

Informed consent is a prerequisite to the commencement of the therapeutic relationship.

Informed consent is a prerequisite to the commencement of the therapeutic relationship. Virtually every mental health profession's ethics code contains provisions requiring therapists to secure potential clients' informed consent before providing any mental health services. The Health Insurance Portability and Accountability Act (HIPAA) Privacy Rule leaves the issue of informed consent to state law. Licensing boards are particularly interested in making sure that clients are thoroughly informed on important matters before consenting to therapy. This is understandable when we realize that consumer protection is one of the primary reasons behind the establishment and continued existence of state licensing boards. Society and the mental health professions desire educated consumers who knowingly and voluntarily consent to mental health care and treatment.

National Guidelines for Informed Consent

American Counseling Association (ACA) Code of Ethics (2005)

A.2. Informed Consent in the Counseling Relationship

A.2.a. Informed Consent

Clients have the freedom to choose whether to enter into or remain in a counseling relationship and need adequate information about the counseling process and the counselor. Counselors have an obligation to review in writing and verbally with clients the rights and responsibilities of both the counselor and the client. Informed consent is an ongoing part of the counseling process, and counselors appropriately document discussions of informed consent throughout the counseling relationship.

American Psychological Association (APA) Ethical Principles of Psychologists and Code of Conduct (2002)

3.10 Informed Consent

(a) When psychologists conduct research or provide assessment, therapy, counseling, or consulting services in person or via electronic transmission or other forms of communication, they obtain the informed consent of the individual or individuals using language that is reasonably understandable to that person or persons except when conducting such activities without consent is mandated by law or governmental regulation or as otherwise provided in this Ethics Code.

National Association of Social Workers (NASW) Code of Ethics (1999)

Section 1.03 Informed Consent

(a) Social workers should provide services to clients only in the context of a professional relationship based, when

(continued)

(Continued)

appropriate, on valid informed consent. Social workers should use clear and understandable language to inform clients of the purpose of the services, risks related to the services, limits to services because of the requirements of a third-party payer, relevant costs, reasonable alternatives, clients' right to refuse or withdraw consent, and the time frame covered by the consent. Social workers should provide clients with an opportunity to ask questions.

Without informed consent, no treatment should be given in the absence of an emergency, in which case consent should be obtained as soon as the client is capable of giving it. Anything short of informed consent leaves the mental health professional vulnerable to a malpractice case and licensing board sanctioning.

What Constitutes Informed Consent?

The meaningful question is not whether informed consent should be obtained but rather what constitutes informed consent. A client has the right to information about many things to properly give consent for treatment. The more information the client receives, the less likely there can be an allegation of improper consent. The ramifications of failing to secure informed consent are varied and serious. It is an ethical requirement to secure informed consent as the previously cited provisions indicate, and the therapist who fails to do so is vulnerable (see Chapter 29, "Professional Vulnerability"). Moreover, without informed consent, the client can argue that he or she is not required to keep the client's end of the bargain (pay for services rendered).

Consider the following general and specific informed consent requirements:

American Association for Marriage and Family Therapy (AAMFT) Code of Ethics (2001)

Principle I: Responsibility to Clients

1.2 Marriage and family therapists obtain appropriate informed consent to therapy or related procedures as early as feasible in the therapeutic relationship, and use language that is reasonably understandable to clients. The content of informed consent may vary depending upon the client and treatment plan; however, informed consent generally necessitates that the client: (a) has the capacity to consent; (b) has been adequately informed of significant information concerning treatment processes and procedures; (c) has been adequately informed of potential risks and benefits of treatments for which generally recognized standards do not yet exist; (d) has freely and without undue influence expressed consent; and (e) has provided consent that is appropriately documented.

When persons, due to age or mental status, are legally incapable of giving informed consent, marriage and family therapists obtain informed permission from a legally authorized person, if such substitute consent is legally permissible.

American Counseling Association (ACA) Code of Ethics (2005)

A.2. Informed Consent in the Counseling Relationship

A.2.b. Types of Information Needed

Counselors explicitly explain to clients the nature of all services provided. They inform clients about issues such as, but not limited to, the following: the purposes, goals, techniques, procedures, limitations, potential risks, and benefits of services; the counselor's qualifications, credentials, and relevant

(*continued*)

(*Continued*)

experience; continuation of services upon the incapacitation or death of a counselor; and other pertinent information. Counselors take steps to ensure that clients understand the implications of diagnosis, the intended use of tests and reports, fees, and billing arrangements. Clients have the right to confidentiality and to be provided with an explanation of its limitations (including how supervisors and/or treatment team professionals are involved); to obtain clear information about their records; to participate in the ongoing counseling plans; and to refuse any services or modality change and to be advised of the consequences of such refusal.

APA *Ethical Principles of Psychologists and Code of Conduct*

10. Therapy

10.01 Informed Consent to Therapy

(a) When obtaining informed consent to therapy as required in Standard 3.10, Informed Consent, psychologists inform clients/patients as early as is feasible in the therapeutic relationship about the nature and anticipated course of therapy, fees, involvement of third parties, and limits of confidentiality and provide sufficient opportunity for the client/patient to ask questions and receive answers. (See also Standards 4.02, Discussing the Limits of Confidentiality, and 6.04, Fees and Financial Arrangements.)

Counselors explicitly explain to clients the nature of all services provided. They inform clients about issues such as, but not limited to, the following: the purposes, goals, techniques, procedures, limitations, potential risks, and benefits of services; the counselor's qualifications, credentials, and relevant experience; continuation of services on the incapacitation or death of a counselor; and other pertinent information. Counselors take steps to ensure that clients understand the implications of diagnosis, the intended use of tests and reports, fees, and billing arrangements. Clients have the right to confidentiality and to be provided with an explanation of its limitations (including how supervisors and treatment team professionals are involved); to obtain clear information about their records; to participate in the ongoing counseling plans; and to refuse any services or modality change and to be advised of the consequences of such refusal.

The best way to document informed consent is with a detailed intake and consent form that provides in clear and easily understood language the information needed to turn a potential client into an informed consumer who can knowingly and intelligently enter into a therapeutic relationship. A signed, detailed intake and consent form, a copy of which is given to the client, ensures there will be little controversy about the information provided to the client and the client's consent to treatment. This form constitutes written evidence of the client's consent to services and becomes part of the client's permanent file. The client will have a difficult time convincing a judge, jury, or licensing board that he or she was not adequately informed before consenting to therapy when confronted with his or her signed, detailed intake and consent form.

The best way to document informed consent is with a detailed intake and consent form that provides in clear and easily understood language the information needed to turn a potential client into an informed consumer.

> **Note:** *The Portable Lawyer for Mental Health Professionals* (Bernstein and Hartsell 2004) contains useful forms for the mental health professional, including a sample Client Information and Consent Form (p. 50).

Constructing an Informed Consent Form

The ethics codes with their general and specific requirements provide direction for creating an intake and consent form that properly documents informed consent. The form should provide the following information at a minimum:

- Intake and consent forms should state the therapist and other professional or staff members who will be involved in the client's care and treatment, including their educational backgrounds, licensing, training, and experience. If a professional under supervision or on probation by a licensing board will participate in the delivery of services, this should be disclosed. Any relationship to an entity (e.g., independent contractor, provider to ABC Managed Care Company, employee of XYZ Counseling Center) should be set out. A client has a right to know and to choose the provider of his or her mental health services.

- Fees for services, including session rates, copays, charges for phone contacts, missed appointments, cancellations, responses to subpoenas and requests for records, testing, report writing, and late payment fees should be specifically addressed. A client should be advised that although third-party payers may be expected to make payment, the client is ultimately responsible in the event payment is refused by a third party. (*Note:* A managed care provider contract may prohibit the charging of any fee to the client except a copay, so a careful reading of all provider contracts and the appropriate tailoring of intake and consent form provisions are critical.)

- Confidentiality and its limitations should be outlined. The client must be informed of exceptions that limit the client's right to confidentiality and the therapist's duty to warn. The legal exceptions to confidentiality should be listed including child abuse, elder abuse, abuse of the physically or mentally disabled, child custody cases, any case in which the mental or emotional health of a party is an issue, sexual exploitation by a mental health professional, criminal cases, fee disputes, malpractice actions, licensing board cases, and imminent physical or emotional danger of the client or a third party (see Chapter 3, "Confidentiality," and Chapter 27, "Duty to Warn," for specific information). Disclosure of client information is not required by law in other instances but is necessary in connection with the client's care and treatment (submitting information to third-party payers, providing services when the therapist is under supervision, staff meetings and consultations with other professionals). Specific consent for disclosure under these circumstances should be obtained on the intake and consent form or in a subsequent consent form.

Confidentiality and its limitations should be outlined.

- Clients should be advised when and how the therapist or the therapist's office might contact them and consent to being contacted in a specified manner and at specific locations and phone numbers, fax numbers, or e-mail.
- The client has the right to be a knowledgeable participant in his or her therapy. The initial goals, purposes, and techniques of therapy should be listed. Any subsequent changes should be documented and signed by the client.
- All available alternative treatments should be disclosed along with information on the relative risks, benefits, and costs, together with the risks of refusing treatment.
- Confidentiality survives the death or incompetence of the therapist as well as the client. A therapist is under an obligation to provide for these contingencies in advance of therapy.

The client has the right to be a knowledgeable participant in his or her therapy.

The *APA Ethical Principles of Psychologists and Code of Conduct* (2002) states:

3.12 Interruption of Psychological Services

Unless otherwise covered by contract, psychologists make reasonable efforts to plan for facilitating services in the event that psychological services are interrupted by factors such as the psychologist's illness, death, unavailability, relocation, or retirement or by the client's/patient's relocation or financial limitations.

- It is unethical for a therapist to become involved in a dual relationship with the client, but the client can violate boundaries with impunity. The client should be advised that boundary violations by either the therapist or the client must be avoided or the therapeutic relationship will be jeopardized. The client should be warned that gift giving, social interaction, and personal or business relationships cannot occur. The form should further state that should the client attempt to draw the therapist into a dual relationship or boundary violation, termination of the therapy and referral to another provider will be the probable result.
- The client should be informed about all testing—the nature and purpose of each test, as well as the identities and credentials of each person involved in the testing process. Consent to the testing and

the involvement of all participants in the testing process should be procured.

- Special circumstances require special disclosure, information, and consent. For example, often a therapist will want to video- or audio-tape a session with a client for self-protection such as with a flirta-tious client or one prone to ignoring competent advice.

The *AAMFT Code of Ethics* (2001) states:

Section 1.12 Marriage and family therapists obtain written informed consent from clients before videotaping, audio recording, or permitting third-party observation.

- Therapy involves risks. Legal disclosure of confidential information in a client's file is just one of the risks. Clients may learn about facts or feelings, or come to realize traits about themselves that they didn't want to admit or face. Clients should be advised of the risk. Nontraditional therapies such as animal therapy involve special and unique risks that the client should be warned about as part of in-formed consent.

The *ACA Code of Ethics* (2005) states:

10. Therapy

10.01 Informed Consent to Therapy

(b) When obtaining informed consent for treatment for which generally recog-nized techniques and procedures have not been established, psychologists inform their clients/patients of the developing nature of the treatment, the potential risks involved, alternative treatments that may be available, and the voluntary nature of their participation.

There are also risks when services are provided via electronic me-dia (i.e., computer and telephone) that should be discussed and dis-closed (see Chapter 1, "Alternative Treatment Methods," for specific information).

This is by no means an exhaustive attempt to list all matters that should be discussed and disclosed to potential clients to ensure that informed consent is secured prior to beginning the therapeutic relationship. Nevertheless, it is representative of the minimal information required by the various ethics codes. The client can never receive too much information where informed consent is concerned. The greater the amount of information disseminated to a potential client, the less chance that the client can establish lack of informed consent in the future.

The client can never receive too much information where informed consent is concerned.

Who Provides Informed Consent?

Consent is useless if it is not obtained from a person with the capacity to consent or the authority to consent for another individual. A person under the influence of alcohol or drugs or a person with diminished mental capacity regardless of cause does not have the mental capacity to give informed consent to treatment. If a person presents himself or herself for therapy while under the influence of alcohol or drugs, informed consent should not be attempted until such time as the person is clearly sober.

If informed consent is not possible because of a person's diminished mental capacity, a therapist should determine if the individual has a legal guardian or someone acting under a lawful power of attorney who can provide informed consent. If there is no legal guardian, the therapist should decline to provide mental care or treatment until one is appointed.

It is not enough to accept the word of the court-appointed guardian. A careful approach requires the therapist to request a copy of the guardian's letter of authority from the court or a copy of the court order appointing the guardian. On receipt, the document should be reviewed to be sure there are no limitations to the guardian's authority to consent for mental health care or treatment. If there is any doubt, a lawyer should be consulted and therapy postponed until such time as the therapist is convinced of the guardian's legal authority to offer consent. Even when clients suffer from diminished mental capacity, mental health professionals should inform them as fully as possible, taking into account the clients' ability to comprehend.

If informed consent is not possible because of a person's diminished mental capacity, a therapist should determine whether the individual has a legal guardian or someone acting under a lawful power of attorney who can provide informed consent.

National Guidelines for Obtaining Informed Consent

American Psychological Association (APA) Ethical Principles of Psychologists and Code of Conduct (2002)

3.10 Informed Consent

(b) For persons who are legally incapable of giving informed consent, psychologists nevertheless (1) provide an appropriate explanation, (2) seek the individual's assent, (3) consider such persons' preferences and best interests, and (4) obtain appropriate permission from a legally authorized person, if such substitute consent is permitted or required by law. When consent by a legally authorized person is not permitted or required by law, psychologists take reasonable steps to protect the individual's rights and welfare.

National Association of Social Workers (NASW) Code of Ethics (1999)

Section 1.03 Informed Consent

(c) In instances when clients lack the capacity to provide informed consent, social workers should protect clients' interests by seeking permission from an appropriate third party, informing clients consistent with the client's level of understanding. In such instances social workers should seek to ensure that the third party acts in a manner consistent with the client's wishes and interests. Social workers should take reasonable steps to enhance such client's ability to give informed consent.

See also *AAMFT Code of Ethics* (2001), Principle I: Responsibility to Clients 1.2 (d) set forth earlier.

Obtaining Informed Consent in Cases of Joint Custody

In today's environment where parents enjoy joint custody of their children, it is increasingly difficult for mental health professionals to determine which parent, or whether each parent, has the right to consent to mental health care or treatment for a minor child. Usually a minor child is defined as a child under 18 and unmarried. In some states, children are considered adults for purposes of consenting to mental health treatment when they marry or when they are emancipated or have their disabilities of minority removed.

As with adult mentally incompetent clients, therapists should insist on reviewing a copy of the most recent custody order before consenting to treat a child if the parents are not married to each other and living together. Therapists should keep a copy of the relevant provisions of the custody decree in the child's file. Again, if there is uncertainty, providers should consult their lawyer before providing services. *Consent in writing given by the wrong person or by a person without legal authority is no consent at all. Consent for treatment of a minor or an incompetent must be authorized by a legally appointed person.*

Consent in writing given by the wrong person or by a person without legal authority is no consent at all.

Obtaining Informed Consent from Minors

In most states, minors can consent to mental health care or treatment in limited circumstances, such as suicide prevention, chemical dependency, and abuse. Therapists working with minors should familiarize themselves with the statutes in their state to be sure they can rely on the informed consent of the minor. When obtaining the minor's informed consent, special care must be given to explaining all the information in terms that the minor can understand.

When obtaining the minor's informed consent, special care must be given to explaining all the information in terms that the minor can understand.

Ethical Flash Points

- Practice statutes require mental health professionals to secure informed consent from each client before providing services.

(continued)

(Continued)

- Ethics codes provide the minimum amount of information that must be disclosed and discussed with a client to establish informed consent.

- Unique treatment methods involve special risks that must be adequately and specifically disclosed. Such methods must be supported by a majority of clinicians or by a learned minority. Before embarking on cutting-edge therapy, assemble a research file to support the methodology.

- Informed consent must be documented. The best way to document informed consent is with a detailed intake and consent form signed by the client.

- Copies of letters of authority, guardianship orders, general and limited power of attorney, and custody orders should be obtained and reviewed with legal consultation if necessary. Only then can you rely on the informed consent of a third party. A legal document file must be maintained for each client where applicable.

Summary

Informed consent is an ethical precondition to the provision of mental health services. The failure to procure informed consent subjects the practitioner to ethics complaints and malpractice actions. Without it, the client's obligation to pay for services is impacted. Informed consent must be obtained from the client or a person legally authorized to consent for the client.

Suggested Research Assignments

1. Locate and discuss any rules promulgated by licensing boards in your state that deal with informed consent.
2. Locate and discuss any state and national professional association ethical guidelines that deal with informed consent. Do you note any differences?
3. Compare and contrast these state licensing board rules with the ethical rules promulgated by the state professional associations.
4. Compare and contrast state licensing board and professional association guidelines with the guidelines of national professional associations.

5. Identify resources/persons you would consult with to safely and ethically obtain informed consent from clients.

6. Research the decisions of your state licensing boards and state and national professional association ethics committees for informed consent related violation sanctions.

7. Research civil case decisions of your state involving a failure to secure informed consent. What damages if any were awarded?

8. Apply the ethical canons of the state licensing board for your discipline to the scenarios at the beginning of this chapter and answer the questions that are posed.

9. Create a set of guidelines for obtaining informed consent from clients that you will implement in your practice.

10. Create an intake and consent form that will document informed consent.

11. Research the law in your state regarding a minor child's ability to consent to mental health treatment.

Discussion Questions

1. What would you tell a new therapist about informed consent and documenting informed consent?

2. What would you tell a stepparent who presents a child for the very first appointment that had been scheduled by the parent?

3. What do you do if a mentally challenged adult patient comes into your office with a brother who asks you to provide services?

4. If a parent presents to you a 12-year-old divorce decree as evidence of her ability to consent to treatment of her 15-year-old daughter, what do you do?

5. What would you do if a client appeared for a first appointment with a strong smell of alcohol on his breath and was slurring his speech?

6. If a minor asks you for treatment because she is having suicidal ideation but asks that you not tell her mother or father, what do you do?

8

Interviewing

Dr. Sweet has practiced for 10 years using traditional "talk" therapy methods. After filling out a mental health history form and a detailed, lawyer-drafted, consent-to-treatment form, clients enter his office and therapy begins. His office is on the outskirts of town near a freeway with relatively easy parking and is convenient to most individuals who seek his services. One day, a new client announces at her first interview that coming to Dr. Sweet's office is not cost-effective for her. In fact, she implies that one-on-one therapy is a relic of the dark ages. It is a pain in the neck and a nuisance. In her firm, almost all communication is electronic, and she wonders why therapy should be different. She is the CEO of a major company, and her hour to visit Dr. Sweet really means an afternoon out of the office when she factors in travel time and waiting at Dr. Sweet's office for her appointment. If she sees Dr. Sweet one hour (50 minutes) each week, she is actually losing two days of productivity every month, since every visit takes one-half day of productive time. She is billed out at $450 per hour. She tells Dr. Sweet that her time is worth more than he charges, and time out of the office is money lost and never regained. She proposes five alternatives:

1. Now that they have met, they could correspond by e-mail when problems arise. She can ask her questions and make her comments at her leisure

and convenience, and Dr. Sweet can respond at his convenience. Not only could they communicate, but there would be a permanent record of the e-mail therapy.

2. *They could continue therapy with regularly scheduled e-mail conferences. At the appointed time, each would log on and carry on a conversation. They would exchange reactions via instant message and the keyboard.*

3. *Each could install a web cam to their computers.*

4. *They could communicate by fax. She will write out the thoughts she has and he will fill in the blanks and respond. They can fax to each other through a secure line that guarantees the confidentiality of the exchange.*

5. *They could continue therapy by telephone. Since both have cell phones, the therapy can continue while he is home with his children and she is in her automobile, boat, or backyard relaxing by the pool.*

As the result of a birth defect, Lucille has always been confined to a wheelchair. This challenging situation has not impeded her scholarship, and this spring she will receive her master's degree. Lucille is seeking online therapy since she finds mobility difficult. Finally she locates a therapist who is willing to treat her using e-mail. The therapist sends Lucille a complete history form and a detailed intake and consent-to-treatment form that Lucille dutifully completes and returns.

The therapy begins, with both Lucille and her therapist corresponding on their AOL accounts. This is a major convenience to them both. Billing is monthly. How might therapy have been different if the therapist could observe the emotion of the moment in addition to the words of the moment? Might the therapeutic modality be different if Lucille participated in face-to-face treatment in addition to e-mail?

We live in an electronic age. In the past, most therapists probably couldn't conceive any acceptable therapy except a personal face-to-face interview in a professional environment. Most would find a telephone session or two acceptable once the therapist-client relationship was established, and such calls would typically be brief and without charge. Certainly the idea of treating clients without meeting them first was not within their comprehension and never occurred in graduate school training. Therapists and clients are now trying to determine how and in what manner modern technology is adaptable to fresh discoveries in technology and how emerging new systems in communication can inure to the therapy profession. The mental health professions are trying to determine unique and innovative therapeutic methods using the whole panoply of equipment available. And this is just today. Considering the speed with which electronic communication is developing, by the time this book is published, new equipment might easily make all of today's innovations historical footnotes.

Traditional Therapy

Traditional mental health services using either talk therapy or medication were based on a personal relationship between therapist and client. Sigmund Freud's statement that his development of the analytic method began with his pioneering analysis of himself highlights the personal connection between the therapist and the client. We cannot imagine Freud sending himself a fax, an e-mail, or using some other electronic method when offering therapy to himself or a client. Nor can we get a mental picture of Freud typing on a laptop while recording notes or providing answers to questions, which are then fed into a computer. Sounds a bit like a subject for a *New Yorker* cartoon, doesn't it? Rather, we think of patients lounging on a couch chatting away while Freud, pencil in hand, is taking notes and responding.

One cannot imagine Freud sending himself a fax, an e-mail, or using some other electronic method when offering therapy to himself or a client.

Advantages of the Face-to-Face Interview

The clinician who interviews the client in person can observe all manner of physical appearances including any disability, nervous habits, body language, and facial and body gestures. The appearance and demeanor of a client can even set the mood of the session. Voice changes of volume, pitch, and resonance can also tell the therapist a great deal about the client that can impact the dialogue. In addition,

Some problems are brought into clearer focus if the therapist knows what the client looks like and how the client reacts to a given question, statement, or inquiry.

some problems are brought into clearer focus if the therapist knows what the client looks like and how the client impulsively reacts to a given question, statement, or inquiry.

Informed consent mandates a certain dialogue between the provider and the client during which, in addition to explaining the intake and consent form, the therapist answers questions concerning fees, goals, and techniques of treatment, limits to confidentiality, whether the therapist will willingly appear in court if needed, and when and how records are available to a client. The interview is important to make certain that the client had ample opportunity to review the forms signed, seek clarification if necessary, and offer informed consent personally to the consultation and continuing therapy.

See Chapter 1, "Alternative Treatment Methods," for the national guidelines regarding the use of technology in therapy.

Risks and Rewards of Technology-Driven Therapy

A blessing of computer-generated therapy is that the client does not have to leave work or comfortable surroundings, drive through traffic-filled streets, and then wait at the therapist's office for the session to begin. Another advantage is that the client can seek advice at the time it is needed or at least when the problem occurs. True, the counseling or therapy may not always be available at convenient times, but neither is that true for one-on-one therapy. No therapy implies a coordination between crisis events and crisis intervention.

A benefit to both therapist and client is that electronic messages can be printed and a hard copy of each question and answer preserved. This is a two-faced coin. On the one hand, all therapy may be reduced to writing; on the other hand, some words take on different meanings when placed on the printed page. If humor is used in therapy, it may look flat, rude, or inappropriate when written down or transcribed on paper. Also, voice inflections, timing, hesitations, volume, pitch, and speed of transmission are all lost or compromised when sent by fax or e-mail. A scowl, which might be important for a therapist to observe, would be lost in a fax transmission.

In one-on-one therapy, the therapist can control confidentiality and the security of what is said and discussed. The therapist can also control what is recorded in the clinical record. The restrictions of the law govern what might be required in court, and other rules might govern what happens if a therapist learns of the unethical conduct of another therapist, but in general the therapist has some control over the dissemination and recording of information received in a therapy session. Most cell phones are not secure. Telephone therapy is similar, although the dangers are not as great. Generally either party in a telephone conversation can easily record the call and keep the recording or reduce it to writing. Federal and state law, however, may preclude surreptitious recording of sessions. Fax transmission is as secure as a local telephone call, but if the wrong digit is pressed, the unintended recipient is under no legal duty to inform the sender that he or she has received confidential electronic information. In truth, the receiver of a wrongly transmitted letter may tell the world, if there is any feeling that the world is interested or might want to know.

Emerging Technology and Ethics

The ethical canons do not prohibit the use of computers in therapy. In fact, the Health Insurance Portability and Accountability Act (HIPAA) Privacy and Security Rules specifically deal with electronic transmission and storage of health-care information. There is no direct general code reference that indicates one-on-one, face-to-face, individual therapy is the only way to offer treatment to a client either. However, there are limitations. The therapist must ensure that the client understands the computer application, what it is used for, and its possible effects. Also, if the computer makes an error, the final ethical and professional responsibility is with the provider, who must establish ethical and technical safeguards to see to the reliability and accuracy of the computer technology.

The provider must also accept responsibility for explaining all the ramifications, good and bad, of computer therapy to the client and structure the relationship so that the computer is an acceptable adjunct to interpersonal therapy. The provider has the responsibility to

The provider has the responsibility to explain to the client all information that clarifies the place, security, and importance of computer use in the therapy.

explain to the client all information that clarifies the place, security, and importance of computer use in the therapy. Finally, the provider needs to caution the client that the very nature of therapy implies that treatment will be less effective unless the therapist and client meet in person at some point or periodically in the therapeutic relationship. An exception to this is in crisis intervention (e.g., a crisis hotline), but in therapy designed to produce long-term results, a personal visit would be warranted and appropriate.

The Texas Licensing Act for Professional Counselors provides a conservative approach:

> Subchapter C. Code of Ethics.
>
> §681.41 General Ethical Requirements.
>
> (g) A licensee shall provide counseling treatment intervention only in the context of a professional relationship. Interactive long-distance counseling delivery, where the client resides in one location and the counselor in another may be used as part of the therapeutic counseling process. Counselors engaging in interactive long-distance counseling must adhere to each provision of this chapter.

Having face-to-face sessions in addition to electronic sessions is advisable. This board has taken the position that they can be used jointly but electronic therapy alone is not acceptable.

The Personal Interview in Forensic Consultations

A question also arises about the use of technology and the absence of a personal interview in forensic consultations. The general rule implied in the ethical guidelines is that a therapist shall not testify concerning a person's ability to function, parent, or cope, nor shall a provider evaluate any individual's mental, emotional, or behavioral condition unless the provider has personally interviewed the individual or the provider discloses with the evaluation that the provider has not personally interviewed the individual (for more information, see Chapter 31, "Forensic Evaluation"). Occasionally, there is a temptation to form opinions based on the input of others such as newspaper reports, magazine articles, information from former spouses or business associates or the children of a marriage without contacting the individual involved and seeking and obtaining a personal interview using commonly accepted therapeutic standards. Nevertheless, professional evaluation, assessment, and appraisal, as well as treatment, diagnosis, and establishing a prognosis require at least one face-to-face interview unless there is a clear documented mental health emergency.

Danger lurks for a therapist who interviews only a former husband (father), stepmother, and child and then testifies that the biological mother is a less suitable parent and that the best interest of the child would be served by father and stepmother rearing the child. Even if this is a correct assessment, failing to interview the natural or birth mother is an ethical violation, especially if she is available, ready, willing, and able to be interviewed. To comment on an individual, that person must be personally interviewed. Indeed, submitting an electronic test or having an e-mail instant conversation is not professionally adequate. An opinion should not be expressed in the absence of some required face-to-face evaluation.

Professional evaluation, assessment, and appraisal, as well as treatment, diagnosis, and establishment of a prognosis require at least one face-to-face interview.

Ethical Flash Points

- Don't worry, mental health professionals will not be replaced by computers.

- Computers are like any other therapy tool or technique. They must be explained to the client, and their use, function, reliability, and position in the scheme of therapy clearly understood.

- Informed consent includes consenting to the use of computers and other types of electronic communications.

- Don't assume the client understands computer use and application. Insert in your intake and consent form some protective language that indicates the client understands the use and function of computers in the therapeutic framework.

- Computer disks, records, printouts, and, perhaps, even hard drives can be subpoenaed into court.

- "Delete" on a computer does not always mean "delete." The words are on the computer hard drive somewhere and a good technician can locate and retrieve them.

(continued)

(*Continued*)

- Therapy has a long history in which conversation was the prime focus. When using computers, tests, or test results, or having the client answer questions on a computer screen, make sure the technique is fitting for this particular client at this time. Make sure you have assembled the literature so that either a majority of practitioners or a learned minority supports the technique used. If the technological process is challenged as being too novel, the therapist is the person who must defend its use. Make no assumptions. Be prepared to defend and document every new technique used.

- Therapists who use modern technology to increase their cash flow or bottom line are cautioned to ensure that the technology being used is appropriate for the type of treatment and the individual being treated.

- Check licensing laws when the client resides or receives information in another jurisdiction. Is your license to practice valid in the recipient's locale, or are you practicing in another state without a license? Get legal and ethical clearance before crossing state lines.

- Therapists are required to keep current with the latest treatment techniques. If an approach is known, available, suitable, and unused, the therapist is involved in an unethical and possibly negligent practice.

- In many cases, the provider is disciplined for failing to do something that might have been done (an act of omission) rather than for doing something that was wrong (an act of commission).

- Any therapist who testifies concerning a client who has not been personally interviewed and observed is skating on very thin ethical ice.

- Complaints will be filed for unethical conduct if an individual loses a court case based on computer-generated opinions stated in court and sworn to from the witness stand. The party who lost the case will often file the complaint.

- Mental, emotional, and behavioral conditions have to be observed. They cannot be detected solely by computer printouts or electronic correspondence. This argues for at least some face-to-face communication in therapy.

- Secondary evidence that might be in a report, such as magazines, newspapers, and interviews with third persons are sometimes helpful, but ultimately clinical objectivity militates that the interview with the client is the definitive factor in determining a diagnosis, prognosis, and treatment plan.

- Technology is evolving at breakneck speed. Its relevance to therapy is gradually improving and will continue to grow and change in the twenty-first century.

Summary

There is a lure to substitute electronics and the time-saving investigative genius of the telecommunication age to accumulate information and make assessments. You should resist this temptation and adhere to the personal interview in all cases where an opinion is sought. When the electronic age is joined with modern developments and a personal interview, the therapist needs documentation to identify the relative weight of all the information gathered. Any opinion formed must include sensible interviewing techniques as well as the benefits gathered from emerging technology. Together, they offer the information needed to reach a defensible assessment, diagnosis, treatment plan, and prognosis.

Any opinion formed must include sensible interviewing techniques as well as the benefits gathered from emerging technology.

Suggested Research Assignments

1. Review and adapt the suggested assignments at the end of Chapter 1.
2. Research communication and compile a list of important verbal and nonverbal communication that a mental health professional might observe in a client interview and what importance each would have on diagnosis and treatment.
3. Select three initial problems clients might present to you during their first session and compile lists of questions that would be appropriate and essential for you to ask during that interview.
4. Develop a list of questions that should be asked at the initial interview, before therapy commences. Which of these questions and what answers would you consider in determining whether you want to treat this particular client, and whether a referral should be made? Keep in mind, the more needy the client, the more difficult termination will be in the future. Questions of abandonment haunt the termination process with the needy, dependent, clingy client.
5. Citing the rules of the state licensing board for your discipline determine whether face-to-face client sessions are required as part of the therapeutic process.

6. Prepare a protocol for providing effective therapy without even one face-to-face session with the client if you determine one is not necessary in your state.

7. What would you need to document to ensure and prove informed client consent to electronic therapy? How would you document informed consent?

8. Identify resources/persons you would consult with to safely and ethically provide electronic therapy?

9. Locate mental health professionals in your area who are providing electronic therapy and find out whether they conduct face-to-face sessions as well. If they do so, find out why, and if they don't, find out why they don't. Also find out what benefits and drawbacks they have experienced with electronic therapy.

10. Research to find any reported malpractice case decisions involving electronic therapy.

Discussion Questions

1. What would you tell a new client who called you by phone and said he did not want to come in for even one face-to-face session?

2. What would you tell a newly licensed mental health professional who tells you she intends to only do electronic therapy and never wants to see clients in person?

3. What would you tell counseling graduate school classes are the risks and drawbacks of electronic therapy from both the client and the therapist's perspective?

4. Is it helpful to know a client's race, physical condition, appearance, and personal oddities?

5. What kinds of information should a mental health professional attempt to gather during a client interview? Is there information you might receive that you would not document in the client's file?

9

Prohibited Clients

Dr. Clean has earned the reputation of a scholar-oriented psychology profes-
sor who is always available to students when they have a problem requiring
therapeutic assistance. Usually the encounters are brief and do not take a lot
of professorial time. Certainly, Dr. Clean does not consider them ''ther-
apy.'' One day, a student approaches him and indicates that her problem
requires more than a brief conversation. Instead, she wants in-depth consul-
tation. Dr. Clean, a licensed professional, is reluctant at first, but later re-
lents and visits with the student. He performs this service without charge.
Would the rules change if Dr. Clean charged a fee for his services? Would
the rules change further if the student was in a program requiring supervision
and Dr. Clean was the supervising therapist? Another question burdened
with subtleties is at what point does a short visit regarding a personal point of
interest change from casual conversation to professional therapy? And when
does an informal conversation become a therapeutic relationship that requires
informed consent, warnings about confidentiality, and dissemination of all
the other information required prior to the commencement of therapy?

Bob, a master's-level licensed professional counselor, is active in the Toast-
master's Club. He often offers presentations to the group to polish his public

speaking skills. One day, he is scheduled to deliver his "Ice Breaker," a talk where the novice speaker offers a biographical sketch of his life to date, his field of interest, and his reason for developing speaking skills. Just as he is about to begin, a guest is introduced to the group. To Bob's horror, the guest is a very troubled woman client. Bob is well aware of the usual therapeutic prohibition against inappropriate self-disclosure. He also knows that an Ice Breaker is full of personal self-disclosure, intimate insights, individual and family experiences, and family history. Information will be shared that a client should not hear. Can Bob proceed? Suppose Bob did not notice that the client was in the room, and she heard it all? And then assume that the client is thrilled because her therapist is also a Toastmaster, and she insists on joining the group. After joining, she maneuvers to sit next to him at every meeting, engaging him in more personal small talk.

Ms. Sweet is the president of the symphony board and also a marriage and family therapist. One of her clients has an interest in this cultural activity and, after a few years' apprenticeship, gradually climbs the ladder to officialdom. She is running for vice president and solicits the support of Ms. Sweet.

There is always a certain amount of small-town politicking going on, and Ms. Sweet's endorsement would be important. Can Ms. Sweet have anything to do with her client's cultural or political ambitions? Must she terminate the therapist client relationship? If therapy is terminated, can Ms. Sweet then promote her client to her friends?

Mrs. O'Reilly is very proud and thankful her daughter has finally graduated from the university with an advanced degree in counseling and is authorized and licensed by the state board to enter into a private practice. As she did with her son, a lawyer, she prepares an announcement list of all her friends, family, acquaintances, and business associates. The proud mother intends to offer her daughter's services and recommend that the individuals and businesses on the list consider her daughter when seeking counseling and therapy. In fact, the list contains the names and addresses of just about everyone Mrs. O'Reilly has ever come into contact with socially or casually. When her daughter discovers that her mother is about to undertake the unabashed wholesale solicitation of clients, should she (a) destroy the list, (b) send out announcements to everyone on the list indicating she is in private practice and soliciting business, (c) send out a bland announcement but nothing else, (d) hire a publicity manager to create literature encouraging new prospective clients to call her, (e) let her mother send out the announcements and then consult with her licensing board, or (f) take some other action?

Identifying Prohibited Clients

The maxim often quoted by lawyers is that the "large print giveth and the small print taketh away." In the case of mental health services, the large print maintains that therapists in a free society may offer services to any person who requests help. The small print, however, places necessary restrictions on therapists against treating certain individuals. A cursory search shows that national ethics codes list several categories of potential prohibited clients who cannot be served, and state guidelines and the professional literature offer others.

Mental health professionals must treat individuals in a context where therapeutic objectivity is not compromised (the only connection between client and therapist is the therapeutic relationship). The therapist cannot achieve this objectivity with current or previous family members, personal friends, or business associates, or any of the other relationships to be mentioned. Certainly, it is impossible to maintain objectivity with past or current sexual partners or individuals with whom the therapist would like to be intimate. The focus on the entire relationship is helping the client, and any activity that derogates from this concentration is inappropriate.

Mental health professionals must treat individuals in a context where therapeutic objectivity is not compromised.

In addition, mental health professionals cannot treat persons currently receiving treatment from another counselor without the other provider's knowledge and consent, because they must coordinate treatment plans and use a unified approach. Also many agencies have, by contract with agents, servants, and employees, as well as independent contractors, rules and internal prohibitions against private practitioners building their practice by diverting clients away from the agencies and into the practice of the private or moonlighting provider. These standards are appropriate and must be honored. Then there are the fuzzy questions: What happens when a long-term

Mental health professionals cannot treat persons currently receiving treatment from another counselor without the other provider's knowledge and consent.

client marries into the family and suddenly becomes an in-law? Or when a business associate with no therapeutic connection sells a business interest to a present or former client, or after weeks or months or even years of effective treatment, the client approaches the therapist with a "by the way, I have been seeing 'X,' another therapist, for a second opinion, and I had actually seen her before I came to see you"? When do formerly acceptable and suitable clients fall within unacceptable ranges or degrees of relationships to the extent that therapeutic objectivity is or can be lost? When this happens, what is the best way to avoid an actual, possible, or perceived ethical infraction?

The Intake Interview

A careful intake interview can prevent many problems with a potential prohibited client. Insightful questioning during the first conference will often uncover current and possibly past and future relationships. When a hint or thread of a conflict appears, fully develop the line of questioning and do not undertake treatment until fully satisfied that the client is ethically eligible. Refusing to begin the client-therapist relationship is easier than terminating it at a later date because of newly discovered information that should have been uncovered in the first session. Do not be reluctant to ask intimate or personal questions. New clients may not understand just why they are questioned concerning relationships, near or far, but the provider has the responsibility to ensure that the current client applicant for therapeutic services is not in one of the prohibited categories. As with all therapeutic contact with clients, actual or potential, the responsibility is on the professional provider to see that all national, state, and local guidelines are honored.

Individuals to Avoid Engaging in Therapy

The ethical canons contain guidelines for accepting clients that affect mental health professionals as they practice their profession. Besides those cited previously, the complete guidelines can be found on the

National Guidelines for Prohibited Clients

American Association for Marriage and Family Therapy (AAMFT) Code of Ethics (2001)

1.3 Marriage and family therapists are aware of their influential positions with respect to clients, and they avoid exploiting the trust and dependency of such persons. Therapists, therefore, make every effort to avoid conditions and multiple relationships with clients that could impair professional judgment or increase the risk of exploitation. Such relationships include, but are not limited to, business or close personal relationships with a client or the client's immediate family. When the risk of impairment or exploitation exists due to conditions or multiple roles, therapists take appropriate precautions.

American Counseling Association (ACA) Code of Ethics and Standards of Practice (2005)

A.5. Roles and Relationships with Clients

A.5.c. Nonprofessional Interactions or Relationships (Other Than Sexual or Romantic Interactions or Relationships)

Counselor-client nonprofessional relationships with clients, former clients, their romantic partners, or their family members should be avoided, except when the interaction is potentially beneficial to the client.

F.3. Supervisory Relationships

F.5.c. Counseling for Supervisees

If supervisees request counseling, supervisors provide them with acceptable referrals. Counselors do not provide counseling services to supervisees. Supervisors address

(*continued*)

(Continued)

interpersonal competencies in terms of the impact of these issues on clients, the supervisory relationship, and professional functioning.

American Psychological Association (APA) Ethical Principles of Psychologists and Code of Conduct (2002)

3. Human Relations

3.05 Multiple Relationships

(a) A multiple relationship occurs when a psychologist is in a professional role with a person and (1) at the same time is in another role with the same person, (2) at the same time is in a relationship with a person closely associated with or related to the person with whom the psychologist has the professional relationship, or (3) promises to enter into another relationship in the future with the person or a person closely associated with or related to the person.

A psychologist refrains from entering into a multiple relationship if the multiple relationship could reasonably be expected to impair the psychologist's objectivity, competence, or effectiveness in performing his or her functions as a psychologist, or otherwise risks exploitation or harm to the person with whom the professional relationship exists.

Multiple relationships that would not reasonably be expected to cause impairment or risk exploitation or harm are not unethical.

(b) If a psychologist finds that, due to unforeseen factors, a potentially harmful multiple relationship has arisen, the psychologist takes reasonable steps to resolve it with due regard for the best interests of the affected person and maximal compliance with the Ethics Code.

(c) When psychologists are required by law, institutional policy, or extraordinary circumstances to serve in more than one role in judicial or administrative proceedings, at the outset they clarify role expectations and the extent of confidentiality and thereafter as changes occur.

3.06 Conflict of Interest

Psychologists refrain from taking on a professional role when personal, scientific, professional, legal, financial, or other interests or relationships could reasonably be expected to (1) impair their objectivity, competence, or effectiveness in performing their functions as psychologists or (2) expose the person or organization with whom the professional relationship exists to harm or exploitation.

3.08 Exploitative Relationships

Psychologists do not exploit persons over whom they have supervisory, evaluative, or other authority such as clients/patients, students, supervisees, research participants, and employees.

American School Counselor Association (ASCA) Ethical Standards for School Counselors (2004)

A.4. Dual Relationships

The professional school counselor:

a. Avoids dual relationships that might impair his or her objectivity and increase the risk of harm to the student (e.g., counseling one's family members, close friends or associates). If a dual relationship is unavoidable, the counselor is responsible for taking action to eliminate or reduce the potential for harm. Such safeguards might include informed consent, consultation, supervision and documentation.

b. Avoids dual relationships with school personnel that might infringe on the integrity of the counselor/student relationship.

(*continued*)

(Continued)

F.1. Professionalism

f. Does not use his or her professional position to recruit or gain clients, consultees for his or her private practice or to seek and receive unjustified personal gains, unfair advantage, inappropriate relationships or unearned goods or services.

National Association of Social Workers (NASW) Code of Ethics (1999)

1.06 Conflicts of Interest

(c) . . . should not engage in dual or multiple relationships with clients or former clients in which there is a risk of exploitation or potential harm to the client. In instances when dual or multiple relationships are unavoidable, social workers take steps to protect clients and are responsible for setting clear, appropriate and culturally sensitive boundaries. (Dual or multiple relationships occur when social workers relate to clients in more than one relationship, whether professional, social, or business. Dual or multiple relationships can occur simultaneously or consecutively.)

The ethical canons contain guidelines for accepting clients that affect mental health professionals as they practice their profession.

web sites for each organization (see Appendix A for a list of web sites for professional organizations). Based on these guidelines, the list of potential clients whom therapists must refer elsewhere include:

- Personal friends
- Financial associates
- Social or organizational acquaintances
- Political associates or cronies
- Clients of an agency with whom you do business if that agency prohibits you from offering private therapy to them
- Students

- Supervisees
- Research participants
- Any individual with whom you customarily barter
- Anyone with whom you have an evaluative relationship
- Employees
- Employers, the employer's wife, children, or family, or close acquaintances
- Former and current sexual partners
- Future contemplated sexual partners
- Family members
- Any person you are not competent to treat

Deciding Who Qualifies as Family

There is no clear definition of who constitutes a family member in the ethics codes. The fluidity of family structure and varying degrees of kinship either directly or through marriage make definite rules hard to evaluate. There are cousins you never see, and "kissing cousins" who are not related by blood but always participate in family activities. When contemplating offering therapy to a close family friend, a family member, or to an individual who may later join the family (e.g., a brother's girlfriend), the conventional wisdom is to make a referral. Yes, everyone has a right to therapy, but not when the therapy might be influenced by emotional relationships or connections or ties that affect the feelings of either the client or the therapist.

Tough Calls

If the presenting client is not specifically mentioned in the previous list but might be *construed* by some to be a member of a prohibited category, it is better not to take a chance. Individuals with whom the therapist's relationship is in a gray area of the ethical guidelines are better referred to another therapist. Remember that questions of impropriety only present themselves when a complaint is filed. At that time, the general feeling is that consumer protectionism would lean toward the complaining member of the public. In this case, it would be the provider's responsibility to prove that the client was not within

Individuals with whom the therapist's relationship is in a gray area of the ethical guidelines are better referred to another therapist.

It is better to lose a potential client than to lose a license!

a prohibited class of clients. The ethical canons also preclude providing therapy to any person who *might or possibly could be* harmed in addition to the specifically identified prohibited clients. It is better to lose a potential client than to lose a license. Keep in mind, when the prohibited relationship comes to the attention of a court or the licensing board, the client feels that he or she has been damaged and is willing to testify to that effect. The provider is now on the defensive. The client can do little that is wrong. It is the professional whose reputation, finances, and treatment plan or prognosis is on the line and must be defended. Should the damaged client be sympathetic, the therapist cannot always expect an objective fact finder.

Occasional Clients

Relationships of any type are by their nature fluid. Therapists cannot control who signs up for a course offered at the university, nor can research participants always be limited or screened to perfection. Indeed, therapists who are active in the community will often bump into present and former clients in the form of students, supervisees selected by a school or agency, or the salesperson who sold the therapist an automobile. In most cases, the ethical concern is easily handled by a referral or an explanation to the client together with documentation of the event and the agreed-on solution. There are few documented cases of ethical violations when therapists used common sense to accept or decline to treat someone. However, this should not minimize the potential problem or the awareness of the provider.

When relationships change to bring the client within prohibited boundaries, proceed with caution. No clinician wants to be the first test case of a possible prohibited client boundary violation (see Chapter 2, "Boundary Violations," Chapter 4, "Dangerous Clients" and Chapter 10, "Risky Clients").

Even though ethical canons might provide some wiggle room (e.g., the provisions of ACA *Code of Ethics*, 2005, under Section A.5. c. and d. that deal with "potentially beneficial" nontherapeutic relationships with clients and former clients; see Chapter 2, "Boundary Violations"), the only safe or relatively risk-managed advice that can be offered is to avoid therapeutic relationships with friends, family members, romantic partners, and supervisees at all cost. For each more remote relationship, contact your lawyer and insurance carrier for definitive advice and get the opinion in writing. Even with people who fall into one of these categories once removed (e.g., the spouse or associate of one of these people), documented consultation is an essential part of the decision-making process. Mental health professionals are insightful people, but they are not mind readers. You can never be certain what a business associate or social acquaintance is thinking. You cannot count on their kind and protective attitude toward you if the therapy goes poorly with the services you provide. If the outcome is poor, you can count on retribution. On careful analysis, the risk presented by treating someone in a gray category will almost always outweigh the benefits to both the person and the therapist.

Ethical Flash Points

- Do not treat a client who falls within the degree of kinship or relationship outlined in this chapter.

- If there is a question concerning whether a client or potential client falls within a prohibited category, consult the canons of ethics first to see if the relationship is specifically prohibited. If concern continues, contact your lawyer, licensing board, malpractice carrier, or a learned colleague. Get clarification and permission in all questionable cases. Seek guidance in writing.

- If there is the slightest potential for harm, or you experience the tiniest twinge of concern regarding your objectivity, refer the person to another mental health professional.

- If a current client marries into the family, tread gingerly and make sure you have obtained and documented informed consent. At least acknowledge that the client was informed and understood the professional guidelines. If at all possible without injuring the client, make a referral and document the rationale for the referral. If appropriate, give the client a copy of the guidelines to help clarify the reason for the referral and offer to cooperate with any future therapist.

(continued)

(*Continued*)

• When in doubt, do not accept the client into treatment.

• Call your professional association or licensing board before proceeding and record their response in the clinical file. Include the presenting problem, the date, the person to whom you spoke, the advice received, and how you complied with it. Be prepared to show a good-faith effort to comply with the published canons of ethics.

• Do not be intimidated by third-party payers. Remember, your license is on the line, not theirs.

• *Note:* In the experience of the authors, one of the major problems therapists have is resisting the temptation to offer free advice to friends and family. Don't!

Summary

Generally, the mental health professional treats individuals in a context where therapeutic objectivity is not compromised, for example, the transaction is arm's length and the only connection between client and therapist is therapeutic. This cannot be realized where current or previous family members, personal friends, business associates, or any of the other relationships previously listed are involved. And certainly, do not treat any past or current sexual partners, nor any you intend to visit in the future (see Chapter 12, "Sexual Misconduct").

In addition, the professional cannot treat an individual currently receiving treatment from another counselor without the other provider's knowledge and consent, as treatment plans must be coordinated and a unified approach used. Conflicting therapies can be disastrous. Also, many agencies have, by contract with agents, servants, and employees, as well as independent contractors, rules and internal prohibitions against private practitioners building their practice by diverting clients away from the agencies and into the practice of the private or moonlighting provider. These standards are appropriate and must be honored.

Then there are the fuzzy questions: What happens when a long-term client marries into the family and suddenly becomes an in-law? Or a business associate with no therapeutic connection sells a business interest to a present or former client, or, after weeks or months or even years of effective treatment, the client approaches the therapist with a "by the way, I have been seeing X, another therapist, for a second opinion, and I had actually seen her before I came to see you"?

When does an acceptable and suitable client fall within unacceptable ranges or degrees of relationships to the extent that therapeutic objectivity is, or can be, lost?

And then, what is the best way to avoid an actual, possible, or the appearance of an ethical infraction? What is the client's perception of what occurred? This chapter suggests some of the options.

Many of the prohibited client problems can be avoided by a careful intake interview. Insightful, thorough, and in-depth questioning during the first conference will often uncover current and possible past and future relationships. When a thread of a prohibition appears, fully develop the line of questioning, and do not undertake treatment until fully satisfied that the client is ethically eligible. Refusing to begin the client-therapist relationship is easier than terminating it at a later date because of newly discovered information that should have been uncovered in the first place.

Suggested Research Assignments

1. Locate and discuss any rules promulgated by licensing boards in your state that list prohibited clients. Generate your own list. Use our suggestions as an informal guide.
2. Locate and discuss any state and national professional association ethical guidelines that deal with prohibited clients. In reviewing ethical guidelines, do you notice any glaring inconsistencies?
3. Can you find any disciplinary actions against mental health professionals in which the relationship was so subtle that creating a prohibited client category was a stretch of logic or good sense?
4. Compare and contrast these state licensing board rules with the ethical rules promulgated by the state professional associations.

5. Compare and contrast state licensing board and professional association guidelines with the guidelines of national professional associations.

6. Identify resources/persons you would consult to safely and ethically make a decision regarding a potentially prohibited client. Create a list of available and trustworthy consultants.

7. Research the decisions of your state licensing boards and state and national professional association ethics committees for prohibited client relationship violation sanctions.

8. Research the civil case decisions of your state related to prohibited client relationships. What damages, if any, were awarded?

9. Apply the ethical canons of the state licensing board for your discipline to the scenarios at the beginning of this chapter, and answer the questions that are posed.

Discussion Questions

1. What would you tell a potential client calling to schedule a first appointment who indicates he got your name from his fiancé whom you treated two years before?

2. What would you tell another mental health professional, who went to graduate school with you, who now has a problem and needs your help?

3. You are sitting alone at a picnic table during a family reunion and a second cousin sits down next to you and begins to tell you about how depressed she is. What do you say?

4. The mother of a child in the school where you serve as a school counselor learns of your side private practice and asks you to counsel with her and her husband and children. What do you say?

5. You sing in your church choir. You stand in the front row. A choir member who stands in the fifth and last row calls for an appointment wanting to initiate therapy with you. What do you say?

10

Risky Clients

Sharon, a licensed professional counselor with 10 years of private practice experience, took a call from a 34-year-old female who wanted to schedule an appointment as quickly as possible. The potential client was very persistent, and Sharon agreed to stay late the following evening to see her. When the client came in for the first session, Sharon had a twinge of uneasiness although the client was respectful and well behaved during the session. The client gushed appreciation when the session ended. Over the next two months, however, the client became increasingly more difficult to deal with. She was insisting on almost daily contact and would become upset if Sharon did not return each call within a short time. The client began to disparage Sharon, first subtly and then directly, with greater hostility. She threatened to sue Sharon for abandonment if she stopped treating her.

Frank, a licensed psychologist, agreed to see Carol, a clinical social worker whose husband had just filed for divorce. Carol had problems with nervousness, sleeping, and anger, and showed signs of depression. They entered into a therapeutic relationship, and as time went on, Carol became confrontational in session and noncompliant with Frank's therapeutic suggestions. When Frank indicated he would not be able to offer favorable testimony if *he were brought in to testify in the divorce case, Carol launched into an attack of Frank and his services, detailing a number of shortcomings that she claimed were violations of the psychologist licensing act. Later when Frank read the licensing act, he realized he had indeed failed to comply with two minor and highly technical rules.*

Deciding Which Clients to Treat

After working with mental health professionals over many years, we began to identify certain types of client who where more likely to file complaints against their treatment providers. As this awareness developed, it also became apparent that mental health professionals were not being appropriately selective with respect to the clients they decided to treat. We felt that by being more selective in taking on clients, the risk of a complaint being filed against the mental health professional could be dramatically reduced.

Even if the practitioner is not in a position to personally select clients, knowledge of the kinds of client that pose greater risk will allow for more careful treatment and more thorough documentation of the services provided to the client. Expect the worst from the client and prepare the best possible record to defend against the complaint.

The first step in selecting clients is to critically and objectively evaluate your professional limitations and strengths. You need to recognize the cases or clients you are personally and professionally better equipped to treat effectively. It might be productive to discuss this with colleagues who know you well or even family members who can provide insightful feedback.

You should attempt to identify the kind of client or problem you really enjoy treating. Which clients offer a pleasing professional experience? It is just as important, however, to recognize the client or problems that you do not like to see come through the office door. Who has the potential to ruin the day?

The second step is to never agree, or allow potential clients to think that you have agreed, to treat them until you have conducted an evaluative session. The potential client should never be allowed to walk into the therapist's office the first time with the understanding that therapy will commence during that session. The potential client should be informed that the first session is solely for the purpose of gathering and sharing information—by *both* the therapist and the client. Explain that therapy is a very personal relationship that is dependent on trust, respect, good communication, and understanding. Both parties must be confident that they are right for each other so the client can achieve the best possible results.

Too many therapists have started therapy with a client they had uneasy feelings about, but like Sharon in the first scenario, they didn't trust their instincts. By making the first session evaluative, the therapist can assess those gut feelings and avoid getting into therapy if the relationship is not good for both parties. You can thus avoid having to go through a contentious and problematic termination if the therapeutic relationship collapses.

The third step is to do a thorough job of gathering information from the potential client during the evaluative session. The discussion of each risky client that follows will include the kind of information that should be solicited from the potential client. A detailed information form should be developed for the client to complete prior to commencement of the evaluative session. The therapist should then review the person's answers with the potential client. Many people will not write down as much information as they should in answering each question. They may not lie, but they don't tell the whole truth. Follow up and flesh out the information that may have been sketchily provided.

A therapist who has to treat a risky client will be motivated to treat the person carefully and fully document the work. Knowing that the client may pose risk, the therapist should establish specific guidelines for the therapy *and for client behavior* for the therapeutic relationship. It should be made clear, in writing, what is expected of the client, and that termination will occur if the client is not compliant. It is helpful in terminating with a client if the therapist can refer the client back to the guidelines and specifically enumerate the lack of compliance. It is also immensely helpful in defending against the complaint the client may file against the therapist posttermination, especially the likely abandonment charge.

Classifying Potentially Risky Clients

Therapy Shoppers and Hoppers

Consumers who have a long history of mental health treatment with multiple providers are risky clients. First, there probably is a reason that they still need services, and it is not because all their prior treatment providers were incompetent. They may be resistant to change or just too difficult to treat. If five or six of your predecessors were unsuccessful, don't count on being the one to make the miracle breakthrough possible.

Second, these clients have picked up a lot of knowledge about therapy—what the rules are—and they know how to write coherent and probable-sounding complaints to the licensing board. They have a basis for comparison. Having seen how other mental health professionals conducted themselves, they will be in a position to be much more analytical and critical of the most recent treatment provider and his or her services.

A person can have valid reasons for going to more than one mental health treatment provider, such as relocations of the client or therapist, changes in insurance coverage, and illness or retirement of therapists. In evaluating a potential client, it is imperative to inquire about prior treatment providers and why and how the therapeutic relationship ended. Secure consent to contact the prior treatment providers before agreeing to enter into therapy. Then contact those treatment providers. Their experiences with the potential client can make your decision to treat or refer much easier. If the potential client refuses to give this consent, then entering into a therapeutic relationship would be an ill-advised move.

Former Mental Health Discipline Students

If the potential client once took psychology classes or started a counseling master's degree program but didn't finish, he or she may show a strong bias about the treating mental health professional. The person may be envious of therapists who successfully reached the goal they didn't or couldn't achieve. They may analyze their therapist while the therapist is analyzing them. They may be critical, thinking they could do a better job than the therapist (e.g., "This is what the therapist could or should have done"; or, "If this had been done, I would have been cured").

Having an interest in the profession, former students may have accumulated a lot of information about therapy, and the rules applicable to it. They can write plausible-sounding complaints that catch the attention of licensing boards. If malevolent and devious enough, they can set a mental health professional up for a complaint.

During evaluation, potential clients should be asked, not just what was their highest level of education, but what courses they took. Specifically ask if the person took any psychology or counseling classes in school. Learning about such coursework may not be enough to persuade a therapist to avoid providing treatment. However, it should at least result in more careful treatment and thorough documentation.

Listen carefully to the vocabulary used. Is it full of psychological terms or jargon? This might indicate a background in one of the mental health disciplines. It may indicate that this potential client has self-diagnosed and is just waiting for confirmation.

Other Mental Health Professionals

If a failed graduate student is risky, just think how much riskier a fully trained and licensed mental health professional can be. This client will most certainly be critically evaluating the treating therapist's services. This client, if not satisfied with the therapy or advice, can and will file a sensible-sounding complaint with specific references to the licensing statute or ethical rules. A few mental health professionals have serious emotional or psychological problems and when riled up can present formidable problems for their treatment providers. They know how and where the most harm can be done.

In the second opening scenario, Frank, the psychologist, received public reprimands from his licensing board after the complaint was investigated. Frank treated the social worker knowing that she was a mental health professional.

Asking potential clients about their occupation may not elicit correct information. Shrewd mental health professionals may lie, knowing that the therapist might be reluctant to treat a mental health professional or fearing the therapist may report them to their own licensing board if they are not competent to practice. Question potential clients about their jobs or occupations, and if your instincts tell you someone is not being truthful, give strong consideration to not treating that person. Just as clients may refuse treatment, providers, subject to limitations, may refuse to treat a particular client. It is easier to refuse to treat than it is to terminate once treatment has begun.

Resist the temptation to want to help a colleague in distress simply because he or she is a colleague. Evaluate this potential client as you would any other client, noting initially the risk presented by the person's profession.

Chronic Complainers

Everyone has encountered the person who always views the glass as being half empty. Mental health professionals encounter more of these types of people than others do. The chronic complainer is the person who blames everyone from their parents, their siblings, their teachers, their coworkers, their bosses, down to the weather and the gods for everything that goes wrong in their lives. They never accept responsibility and are quick to lay blame elsewhere. Is it hard to imagine that this person will not get around to blaming his or her therapist when life doesn't get better? Chronic complainers often are quick to file complaints and lawsuits against professionals and service providers they engage when they are dissatisfied with the services they receive. In reality, they are never satisfied. They confuse competent therapy with unrealistic anticipated results.

To ferret out the complainers, a mental health professional should ask the following questions: "Have you ever filed a lawsuit against a person or company?" "Have you ever filed a complaint against a professional?" "Have you ever lodged a complaint against a coworker?" If the answer is yes, follow up with additional questions. Try to ascertain if this is a pattern. Can a therapist safely assume that a person who has filed lawsuits or complaints against other service providers will not do so against him or her? Of course not. Chronic complainers will continue to complain and should be avoided if at all possible.

Disgruntled Family Law Litigants

An increasing number of complaints are being filed against mental health professionals by clients or former clients who are unhappy with the outcome of their custody or divorce cases. Typically, one party and sometimes both parties are angry about a case outcome. Judges have judicial immunity, lawyers can hide behind the facts and the judge's ruling, but mental health professionals who testify or provide records are sitting ducks for the angry litigants.

It is impractical to think a therapist can avoid treating every client who potentially could become involved in a divorce or custody case. The practice would have to be limited to single people who never intend to marry and who are unable to procreate or adopt a child. However, it is not impractical to inquire about the possibility of such matters when the client presents for an evaluation. Ask about marital status, separations, children, and so on to determine if a family law case is imminent or probable. If it is and the therapist is not comfortable with the prospect of becoming involved in such a lawsuit, the potential client should be so advised and referred elsewhere.

If one parent is presenting a child for treatment, you should condition providing treatment on the presenting parent's agreement for you to contact the other parent. Seek to gather information from and to involve that other parent in the child's therapy when appropriate. Too many times, a therapist is given false or distorted information about the absent parent in an attempt to influence the therapist. Chapter 31, "Forensic Evaluation," discusses some of the hazards of forensic work. In the context of this chapter, if a parent refuses to allow contact with the other parent, the evaluating mental health professional should strongly consider not accepting the case. Keep in mind that a treatment provider cannot testify or offer an unqualified opinion concerning the "best interest of a child" unless the professional has evaluated all persons who seek custody or conservatorship.

Clients with Borderline Personality Disorders

Every time we asked a group of mental health professionals who is the most risky client to treat, the response was always an emphatic "borderlines!"

Once, in discussing clients with borderline personality disorders with a state board investigator, the investigator summed these people up in this manner, "Pit Bulls." Persons suffering from borderline personality disorder or similar disorders are sometimes characterized as persistent, confrontational, intelligent, demanding, and threatening. *DSM IV* 301.83 defines Borderline Personality Disorder as:

> A pervasive pattern of instability of interpersonal relationships, self-image, and effects, and marked impulsivity beginning by early adulthood and present in a variety of contexts, as indicated by five (of nine) diagnostic criteria. Three criteria are:
>
> 1. Frantic effort to avoid real or imagined abandonment.
> 2. A pattern of unstable and intense interpersonal relationships characterized by alternating between extremes of idealization and devaluation . . .
> 8. Inappropriate, intense anger or difficulty controlling anger . . .

It is not hard to imagine a client with a borderline personality disorder gushing appreciation and praise for a therapist early on and subsequently becoming disparaging and then frantic when the therapist threatens termination. If a therapist follows through with termination, then the client may express anger through a complaint to a licensing board, an employer, a managed care or insurance company, the Office of Civil Rights and, probably, with all these entities. The person with borderline personality disorder will attempt to inflict as much harm as possible on the therapist through legal means and in rare cases through illegal activity such as repetitive and harassing phone calls, trespass, and threatening e-mails.

With these universally recognized difficult clients, it is a good idea to ask potential clients about any diagnosis they may have been given in the past even if they feel it was incorrect. If a therapist suspects a potential client suffers from borderline personality disorder and the therapist is not comfortable in treating this disorder, then declining to provide treatment after an evaluation session is much easier than terminating with the client after therapy has commenced.

On several occasions, we have been asked if it is unethical to knowingly refuse to treat people with this disorder. Recently a group of psychologists cited the APA *Ethical Principles of Psychologists and Code of Conduct* (2002) provision that states:

3.01 Unfair Discrimination

In their work-related activities, psychologists do not engage in unfair discrimination based on age, gender, gender identity, race, ethnicity, culture, national origin, religion, sexual orientation, *disability*, socioeconomic status, or any basis proscribed by law.

We do not believe a personality disorder constitutes a "disability" as that word is used in this section of the APA Ethics Code. In this context, disability is being used in a legal sense such as physical or mental impairment that would entitle a person to specific protection from discrimination. People with borderline personality disorders are not considered a protected class of citizens requiring specific statutory protection.

The APA Ethics Code also states:

2.01 Boundaries of Competence

(a) Psychologists provide services, teach, and conduct research with populations and in areas only within the boundaries of their competence, based on their education, training, supervised experience, consultation, study, or professional experience. (See Chapter 4, "Dangerous Clients," and Chapter 11, "Repressed and Recovered Memories," for other National Guidelines on competency.)

It is appropriate to refuse to take on clients whom a therapist does not feel competent to treat. A marriage and family therapist would feel no hesitancy in referring a spouse with a serious alcohol problem to a chemical dependency counselor. Because people with borderline personality disorders are so difficult, not every therapist is going to feel competent to handle their care. We know of very few mental health professionals who seek specialized training to treat this disorder. They exist thankfully, and all mental health professionals should learn who they are in their area so they can make referrals of known or possible clients with borderline personality disorder to these specially trained and experienced treatment providers.

A careful and prudent therapist who declines to enter into therapy with such a client is not being discriminatory but is making an objective decision that he or she is not the best option for treatment of that person. There is a duty then to refer the client to a therapist who can best provide treatment. A wise provider should always have an available list of licensed, capable, specialized professionals who accept referrals. They should be competent and also have professional liability insurance in case the client is dissatisfied for any reason. Such liability insurance should be verified prior to making the referral.

People with borderline personality disorders have the capacity to be very squeaky wheels with licensing boards. On intake, press for information about a prior diagnosis and talk to previous treatment providers before starting therapy. In the first scenario, Sharon failed to trust her instincts, did not question her client about prior diagnosis, and failed to contact the client's prior treatment providers. She learned a very tough lesson and ultimately had to secure a restraining order against the client. Fortunately for Sharon, this client obeyed the order. We have encountered a few severely ill clients of mental health professionals who ignored a restraining order and did not feel obligated to respect the orders issued by a judge. It was necessary to pursue subsequent criminal action that resulted in the clients being sent to jail. Now these therapists are wondering what will happen when these clients are released.

Attorneys

After working recently with several mental health professionals who had complaints filed against them by attorney clients or attorney parents of children they treated, we have added attorneys to our list of risky clients. The risk is pretty obvious. Attorneys can be smart, narcissistic, arrogant, combative, devious, and relentless—adding up to a nightmare for the therapist.

Attorneys know how to research and draft complaints. They can be technical and legalistic. Given the incentive (getting back at the therapist), they will scour the licensing act for support or substance for their complaints. They are generally not afraid of confrontation and may thrive on it. They will expend great amounts of time and energy in proving that they are correct and the therapist should be sanctioned.

Recently, one of the authors underwent an emergency appendectomy and recalled the look of fear on the anesthesiologist's face when hearing the response to his question, "What do you do for a living?" It would be wise for a mental health professional to have a similar reaction when learning that the potential client is a lawyer. As previously stated, ask about employment and occupation history. Ask what their spouse does for a living. The attorney spouse can be just as problematic for the treatment provider. When learning that a potential client or the client's spouse is a lawyer, ask what kind of law they practice. Litigators will be far riskier than a lawyer who specializes in wills and trusts.

Ethical Flash Points

- Therapists should resist their impulse to want to help everyone who comes in for help.

- It is true that certain people present greater risk for a therapist than others. Develop a mental list of those cases or people you believe could be problematic.

- Mental health professionals should objectively analyze their own strengths and weaknesses before treating clients.

- Structuring a practice so that initial sessions with clients are evaluative will allow for better information gathering and time for reflection before offering treatment.

- A potential client should never have the expectation of treatment, absent an emergency, when he or she first inquires about treatment or comes into the office. The potential client should be informed that the first session is solely for the purpose of gathering and sharing information, by both the therapist and the client.

- If a potential client admits to prior mental health treatment, ask about diagnosis and the identities of the treatment providers. Then get permission to talk to these professionals and do not agree to enter into treatment until you have consulted them.

(continued)

(*Continued*)
- Develop a detailed information form for each potential client to complete and then review it and discuss it with the person, fleshing out vague or incomplete responses.

- If the employment situation prevents client selection, use the same process outlined here to identify risky clients so more careful treatment can be provided and more thorough documentation recorded of the treatment.

- If a risky client is to be treated, develop and provide the client with specific written guidelines for the therapy and client behavior. The client should be informed that lack of compliance will result in termination of the therapeutic relationship.

Summary

Identifying clients who pose risk to the therapist should lead to a more selective process in choosing which clients to treat. Eliminating the riskier potential clients from the practice should lead to fewer complaints for the therapist to defend. Eliciting greater and better information from potential clients and making the first session evaluative only is not enough, however. Therapists should objectively analyze their own strengths and weaknesses as well and determine what types of problems or clients they are most competent to treat. Knowing yourself well is as important as knowing the potential client.

The authors can give no better advice than to urge therapists to trust their instincts. It does no good to be able to say later, "I knew this client would be a problem." Or, "I had a bad feeling about that client." Mental health professionals cannot effectively treat every person who walks in the door, nor are they required to treat every person who seeks help. Better client selection will lead to fewer complaints, peace of mind, and better overall quality of life and practice.

Suggested Research Assignments

1. Locate and discuss any rules promulgated by licensing boards in your state dealing with client selection, client intake, and client referral.

2. Locate and discuss any state and national professional association ethical guidelines that deal with client selection, client intake, and client referral. In reviewing ethical guidelines, do you notice any glaring inconsistencies?

3. Compare and contrast these state licensing board rules with the ethical rules promulgated by the state professional associations.

4. Compare and contrast state licensing board and professional association guidelines with the guidelines of national professional associations.

5. Identify resources and persons you would consult with to safely and ethically make a decision about a potentially risky client.

6. Research the decisions of your state licensing boards and state and national professional association ethics committees for client selection, client intake, and client referral violation sanctions.

7. Apply the ethical canons of the state licensing board for your discipline to the scenarios at the beginning of this chapter and answer the questions that are posed.

8. Develop an intake form that elicits the most relevant information concerning the client to determine whether the client should be accepted into therapy.

9. Talk to practicing mental health professionals in your area about who they perceive as risky clients and how they handle these situations.

Discussion Questions

1. A client expresses dissatisfaction with your therapy. What do you say? Role-play a scenario wherein you mollify the unhappy client without admitting negligence or unethical practice, and yet mediate in such a way that both you and the client are satisfied.

2. What do you say to a potential client who refuses to complete your intake form and provide information regarding prior mental health treatment and the professionals who provided the treatment?

3. A potential new client has come into your office for the first session (evaluative only). The client has a menacing and frightening appearance, and he lets you know that he served 10 years in the state

penitentiary for sexual assault and attempted murder. What do you do and say to this person?

4. The mother of a 10-year-old girl wants you to treat her daughter, indicating something is going on at her father's home during visitations (parents are divorced), but she is not sure what. She just knows her daughter cries when she has to visit with her father. The mother does not want you to contact the father under any circumstances. What do you say and do?

5. Taking into account your own personality and professional strengths and weaknesses, what types of client would you consider too risky for you to treat?

11

Repressed and Recovered Memory

A mature woman visits a therapist. Under hypnosis, or perhaps after prob-
ing questions, she vaguely remembers being touched inappropriately by her
uncle when she was very young. As the therapy visits continue, the touching
gradually comes more clearly into focus. Finally, as a result of the progres-
sively increasing intensity of the memories, she cuts off all contact with her
uncle and his family and extended family. The family system is now chaotic,
and what was once a loving family is totally estranged. Three years after the
therapy terminates, she concludes (correctly or incorrectly) that the therapist
implanted the idea of the inappropriate touching in her mind. She recants,
but by now, the family damage is complete. The relationship can never be
restored. She complains to the licensing board about the therapist and indi-
cates she was led to inappropriate, incorrect, and damaging conclusions. Or,
her uncle, having been cleared of any wrongdoing, feels cheated out of years
of uncle-niece love and affection. He files a complaint with the licensing
board. Fast-forward to the trial for negligent diagnosis, which occurs sepa-
rate and distinct from the hearing before the licensing board. The mature
woman is now in court. A parade of expert witnesses testify, with ponderous
tomes to back them up, that repressed and recovered memories are in fact
valid theories and capable of being discovered, diagnosed, and treated.

At the same time, another group of expert witnesses testify (after affirming or swearing on a Bible) that repressed and recovered memories, no matter how they come to the surface, are not reliable. Who decides which theory is correct? In a trial, it is the judge, usually a lawyer, or a jury of laypeople chosen from the community. The fact finder or decision maker is not a mental health professional, but a lay individual. In a complaint to the licensing board, the fact finders are usually coprofessionals with mental health backgrounds who understand the concept of repressed and recovered memory, together with the method of diagnosis and treatment. However, this is not to imply that professional boards are without prejudices. A casual survey would indicate that there are militant advocates and contrary opinions. Therefore, exercise caution when diagnosing a recovered or repressed memory. The reputation you save may be your own.

Professional Liability Today

"Periodically, therapists get an urgent wake-up call about specific dangers concerning particular professional liability issues. In the 1970s, the *Tarasoff* case pointed out risks when therapists fail to warn potential victims about patients' threats to identifiable intended victims. In the '80s, multimillion dollar awards in sexual misconduct cases forced providers to rethink their conduct—and pay higher insurance premiums. Now, a tide of repressed memory lawsuits are roiling the liability waters" ("Special Report" 1998). On September 3, 1999, the *Wausau Daily Herald* reported that a jury awarded $825,000 to the wife of a former mayor in a suit she filed against her psychiatrist. The psychiatrist allegedly implanted memories of childhood sexual abuse and satanic rituals in her mind. The article quoted Dr. Sionag Black, a three-year member of the American Psychological Association's Ethics Committee, as saying, "It's [treating a patient for multiple personality disorder] been pretty clear that's a very dangerous thing to do. It opens therapists up to exactly what happened to this man." In referring to relaxation and discipline over bad habits, Dr. Black stated, "Hypnosis can be a very valuable tool in other areas. But to use as a form of, 'Let's use it to see what your past is,' is a very risky thing to do. This is another scary case that shows us that." The article further reported that in 1997 an Appleton, Wisconsin, resident settled out of court for $2.4 million in a similar suit against a Montana psychiatrist. (This information can be accessed through the *Wausau Daily Herald*'s archives found at www.wausaudailyherald.com.) As mental health and legal scholars debate whether repressed memory is a valid scientific theory, juries have made it clear that they don't like it and are assessing large damage awards; insurance companies are demonstrating they are afraid of it, settling cases for substantial sums. In *Shazade v. Gregory*, 923 F. Supp. 286 (D. Mass. 1996), Judge Edward F. Harrington wrestled with the admissibility of evidence and testimony regarding repressed memory. The judge reviewed prior case decisions that disallowed repressed memory evidence and testimony on the basis that the theory was not widely accepted in the field of psychology. Citing that the *Diagnostic and Statistical Manual of Mental Disorders* (DSM-IV; American Psychiatric Association 1994) recognizes the concept of repressed memories, and psychological studies, Judge Harrington made the following findings:

As mental health and legal scholars debate whether repressed memory is a valid scientific theory, juries are making it clear that they don't like it and are assessing large damage awards.

- The theory has been the subject of various tests.
- The theory has been subject to peer review publication.
- Repressed memory, as is true with ordinary memories, cannot be tested empirically, and may not always be accurate; however, the theory itself has been established to be valid through various studies.
- The theory has attained general acceptance within the relevant scientific community of clinical psychiatrists.

Judge Harrington ruled in favor of allowing evidence and testimony based on the recovered memories of the victim. Other courts have declined to allow the evidence and testimony on the basis that repressed and recovered memories have not been shown to be scientifically reliable (see Chapter 16, "Challenging the Expert Witness: The *Daubert* Case," *The Portable Guide to Testifying in Court*, Bernstein and Hartsell 2005). When that happens, it is not hard to understand how courts and juries can find against a therapist who considers the repressed memory concept and diagnosis as scientifically reliable and embarks on a course of treatment consistent with that belief.

There is ample support for the concept or theory of recovered memories. The web site for the Recovered Memory Project lists 101 corroborated cases of recovered memory including 43 cases from legal proceedings (www.brown.edu/Departments/Taubman_Center/ Recovmem/archive.html).

In 1993, the American Psychiatric Association issued its "Statement on Memories of Sexual Abuse" noting: "Children and adolescents who have been abused cope with the trauma by using a variety of psychological mechanisms. In some instances, these coping mechanisms result in a lack of conscious awareness of the abuse for varying periods of time. Conscious thoughts and feelings stemming from the abuse may emerge at a later date."

As the acceptance of repressed memory theory has grown, there has not been equal acceptance or agreement on treatment methodology. Until mental health professionals achieve a consensus on how best to treat patients with repressed and recovered memories, there will continue to be an abundance of claims and lawsuits. It is worth noting that while repressed or recovered memory might, in time, become a reliable and substantiated diagnosis, the witness who has to defend this diagnosis and who offers a treatment plan has the burden of proving that the both the diagnosis and plan are valid and accurate psychological tools. "Because I say so" is not mental health proof. Academic evidence must be proffered to the court.

You must always keep in mind that clinical information concerning psychotherapy cannot be obtained from TV sound bites, magazines, or newspapers. Often the sound bite, though accurate, is misleading, and newspapers and magazines cannot be relied on to convey accurate therapeutic or legal advice or opinions. They don't necessarily lie, but the goal is to sell newspapers or to hold the attention of the radio or TV audience. For reliable research, consult learned treatises, professional journals, or complete published cases. A newspaper is perfectly honorable if it publishes a current case result. It is not ethically bound to publish the results if the case is reversed, nor it is obligated to give the reversal equal space.

When quoting case precedents, always verify and evaluate the source.

The Role of Informed Consent in Repressed Memory Cases

Failing to secure informed consent has been a theory of negligence for which juries have consistently found therapists liable in malpractice cases, including repressed memory cases. *Psychotherapy Finances* ("Special Report" 1998) reported that in a Texas case, lack of informed consent helped convince a jury to award a patient $5.8 million after the patient spent 5 years in therapy with little improvement.

Mental health professionals should learn from repressed memory lawsuits that informed consent requires disclosure and consent on the type of treatment given, the risks and benefits of the type of treatment presented and, just as important, the alternative treatment methods available.

Informed consent provisions can be found in most ethical codes (see Chapter 7, "Informed Consent"). Many therapists think that as long as they discuss confidentiality and fees with a client they have satisfied their informed consent obligation. Mental health professionals should learn from repressed memory lawsuits that informed consent requires disclosure and consent on the type of treatment given, the risks and benefits of the type of treatment presented, and—just as important—the alternative treatment methods available as well as the risks of forgoing treatment. It is critical to document informed consent. Failure to provide this information is an ethical violation and can result (and has) in a substantial jury award. Written information that the client signs or acknowledges receipt of in writing can go a long way in litigation when defending against an allegation of a lack of informed consent.

Informed Consent and Experimental Therapies

New or experimental therapies have often been attacked in lawsuits by former clients and patients and their attorneys (e.g., aggressive reparenting where adults crawl around on the floor drinking from baby bottles; psychic surgery; past-life regression, entity releasement; life regression, trust falls, and hitting with foam bats). Securing informed consent when using new and cutting-edge therapy may be difficult to establish for the typical juror who is predisposed to view mental health care with skepticism. Without published studies and research to document the effectiveness of a type of therapy, it may be impossible to advise clients on the risks and benefits, thereby precluding the informed consent ethical codes require. Whenever using a treatment that is *generally* accepted but not *universally* accepted, such as therapy to uncover repressed and recovered memory, the therapist should draft an appropriate consent form in which the client consents, in writing, to the treatment and then send it to a lawyer knowledgeable in mental health law for review. If one reviews the consent forms that hospitals and some physicians and dentists require their patients to sign, the advantage of a provider form becomes obvious. Therapists can never be protected from all risks in our litigious society, but consent forms that inform the client generally and specifically of the risks involved in therapy can afford some protection from litigation and complaints to licensing boards. Gone are the days of the one-sentence or one-paragraph consent form. After a lawyer approves the form, the therapist should ask each potential client to sign and date it, and give the client a copy. Written consent serves as a bulwark against a client who later claims, "I was not informed of the nature of the treatment, the consequences, nor the techniques." The information should be spelled out in clear and lay language for the client to read, question, and discuss. A thorough, lawyer/therapist-drafted informed consent form is the first line of defense in any claim for either an ethics violation or a malpractice suit.

Without published studies and research to document the effectiveness of a type of therapy, it may be impossible to advise clients on the risks and benefits, thereby precluding the informed consent that ethical codes require.

The Role of Therapist Competence in Repressed Memory Cases

The question of the mental health professional's competence as indicated by learning, training, education, experience, or license often plays a large role in a repressed memory lawsuit. These suits frequently involve a dissociative identity disorder diagnosis. Lack of adequate professional training and experience in this area can certainly doom a lawsuit to a poor and possibly tragic result for a therapist emotionally, professionally, and financially. Ethically, mental health professionals are strictly admonished to provide services only within the scope of their demonstrated competency.

Do not exceed your level of competence. It sounds simple, but mental health professionals who are sincerely motivated by their desire to help clients often let their hearts cloud their judgment. A professional mental health license or a university degree does not make a therapist competent to handle clients with difficult problems such as those presented by repressed memory and dissociative identity disorder. Know your limits. When the client or the client's problems exceed the level of individual competence, a mental health professional is ethically obligated to terminate and refer the client to another provider better able to provide treatment. Because professionals dispute the validity of repressed memories and uncertainty exists regarding what treatment techniques should be used, only the most careful, educated, trained, and experienced therapists should attempt to treat clients in this area. Unless the therapist fits this description, a referral is the only ethical option. Every professional has personal standards of formal and informal sources of continuing education, with workshops, seminars, classes, individual research, and personal readings providing important information that increases the provider's individual competence. Therapists should document every course, seminar, workshop, and individual study and reading they undertake. Thus, if challenged in court or by a disciplinary committee, the therapist could show evidence of learning, training, and experience (competence) by demonstrated background on the subject at hand.

Consider the following scenario: Suppose a therapist, through hypnosis or in the course of numerous visits, uncovers a repressed memory that affects the client in a serious and negative manner. Then the therapist elects to make a referral (realizing a level of competence has been exceeded) and there is no one in the community who will accept this kind of referral because of the risks involved. Then what? Abandonment?

Do not exceed your level of competence.

Because professionals dispute the validity of repressed memories and uncertainty exists regarding what treatment techniques should be used, only the most careful, educated, trained, and experienced therapists should attempt to treat clients in this area.

National Guidelines for Therapist Competency

American Association for Marriage and Family Therapy (AAMFT) Code of Ethics (2001)

3.11 Marriage and family therapists do not diagnose, treat, or advise on problems outside the recognized boundaries of their competencies.

American Counseling Association (ACA) Code of Ethics (2005)

A.11 Termination and Referral

A.11.b. Inability to Assist Clients

If counselors determine an inability to be of professional assistance to clients, they avoid entering or continuing counseling relationships. Counselors are knowledgeable about culturally and clinically appropriate referral resources and suggest these alternatives. If clients decline the suggested referrals, counselors should discontinue the relationship.

National Association of Social Workers (NASW) Code of Ethics (1999)

1.04 Competence

(a) Social workers should provide services and represent themselves as competent only within the boundaries of their education, training, license, certification, consultation received, supervised experience, or other relevant professional experience.

(b) Social workers should provide services in substantive areas or use intervention techniques or approaches that are new to them only after engaging in appropriate study, training, consultation, and supervision from people who are competent in those interventions or techniques.

Hypnosis and Relaxation Techniques

Hypnosis and its functional equivalent, relaxation and visualization techniques, have come under attack in repressed memory and other types of damage suits. In *Borawick v. Shay* (842 F. Supp. 1501 (D. Conn. 1994); aff 'd 68 F.3d 597 (2d Cir. 1995), certiorari denied 116 S. Ct. 1869, 134 L. Ed. 2d 966 (1996)), the federal court ruled that a victim could not testify because her recollection had been rendered unreliable by the past use of hypnosis for therapeutic purposes. A noted side effect of hypnosis is the creation of memories that may not be accurate: the phenomenon of false and implanted memories. Failing to advise the client of this side effect and the failure of the therapist to recognize that a "recovered memory" of abuse may not be true and to seek corroboration has resulted in a finding of negligence. If mental health professionals are going to use hypnosis, it is critical that they be thoroughly trained and experienced and closely follow the guidelines of the American Society for Clinical Hypnosis (www.asch.net).

A noted side effect of hypnosis is the creation of memories that may not be accurate: the phenomenon of false and implanted memories.

Ethical Flash Points

- Beware of the client who reveals repressed memories.

- Repressed memory cases have resulted in substantial jury awards and settlements in favor of complaining clients/plaintiffs.

- The lack of universal acceptance of the validity of repressed memory as a scientific theory with appropriate treatment techniques makes this an attractive and fertile area for malpractice suits as well as ethical complaints.

- Failing to adequately secure informed consent is an ethical violation and a common allegation in repressed memory lawsuits. Remember, clients are entitled to an explanation of alternative treatments as well as an explanation of the risks of forgoing treatment.

- Informed consent includes advising clients of alternative forms of treatment, not just the benefits and risks of the treatment used.

(continued)

(*Continued*)

- Therapist competence is critical in treating clients with repressed memory or when employing hypnosis and other less conventional types of therapy.

- A wise therapist maintains a comprehensive log of all training received as well as personal readings, research, and studies.

- Always attempt to corroborate recovered memories and never accept them as accurate without corroboration.

- Failure to terminate and refer when a therapist lacks the education, training, license, and experience to treat a client's problem is an ethical violation and a basis for establishing professional negligence.

- Hypnosis can cause false memories, and the client should be advised of this as part of informed consent to this type of treatment.

- New or unconventional types of therapy may be so unproved that they defy informed consent.

- Treatment modalities are constantly evolving. A theory accepted today might be invalidated tomorrow, and a theory rejected today might, after additional professional input, be generally accepted tomorrow.

Summary

Even though a therapist may secure the education, license, training, and experience that would allow other mental health professionals to view him or her as competent with respect to certain types of therapy, it does not ensure that the complaints committee of a disciplinary board or a jury will look on his or her competence, treatment, and services favorably. Debated and unproved theories and types of treatment make the kind of informed consent required by ethics codes difficult to obtain. Explaining a theory may also be difficult, and ensuring that the client understands the explanation is still more difficult.

Repressed memory and repressed memory treatment fall into this category and should cause mental health professionals to seriously reflect on whether they wish to become professionally involved with a repressed memory client. When a client reveals a repressed memory, a therapist should be wary not only about the accuracy of the memory but also about the therapist's ability to treat the client. A referral may be a better course of action.

Suggested Research Assignments

1. Locate and discuss any rules promulgated by licensing boards in your state dealing with competency.
2. Locate and discuss any state and national professional association ethical guidelines that deal with competency. In reviewing ethical guidelines, do you notice any glaring inconsistencies?
3. Compare and contrast these state licensing board rules with the ethical rules promulgated by the state professional associations.
4. Compare and contrast state licensing board and professional association guidelines with the guidelines of national professional associations.
5. Identify resources and persons you would consult with or train with to become competent in the areas of recovered memories and hypnosis.
6. Identify colleagues available for consultation and referral if deemed necessary when difficult or incredibly challenging cases arise. Determine if they are available to current clients, the cost, and whether they have current malpractice or professional liability insurance in force.
7. Research the decisions of your state licensing boards and state and national professional association ethics committees for competency violation sanctions.
8. Research legal case decisions for your state that involve recovered memory, hypnosis, or failure to obtain informed consent.
9. Develop an intake form that adequately documents informed consent for hypnosis.
10. Talk to practicing mental health professionals in your area who treat clients with recovered memories or through the use of hypnosis and report back on what you learned from these practitioners.
11. Review some of the literature published by national organizations that deal with recovered and repressed memories. What is their point of view?

Discussion Questions

1. A client you have been treating for depression advises you that she has a recurring dream of her father sexually abusing her when she was young. She asks you if this could mean it really happened. What do you say and do?

2. You have completed hypnosis training and want to implement this treatment option in your practice. What should you do before offering this treatment?

3. A local judge calls and asks, off the record, how reliable are recovered memories. What do you tell him?

4. A 32-year-old client reports that she has begun getting "flashbacks" of being raped when she was 10 or 11 years old. You do not feel competent to deal with this problem. What do you say and do? What do you document?

5. What is the history of recovered memory cases? Is it worth the risk to take on these problems as a treating mental health professional?

12

Sexual Misconduct

Mickey, a tall, attractive woman, checked herself into the charity hospital emergency room. Randy, the psychiatric intern on call, was compassionate, understanding, and single. As soon as Mickey saw him, her spirits soared. She insisted he treat her personally and later came to his office in the medical school wearing a miniskirt, spiked heels, and flattering makeup. She captivated Randy, and after a few months of outpatient treatment, they met for coffee in the medical school cafeteria. Later they met for a movie, then a few drinks, and finally they began an affair. This was heaven to Mickey as long as she received Randy's undivided attention, but as any professional can imagine, her underlying problems did not go away. Finally the intern called Mickey to terminate both their social and professional relationship. Mickey was mortified. She felt this was another male rejection made by the man she trusted most. Devastated, she took an overdose of sleeping pills and found herself back in the emergency room, where she discussed her relationship with Randy with another intern. It all became part of the medical school psychiatric clinical file. Still angry, Mickey called a lawyer. Randy lost his medical license, and Mickey gained a substantial settlement. Why would educated, intelligent people allow themselves to be seduced in a situation so clearly dangerous, destined to fail, and unethical?

Note: *Some literature and case law suggest that if an affair occurred between the patient/client and another medical staff member, but not the actual treating physician, it would still constitute an ethical infraction and liability. No one on the professional staff who meets Mickey as a result of her seeking therapeutic help should change the relationship from therapeutic to social. A high boundary wall surrounds Mickey and protects her from everyone she encounters in the hospital as a result of her quest for professional treatment.*

Thelma, a social worker, led a lesbian therapy group. One woman attended the first session and then dropped out. Later, she called to invite Thelma to lunch. Soon after, they started dating and ultimately moved in together. Another group member observed the one-time visit in group therapy and later saw the two women together in an apparently affectionate situation. Jealous, she investigated and determined that the relationship was unethical and forwarded her findings (a summary of community gossip) to the licensing board. The facts were admitted, and the board took disciplinary action. There was no way to justify the relationship between Thelma and any person whose introduction occurred in a therapeutic framework and who was listed on the group roster as a person receiving or participating in a group therapy session she facilitated.

John, a therapist, and Susan, his client, met in Massachusetts while he was pursuing his doctorate in counseling psychology. He treated her under the supervision of a clinical professor when she sought help from the counseling center where he was enrolled in a practicum. After graduation, he remained in the same city where he occasionally saw Susan in church, but nothing ever happened between them except a friendly "hello" and a nod. Later John relocated to California, and five years later by complete coincidence Susan moved to the same town and joined his church and Sunday school class. This time they began dating, but he later broke things off with her. Susan was furious and filed a complaint. She said she had fantasized about John for the past 5 years, that he knew about her fantasies, and in dating her took advantage of their former intern-client relationship. In her complaint, she indicated she was so emotionally damaged by the social relationship that she would never recover. John was subject to disciplinary action by his licensing board. The board concluded that he should have resisted becoming involved with Susan because their relationship had a tendency to be exploitative. John, as a mental health professional, was the responsible party.

Prevalence of Sexual Misconduct

Engaging in sexual misconduct with clients is more prevalent among mental health professionals than we might imagine. A quick review of sanctions published by licensing boards in any state will reveal a significant number of mental health professionals who have committed sexual improprieties with clients or former clients.

We have lectured throughout the country urging mental health professionals to maintain an effective clinical distance between themselves and their clients and former clients. The danger legally and ethically of dual relationships and boundary violations, particularly those involving sexual misconduct, causes much grief, anxiety, and concern for mental health professionals and the consumer-oriented boards who enforce the rules. Nevertheless, somewhere in the nation at any given time therapists are busily engaging in such activities, whether they pursue a client sexually or intimately, or a client pursues them and they cannot resist the temptation. Either way, it is the mental health professional who ultimately loses. If caught, providers may be dismissed from their national organizations, terminated from their professional employment, found guilty of a felony in some states, and certainly risk having their licenses revoked for committing an unethical act. Considering that most professional organizations and licensing boards have a zero tolerance level for sexual intimacies with a client, why does it happen?

There is no therapeutic modality or school for training mental health providers that permits sex with a client and no accepted literature that in any way condones such a relationship. Indeed, schools, the literature, the pundits in the field, and every speaker we have ever heard condemn the practice. Yet, sex with a client continues to disturb therapeutic relationships and causes physical, psychological, and emotional damage. There is nothing right about having sex with a client. Sexual misconduct with a client is ethically, legally, and criminally wrong.

Sexual misconduct with a client is ethically, legally, and criminally wrong.

Consider the big picture. When a mental health provider is caught having sex with a client, he or she destroys the reputation of helping professionals in general. Many cases of sexual exploitation lead to media exposure that fans the flames of public cynicism against the mental health field and destroys or at least minimizes the excellent work that the vast majority of helping professionals offer to the community in general and individuals and families in particular.

Rarely does sex with a client happen quickly. Usually, an honest clinical relationship first develops between the therapist and the client. We have had a client who wanted to file a complaint because the therapist exhaled too hard in the client's ear and the client thought he was panting with excitement over the client!

The therapist knows that to cross clinical boundaries is wrong and initially resists any other relationship. Gradually, however, the barriers break down, and one activity leads to another. The offense compounds itself. If the relationship sours, the client may feel hurt, humiliated, exploited, or taken advantage of, and may go so far as to file a licensing board complaint or malpractice suit, or both. It is not uncommon for a complaint to be filed with a licensing board or national organization while, simultaneously, litigation is pursued.

Of course, some therapist-client relationships do last. There are numerous cases where the parties have married, but this does not make the therapist's conduct ethical. Marriage is not a cure or panacea for unethical conduct. If either the therapist or the client is married or was in a significant relationship when the affair began, the client's or therapist's significant other or both are sure to at least consider reporting the unethical liaison. Jilted spouses do not take kindly to therapist-client sexual relationships that break up marriages. The natural inclination is to file a complaint and let the professional boards do the investigating and take appropriate action.

Marriage is not a cure or panacea for unethical conduct.

Therapists who are guilty of sexual misconduct with clients, except for a few very rare exceptions, are not sexual predators. In fact, most proved to be competent and caring professionals who crossed a line they knew they should not have crossed. Usually, at the time the therapist made the mistake or entered into the relationship, bad things were happening or had recently occurred in the therapist's life. The therapist may have recently experienced a divorce, death of a family member, substance abuse or addiction, a relationship breakup, financial problems, job termination, or illness. The therapist was vulnerable to a predatory or unprincipled client. The issues in their personal lives rendered them more vulnerable to having sexual or intimate contact with a client or former client. This does not excuse or condone the action. A therapist who is impaired in any way should not be treating clients. It is imperative for mental health professionals to get help when personal problems arise and to take stock of their vulnerability and ability to competently treat clients while receiving the assistance.

The ethics codes of mental health disciplines are remarkably similar relating to sex with clients, sexual intimacies, or any social or sexual relationship. Every code contains some restrictive language that prohibits sex with a client, a former client, or anyone who might consider him- or herself to be a client.

National Guidelines for Sexual Misconduct

American Association for Marriage and Family Therapy (AAMFT) Code of Ethics (2001)

1.4 Sexual intimacy with clients is prohibited.

1.5 Sexual intimacy with former clients is likely to be harmful and is therefore prohibited for two years following the termination of therapy or last professional contact. In an effort to avoid exploiting the trust and dependency of clients, marriage and family therapists should not engage in sexual intimacy with former clients after the two years following termination or last professional contact. Should therapists engage in sexual intimacy with former clients following two years after termination or last professional contact, the burden shifts to the therapist to demonstrate that there has been no exploitation or injury to the former client or to the client's immediate family.

(continued)

(Continued)

American Counseling Association (ACA) Code of Ethics (2005)

A.5. Roles and Relationships with Clients

A.5.a. Current Clients

Sexual or romantic counselor-client interactions or relationships with current clients, their romantic partners, or their family members are prohibited.

A.5.b. Former Clients

Sexual or romantic counselor-client interactions or relationships with former clients, their romantic partners, or their family members are prohibited for a period of 5 years following the last professional contact. Counselors, before engaging in sexual or romantic interactions or relationships with clients, their romantic partners, or client family members after 5 years following the last professional contact, demonstrate forethought and document (in written form) whether the interactions or relationship can be viewed as exploitive in some way and/or whether there is still potential to harm the former client; in cases of potential exploitation and/or harm, the counselor avoids entering such an interaction or relationship.

American Psychological Association (APA) Ethical Principles of Psychologists and Code of Conduct (2002)

10. Therapy

10.05 Sexual Intimacies with Current Therapy Clients/Patients

Psychologists do not engage in sexual intimacies with current therapy clients/patients.

10.06 Sexual Intimacies with Relatives or Significant Others of Current Therapy Clients/Patients

Psychologists do not engage in sexual intimacies with individuals they know to be close relatives, guardians, or significant others of current clients/patients. Psychologists do not terminate therapy to circumvent this standard.

10.07 Therapy with Former Sexual Partners

Psychologists do not accept as therapy clients/patients persons with whom they have engaged in sexual intimacies.

10.08 Sexual Intimacies with Former Therapy Clients/ Patients

(a) Psychologists do not engage in sexual intimacies with former clients/patients for at least two years after cessation or termination of therapy.

(b) Psychologists do not engage in sexual intimacies with former clients/patients even after a two-year interval except in the most unusual circumstances. Psychologists who engage in such activity after the two years following cessation or termination of therapy and of having no sexual contact with the former client/patient bear the burden of demonstrating that there has been no exploitation, in light of all relevant factors, including (1) the amount of time that has passed since therapy terminated; (2) the nature, duration, and intensity of the therapy; (3) the circumstances of termination; (4) the client's/patient's personal history; (5) the client's/patient's current mental status; (6) the likelihood of adverse impact on the client/patient; and (7) any statements or actions made by the therapist during the course of therapy suggesting or inviting the possibility of a posttermination sexual or romantic relationship with the client/patient.

(continued)

(Continued)

National Association of Social Workers (NASW) Code of Ethics (1999)

1.09 Sexual Relationships

(a) Social workers should under no circumstances engage in sexual activities or sexual contact with current clients, whether such contact is consensual or forced.

(b) Social workers should not engage in sexual activities or sexual contact with clients' relatives or other individuals with whom clients maintain a close personal relationship when there is a risk of exploitation or potential harm to the client. Sexual activity or sexual contact with clients' relatives or other individuals with whom clients maintain a personal relationship has the potential to be harmful to the client and may make it difficult for the social worker and client to maintain appropriate professional boundaries. Social workers—not their clients, their clients' relatives, or other individuals with whom the client maintains a personal relationship—assume the full burden for setting clear, appropriate, and culturally sensitive boundaries.

(c) Social workers should not engage in sexual activities or sexual contact with former clients because of the potential for harm to the client. If social workers engage in conduct contrary to this prohibition or claim that an exception to this prohibition is warranted because of extraordinary circumstances, it is social workers—not their clients—who assume the full burden of demonstrating that the former client has not been exploited, coerced, or manipulated, intentionally or unintentionally.

(d) Social workers should not provide clinical services to individuals with whom they have had a prior sexual relationship. Providing clinical services to a former sexual partner has the potential to be harmful to the individual and is likely to make it difficult for the social worker and individual to maintain appropriate professional boundaries.

1.10 Physical Contact

Social workers should not engage in physical contact with clients when there is a possibility of psychological harm to the client as a result of the contact (such as cradling or caressing clients). Social workers who engage in appropriate physical contact with clients are responsible for setting clear, appropriate, and culturally sensitive boundaries that govern such physical contact.

Is Sex with Clients or Former Clients Ever Okay?

To tell mental health professionals of any discipline that sex with a client is prohibited seems redundant. Every practitioner in the field knows that exploitative behavior is not tolerated in the profession, and dual relationships, boundary violations, and sex with clients are clearly unethical. Yet, a reminder is necessary because therapists continue to disregard this prohibition. Disciplinary actions appear in the publications monthly that relate episodes of inappropriate intimacy between professional providers and clients. In most cases, the provider knew better. Disciplinary committees are not sympathetic to violators of sexual prohibitions. A complex defense on behalf of the therapist will not be tolerated. In this case, "thou shalt not" means exactly what it says. There is no wiggle room. Ethics codes generally prohibit sexual contact with any client or former client. Some codes provide that sexual contact with a client is prohibited during the clinical relationship and for 2 or 5 years thereafter. After the prescribed period of zero contact, some codes allow a social or sexual relationship between therapists and clients as long as the client is no longer emotionally dependent on the therapist. The burden is on the therapist to prove lack of emotional dependence and the absence of exploitation by the therapist. The burden is so high that we struggle to think of a case when this burden can be met if it is the client or former client who is complaining. The cases we were personally involved in as attorneys in which the therapist could meet his or her burden were brought by a third party, an ex-spouse or lover of the client or former client. In those cases, the romantic relationship was still strong between the therapist and the client or former client who supported the therapist in defense of the case. Often the client and therapist were married. However, if the client is coming after the therapist, that professional is most likely going to be sanctioned by a licensing board and have a malpractice judgment entered against him or her in favor of the client or former client.

Mental health professionals should not engage in sexual contact with an intern the professional supervises, a student at an educational institution at which the professional provides professional or educational services, or close friends or relations of clients or former clients.

To be safe, we advocate that mental health providers should never engage in anything other than a clinical relationship with clients or former clients. Furthermore, mental health professionals should not engage in sexual contact with an intern the professional supervises (AAMFT *Code of Ethics*, 2001, 4.2), a student at an educational institution which the professional provides professional or educational services (ACA *Code of Ethics*, 2005, F.10.a.), or close friends or relations of clients or former clients (APA *Ethical Principles of Psychologists and Code of Conduct*, 2002, 10.06). It is not an adequate defense to say the sexual contact, sexual exploitation, or therapeutic deception with the person occurred with the person's consent, outside the person's professional counseling sessions, or off the premises regularly used by the provider for the professional counseling sessions. Besides sexual intimacy, other prohibited acts include sexual harassment, creating a hostile environment, making improper comments or gestures, requesting sexual details beyond those needed for the client's therapy, and requesting a date. Some state licensing acts mention with particularity all the parts of the client's body professionals should not touch.

Ethical Flash Points

- Every mental health discipline prohibits sexual intimacy with clients.

- Intimacy means anything that a client could interpret to be either sexual or intimate.

- Sexual intimacies are a common problem in the mental health field judging by the number of complaints filed in this area. Malpractice insurance policies generally limit coverage in this area because of the number of reported incidents. Most policies contain specific monetary limits for sexual misconduct cases. Read your policy. And keep in mind that if you work for an agency with a malpractice or liability insurance policy, the coverage might be limited to the agency and may not cover individual employee practitioners.

- Malpractice coverage for representation before a disciplinary board is even more limited. Therapists are responsible for all fees incurred beyond their deductible. Read your policy.

- The "two or five years after termination" permissive language in some ethics codes is usually drafted to shift the responsibility to the therapist to ensure that no harm befalls the client.

- Some guidelines require that therapists who discover or receive knowledge of another therapist's inappropriate sexual contact with a client are ethically bound to report it or their own license is in danger.

- Most disciplinary boards usually ignore convoluted explanations (sometimes called fairy tales) to justify unethical sexual misconduct.

- Sex with clients is one of the top two or three major ethical infractions committed by therapists of all disciplines.

- When sex between a therapist and client takes place, the therapist has no legitimate defense. The therapist only has unbelievable, ill, and hastily conceived excuses that any ethics board will discount.

- In a "he said" versus "she said" swearing match, the therapist is usually discounted and the consumer of mental health services is believed unless there are unusual circumstances (e.g., the encounter could not have taken place the way the consumer/ client narrated the story; the consumer/client has repeated the story several times, and

(continued)

(Continued)

each time there are significant differences and sufficient inconsistencies to make the tale unbelievable; the consumer/client has made the same accusation against so many therapists in exactly the same manner that the narration is not believable).

- Be aware that good therapists have made mistakes when they were experiencing their own serious personal problems. Get the professional help you need before trying to help clients.

- Sex = exploitation.

Summary

The good news is that all mental health professionals know on some level that sex with a client is bad. The bad news is that sexual exploitation continues to be a constant source of client complaints and irritation to licensing boards and national organizations, not to mention damage to the exploited client. When the therapist feels, clinically, that a client has more than a professional interest, the problem has to be brought to the surface, discussed, and handled. The client must be made to understand the professional's ethical guidelines and told that such activities are prohibited (providing a copy of the guidelines if needed). The method of diffusing a possible explosive situation must be documented. Remember, the client may feel rejected, and some anger may result. Handle clients who appear to be interested sexually as a clinical problem of transference. But the end result must always be to just say no!

Handle clients who appear to be interested sexually as a clinical problem of transference.

If the therapist realizes that he or she has more than a therapeutic interest in the client, an immediate response must take place. Introspective analysis of the issue and what is taking place in the therapist's personal life may be sufficient to put the improper interest to rest. If not, seeking assistance from a competent therapist or a referral of the client may be warranted. Again, the end result must always be to just say no!

Suggested Research Assignments

1. Locate and discuss any rules promulgated by licensing boards in your state dealing with sexual misconduct.
2. Locate and discuss any state and national professional association ethical guidelines that deal with sexual misconduct. In reviewing ethical guidelines, do you notice any glaring inconsistencies?
3. Compare and contrast these state licensing board rules with the ethical rules promulgated by the state professional associations.
4. Compare and contrast state licensing board and professional association guidelines with the guidelines of national professional associations.
5. Identify resources and persons you would consult to learn more about the issue of sexual misconduct by mental health professionals and why it occurs.
6. Research the decisions of your state licensing boards and state and national professional association ethics committees for sexual misconduct violation sanctions.
7. Research legal case decisions for your state that involve sexual misconduct by mental health professionals.
8. Talk to practicing mental health professionals in your area and ask them how they handle clients who attempt to initiate romantic or sexual relationships with them. Develop a response to the aggressive client that allows the therapy to continue without giving in to the improper advances.
9. Develop a protocol for dealing with a client who attempts to initiate a romantic or sexual relationship with you.
10. Develop a protocol for dealing with your own romantic or sexual interest in a client.

Discussion Questions

1. A client you have been treating for depression advises you that he has been having a recurring dream in which he has sensational sex with you. What do you say and do? What do you document?

2. A colleague and close friend working with you in an agency that provides mental health services to children advises you that the divorced father of one of her child clients wants to take her on a trip to Cozumel for the weekend. What do you advise?

3. Ten years after you ended successful therapy with a client, you run into her at a health club. She tells you that subsequent to your wonderful therapy she built a small company that she just sold for $10 million. She says that she is in terrific health, mentally, physically, and financially and would love to have dinner with you. What do you do?

4. You find yourself being attracted to one of your clients, and this attraction is distracting you during the counseling sessions with the client. What do you do? What, if anything, do you document?

13

Terminating Therapy

Susan had been in therapy with Dr. Smith for about 5 months and was feeling better about herself, her family, and her environment. In fact, Dr. Smith told Susan that the time had come to end therapy. The next visit would be an exit interview, where they would recapitulate the treatment plan, review how it had been successful, and terminate their professional relationship. Of course, Susan could contact Dr. Smith again should another problem occur, but for now she no longer required regular visits with him. Susan was a private pay client and did not claim managed care benefits nor did she process an insurance claim. Although Dr. Smith indicated that further therapy was unnecessary at this time, Susan said she was willing to continue to pay Dr. Smith weekly for the opportunity to visit and talk to him because he was the only person who would listen to her without interruption. Should a therapist continue to see a client who just wishes to chat? Could it be considered abandonment to refuse to see a client who wants to continue the client-therapist relationship after the therapist has indicated the client can function normally without further therapy or treatment?

Jack had been in therapy for about a year without measurable improvement. He did not feel better, nor did he feel worse. The therapist tried various treatment techniques, none of which seemed to bring about any positive change in the presenting problem. The therapist wondered if the therapy was not working or if there was a problem with the therapist-client relationship, some unknown circumstance, or possibly some client-centered but undiagnosed problem. The therapist asked herself if ethically, the client's situation must always improve with therapy for it to be considered successful, or if therapeutic success might be claimed also when a client's condition doesn't deteriorate. In either case, should the therapist continue the therapy even though the client's presenting condition is not measurably improved?

Joan had been in therapy for about a year with excellent results. After discussing terminating treatment with the client, the therapist and client agreed to conclude therapy. The client left the office feeling happy with the therapy, happy with the therapist, and happy with herself. The first day of the rest of her life was going to be a glorious reawakening of new opportunities. But how does the therapist close the file? Is it automatically closed because no appointments are scheduled and the client does not, at this point, intend to return? What does the client have in writing—only a canceled check marked "paid in full"? Is that adequate?

John had been in therapy off and on for several years. When he needed a consultation, he called Susan, his social worker, made an appointment or appointments as needed, and then waited until the next stress period before he called again. On one of these occasions, after a mutually satisfactory three-session series, John mentioned that he was being transferred and would be leaving town in about a month to accept a promotion 1,000 miles away at company headquarters. Susan said "Congratulations," and John left. That brief dialogue served as the termination interview. Susan later heard through the grapevine that John had become overwhelmed in his new position and was subsequently dismissed. He was now unemployed, very distressed, and unsuccessfully seeking gainful and appropriate employment. Does ethical follow-up mandate that therapists who casually hear a rumor of unhappiness contact a former client and suggest continuing therapy?

Earnest was hostile and angry. At the end of his last session, he made malicious but indirect threats, suggesting dangers to himself and others, before

*storming out of the therapist's office. He did, however, make another ap-
pointment for the next week before leaving. His next appointment came and
went, but Earnest did not appear. He was simply a no-show. His therapist
could not locate him by phone, and letters to his last known address were
returned unopened. In a sense, Earnest had unilaterally terminated the therapeutic relationship. Does such an act serve to terminate the therapeutic relationship, or does an ethical responsibility bind the therapist to the client
until there is a formalized termination? Do a no-show and a "can't locate"
signal an official termination? And, ethically, what happens next?*

*Sam had been a client on and off for 5 years when he and his therapist mu-
tually agreed to terminate treatment. Over the next few years, Sam's life
turned downward. He had family and domestic problems, the upward trend
of his career leveled out and was less rewarding spiritually and financially,
and in general, he thought his life was in decline. On reflection, he feels the
therapist "should have" and "could have" done more for him. In a fit of
pique, he calls his former therapist.*

The Therapeutic Relationship

Therapy begins with an express or implied contract between clients
and therapists, in which therapists represent that they will provide
competent treatment to their clients; and clients, advised of the various ramifications of therapy, give informed consent to the treatment
offered. With that offer and acceptance, the therapy begins. It is advisable to have a lawyer draft and the therapist approve an intake and consent form that is signed by both parties and inserted in the clinical file.

Therapy ends when the treatment is terminated. Final or temporary
termination can happen for various reasons. Treatment can end when
the client simply stops keeping appointments and disappears into ob-
livion despite the therapist's best efforts to make contact. It can also
end by mutual agreement or because the third-party payer declines further payment and the client cannot afford additional sessions without
such reimbursement. At such times, therapists usually inform clients
of available community resources and wish them well. Therapy may

also be terminated when clients are transferred or when the therapist retires, becomes ill, moves, or terminates with the current association or agency and another therapist is assigned to the file. Therapy can end when it clearly is no longer benefiting the client, or when the client or therapist, for whatever reason, is no longer comfortable with the treatment plan. Often therapy terminates when the client and therapist mutually agree that the treatment goals have been realized and further treatment is no longer appropriate. The goal of effective therapy has been attained.

When to Terminate Therapy

The therapist-client relationship should be terminated when:

- The future services needed are not within the provider's professional competency.
- The provider is or becomes impaired due to physical or mental ill health or the use of medication, drugs, or alcohol.
- Continued service is not in the client's best interest.
- Professional ethical canons are violated because of relationships within or outside the provider's control.
- In the professional's opinion, the client is not benefiting from those services offered. *When services to the client are still indicated, the provider should take reasonable steps to facilitate the transfer to an appropriate source of care.*
- A person who needs a license to practice has the license revoked, suspended, or otherwise limited or canceled.
- A client joins the same church and sits next to you in the choir, marries your sister, threatens to sue you, threatens to harm you, or otherwise expresses forceful displeasure with you, your treatment, or your profession.
- For whatever reason, the continued therapy violates a published canon of ethics.

Every mental health discipline has published ethical guidelines concerning appropriate termination and the procedures for such termination. State or national licensing boards have disciplined many mental health professionals because they did not strictly follow their published guidelines, did not properly document that the guidelines were followed, or both. Chapter 15 indicates that ethical guidelines, when not followed, may be introduced as evidence in a malpractice suit to indicate minimum standards of practice. Termination with less than minimum standards might indicate civil negligence. Appropriate termination is part of documented, ethical, risk-free treatment.

National Guidelines for Terminating Therapy

American Association for Marriage and Family Therapy (AAMFT) Code of Ethics (2001)

1.9 Marriage and family therapists continue therapeutic relationships only so long as it is reasonably clear that clients are benefiting from the relationship.

    1.10 Marriage and family therapists assist persons in obtaining other therapeutic services if the therapist is unable or unwilling, for appropriate reasons, to provide professional help.

    1.11 Marriage and family therapists do not abandon or neglect clients in treatment without making reasonable arrangements for the continuation of such treatment.

American Counseling Association (ACA) Code of Ethics (2005)

A.11.b. Inability to Assist Clients

If counselors determine an inability to be of professional assistance to clients, they avoid entering or continuing counseling relationships. Counselors are knowledgeable about culturally and clinically appropriate referral resources and

(continued)

(*Continued*)

suggest these alternatives. If clients decline the suggested referrals, counselors should discontinue the relationship.

A.11.c. Appropriate Termination

Counselors terminate a counseling relationship when it becomes reasonably apparent that the client no longer needs assistance, is not likely to benefit, or is being harmed by continued counseling. Counselors may terminate counseling when in jeopardy of harm by the client, or another person with whom the client has a relationship, or when clients do not pay fees as agreed upon. Counselors provide pretermination counseling and recommend other service providers when necessary.

A.11.d. Appropriate Transfer of Services

When counselors transfer or refer clients to other practitioners, they ensure that appropriate clinical and administrative processes are completed and open communication is maintained with both clients and practitioners.

American Psychological Association (APA) Ethical Principles of Psychologists and Code of Conduct (2002)

10.10 Terminating Therapy

(a) Psychologists terminate therapy when it becomes reasonably clear that the client/patient no longer needs the service, is not likely to benefit, or is being harmed by continued service.

(b) Psychologists may terminate therapy when threatened or otherwise endangered by the client/patient or another person with whom the client/patient has a relationship.

(c) Except where precluded by the actions of clients/patients or third-party payors, prior to termination psychologists provide pretermination counseling and suggest alternative service providers as appropriate.

National Association of Social Workers (NASW) Code of Ethics (1999)

1.16 Termination of Services

(a) Social workers should terminate services to clients and professional relationships with them when such services and relationships are no longer required or no longer serve the clients' needs or interests.

(b) Social workers should take reasonable steps to avoid abandoning clients who are still in need of services. Social workers should withdraw services precipitously only under unusual circumstances, giving careful consideration to all factors in the situation and taking care to minimize possible adverse effects. Social workers should assist in making appropriate arrangements for continuation of services when necessary.

(c) Social workers in fee-for-service settings may terminate services to clients who are not paying an overdue balance if the financial contractual arrangements have been made clear to the client, if the client does not pose an imminent danger to self or others, and if the clinical and other consequences of the current nonpayment have been addressed and discussed with the client.

(d) Social workers should not terminate services to pursue a social, financial, or sexual relationship with a client.

(e) Social workers who anticipate the termination or interruption of services to clients should notify clients promptly and seek the transfer, referral, or continuation of services in relation to the clients' needs and preferences.

(f) Social workers who are leaving an employment setting should inform clients of appropriate options for the continuation of services and of the benefits and risks of the options.

The Termination Process

In a sense, the complete termination process begins with a detailed intake form that becomes an important part of the clinical file and ends with the documented final session. Prior to commencing treatment, be sure to obtain one or two addresses and phone numbers, and—most important—explicit written consent to contact the client at the phone numbers and addresses furnished. (The fact that the client has given the therapist an address and phone number does not specifically indicate that the client has given permission to be called, contacted by mail, or otherwise communicated with at that address or number.) It is also important to periodically update this information because numbers and addresses change from time to time. Since termination has ramifications both ethically and as a malpractice risk, the therapist should take certain additional precautions whenever terminating a client-therapist relationship.

First, be sure to document the rationale for termination: why it is taking place, and how it is in the client's best interest.

First, be sure to document the rationale for termination: why it is taking place, and how it is in the client's best interest. Therapists are usually held liable for something they failed to do, not something they did. Thus, it is a good idea to have a termination process and procedure in place in which therapists inform clients of all further treatment they might need, and the means they might utilize to obtain further treatment. The checklist is for use at termination. All the items are essential to protect the provider from an ethical infraction. Some procedures will be more rigorous than ones you may be currently using, but that is the point. Malpractice suits and ethical complaints to the licensing boards are the new American pastime.

Termination is always a potential problem—even when the decision at the time is mutual and friendly. If the proper steps are not followed, the termination can come back to haunt you—even years later. Relationships are fickle. At one time, most clients were satisfied clients. Then an event occurred such as a voluntary opinion from a friendly mental-health-discipline graduate student, or one that evolves from a conversation with another person in therapy, and suddenly the hero becomes the object of rejection and invective, criticism, or abuse. The tables and attitude have turned. Yesterday's hero is today's villain. Protective documentation is the first defense to this change in attitude.

Checklist for Terminating Therapy

☐ Schedule an exit session or termination interview to make sure clients understand: (1) what is taking place, (2) the reasons behind it, and (3) any recommendations you have.

☐ Prepare a termination letter (see Figure 13.1 and the Termination Letter Checklist that follows, as shown on pp. 186–188) ahead of that session. Review the letter with the client, then have the client sign it, and insert a copy in the client's file.

☐ If you feel further treatment is advisable or necessary, make that explicit both in your interview and in the letter. Psychiatrists need to tell patients who are on medication to continue their medication subject to medical controls. Patients must understand that a psychiatrist has to review the medications periodically to determine if they are still appropriate or if they should be discontinued. Limitations must be placed on prescriptions. It is often advisable to advise a terminating client to consult a psychiatrist if the problem persists, or if the client is visiting with a psychiatrist, then that treatment should continue until the patient is terminated or discharged.

☐ If the client is moving to a place where no mental health professional is available, contact the client periodically to make sure the client is doing well. Clients should agree in writing that if a problem arises, they will contact a professional, or call an emergency number before hurting themselves or others.

☐ Be persistent in trying to reach a client, especially one who simply fails to show up or make another appointment. If a face-to-face termination interview isn't possible—because the client refuses, or for any other reason—a phone conference should be attempted. A copy of the termination letter should be sent to an authorized mailing address (an address where the client has said the therapist may send correspondence), especially if you believe the person *needs* further treatment. Be sure to explain in detail the need for continuing mental health treatment. Recommend at least three other therapists or referral sources in the letter. If the client can't be reached, two copies of the termination letter, including a self-addressed, stamped envelope, should be sent by certified mail with return receipt requested. Two copies should also be sent by standard mail in the event the client chooses not to accept and sign for the certified mail that often involves a trip to the local post office. Ask the client to sign both copies and return one to you. Recommend to the client that the termination letter be delivered to any subsequent therapist.

☐ Review the ethical guidelines of your profession concerning termination. Make sure you have scrupulously followed them. Many providers belong to several national organizations and have multiple licenses. A provider who has a license or belongs to a national organization is bound by the ethical code of that specific organization or all organizations in which he or she has a membership. If the provider belongs to a subspecialty group within an organization, the guidelines of the subspecialty group also bind the provider. Where there are multiple guidelines, use the most restrictive, and comply with the most severe; if one states that termination may be oral and another requires written communication, get it in writing.

Termination Letter Checklist

☐ Include the client's name (no "Dear Client" form letters).
☐ Identify the date when the therapy actually began.
☐ Note the termination date.
☐ Include the primary and secondary diagnosis.
☐ Describe the reason for termination.
☐ Summarize treatment, including any need for additional services.
☐ List three or more referrals or referral sources, including addresses and phone numbers. Verify that they are still current. (Nothing is worse than referring to a crisis hotline when the number has been disconnected.)

Anthony Kindheart, LPC

6894 Forest Park Drive
Suite 268
Dallas, Texas 75206
July 17, _____

Mr. Kevin Jones
1425 Centenary
Dallas, Texas 75210

Re: Termination of Treatment

Dear Mr. Kevin Jones:

It has become necessary, for the reasons stated below, to terminate our professional and therapeutic relationship. I will maintain your records for the period required by law and will make copies of your records available to you upon written request. You may be charged a reasonable fee for the cost of duplicating the records.

Our work together began on July 1, _____, and ended on this date. During this time, we worked on improving your occupational and social functioning and alleviating your depression by addressing factors that may have caused, contributed to, or aggravated your depression.

In the exercise of my professional judgment, I have concluded that you have not made satisfactory progress in improving your social and occupational functioning and with your depression. I believe you are in need of additional mental health services for treatment of your depression and possible chemical dependency. These services can be best provided to you by one of the following:

Richard Lewins, MD, (214) 489-3624, 1900 Main Street, Suite 120, Dallas, TX 75201
Sylvia Jones, LCDC, (972) 270-9142, 689 LBJ Freeway, Suite 410, Dallas, TX 75214
Harold Jones, PhD, (214) 814-3621, 48764 Mockingbird, Suite 206, Dallas, TX 75206

I recommend you contact one of these providers, or another provider of your choosing, as quickly as possible to schedule an appointment. With your written consent, I will consult with any professional of your choosing and will forward the file or a summary of your treatment to my successor.

Your primary discharge diagnosis is: 296.32 Major Depression, recurrent.

(continued)

(Continued)

This termination is not due to any personal reasons but solely due to my desire for you to achieve the highest possible level of mental health wellness and social and occupational functioning. I believe referring you to one of the providers listed above presents the best possibility for this to occur. I wish you success and want you to know that I will make myself available for consultation with anyone you choose to work with, in order to make this transition as easy as possible.

Sincerely,

_____

Anthony Kindheart, LPC

I acknowledge receipt and review and accept and understand the terms of this termination letter, dated the 17th day of July, 20____ .

_____   _____

Kevin Jones   Date

                                 _____

                                 Social Security Number

Figure 13.1 Sample Form: Client Termination Letter

☐ Draft a statement that the client understands what termination of treatment is, and accepts the responsibility to personally seek further treatment if appropriate.

☐ Use language that indicates the client accepts the consequences of the client's failure to follow up in securing further treatment.

☐ Include signature lines for both the therapist and the client, with a date line for each signature.

☐ If mailing, include two copies with a self-addressed, stamped envelope. Indicate "Enclosure" at the bottom of the termination letter. Be sure the client understands that one copy is to be signed and returned.

Even in the unusual situation where termination occurs due to threats of harm to the therapist made by the client or a person in a close relationship with the client and a face-to-face termination session is not advisable, a termination letter as outlined here should be prepared and sent. It brings closure to the therapeutic relationship and represents documentation of the completion of the therapist's ethical duty to the client. File a copy of the letter in the client's file.

Maintaining the Clinical File

A carefully drafted intake and consent form (perhaps lawyer-drafted to protect the therapist, or at least lawyer-approved) sets out the steps and procedures for termination and authorizes the mental health professional to contact the client should termination occur by any means other than a mutual agreement and exit interview. Then, as the final notation in the file, the clinical case notes must reflect the circumstances of termination, the termination process, and if appropriate, the fact that therapy has been successfully concluded before the file is officially closed.

After the participatory therapist-client relationship has been terminated, the file must be properly stored and preserved for the length of time required by both statute and ethical canons for adults and minors. In many cases, the client may return for future therapy, and the current clinical file will be of tremendous value. In this sense, termination does not really mean termination; it means abatement. The client is on therapeutic hold. The file will be preserved in a safe, secure, and confidential manner for at least as long as required by law and as set forth in state ethical codes. If sufficient storage facilities are available, perhaps it will be stored forever.

Is Termination the End of Therapy?

Once the therapist and client mutually agree to end therapy and the file is closed, what happens? Theoretically, the therapist could move, retire, leave the profession, or change from private practice to another means of making a living. Does the phrase or maxim "once a client, always a client" hold true in these situations? Probably not, but licensing boards have strange and variable statutes of limitations. Should an

Clinical case notes must reflect the circumstances of termination, the termination process, and the fact if appropriate, that therapy has been successfully concluded before the file is officially closed.

After the participatory therapist-client relationship has been terminated, the file must be properly stored and preserved for the length of time required by both statute and ethical canons for adults and minors.

unhappy client, as evidenced by Sam earlier in the chapter, call the therapist years later, the situation should be confronted rather than ignored. Probably, the pique can be ameliorated or defused with a minimum of effort, leaving a content former client. Joining in combat might create a licensing board complaint. When this happens, the board usually has state or national resources behind the complainant, the former client, whereas the mental health providers are on their own, financially and emotionally.

Continuing obligations might be (a) to make a referral if needed, to the client who calls years later requesting continuing therapy, (b) having the file available for the necessary number of years required by either statute or licensing board rules and being able to produce a copy for the client on request, (c) being available to consult with any subsequent therapist concerning the client or, (d) being subject to orders of a court for either deposition, interrogatories, or testimony in the event of litigation regarding the client or the client's estate.

Malpractice versus Ethical Violations Regarding Termination

A malpractice suit is litigation for money damages filed in the civil justice system.

A malpractice suit is litigation for money damages filed in the civil justice system. Such damages may be awarded by a judge or jury who determine what amount of money, if any, will compensate the plaintiff (former client) for the damages caused by, in this case, the defendant's (the therapist) negligent termination of the therapeutic relationship.

An ethical violation begins with a complaint filed with a licensing board.

An ethical violation, on the other hand, begins with a complaint filed with a licensing board. The board considers the complaint and, if it is justified, can revoke or suspend a license or put restrictions on the practitioner. The result can ruin a career, especially if a license is absolutely necessary to establish and maintain a practice or treat clients.

Malpractice is determined by a judge, jury, or both. An ethics violation is determined by a licensing board or, if the complaint is submitted to a national organization, to the complaints committee of the national organization. As stated elsewhere in this book, the profession's ethics code can be introduced into evidence in either case to indicate the minimum standards of the profession. Practitioners must justify any deviation from these standards, especially if some harm damages a client. Malpractice insurance can protect the therapist from the financial ramifications a malpractice suit (see Chapter 24, "Malpractice Insurance"). If there is coverage for licensing board cases, the malpractice insurance policy will cover attorneys' fees to defend against an ethical complaint, but the provider cannot be protected by insurance against the financial losses due to revoked license.

Malpractice insurance can protect the therapist from the financial ramifications a malpractice suit.

There is no ethics violation insurance.

Ethical Flash Points

- When therapy is no longer benefiting the client, the therapeutic relationship must be terminated.

- Therapy has to be reviewed and possibly terminated when the technique used is not working. It might be the therapist-client mix, some hidden or subtle agenda of the therapist or client, or something else. Not every therapist can successfully treat every client who makes an appointment. And the factors for an unsuccessful client-therapist relationship may not be obvious to either party. The initial interview is helpful when determining the mix. Sufficient time should be allowed so that both parties are satisfied that the therapy can proceed with each party knowledgeable concerning the expectations of the other and what is expected of them.

- Ethical termination requires meticulous attention to the details of a termination interview and letter, which the therapist and client should sign. Use of a termination checklist is advised.

- The therapist should always offer to be available personally or to cooperate with a subsequent professional if needed.

- Document carefully the circumstances of every termination, but be especially diligent whenever a client is angry, confrontational, or threatening. Offer help and referrals. Defuse the situation and document the actions taken. Be kind. Be sensitive. Be constantly aware.

- Consult the canons of ethics in your jurisdiction together with any national organizations to which you belong. Make sure you have complied with all the requirements of

(continued)

(*Continued*)
local codes and national guidelines. If they are in conflict, adhere to the most restrictive guidelines.

- Review the checklist and termination letter carefully at least twice to make sure nothing has been omitted. Have a lawyer review the letter and your procedures as well to save yourself a headache down the road. Always remain aware that clients' attitudes can whimsically change.

- Consider termination the final but necessary and eventual step in the treatment plan.

- Review the ethical circumstances of appropriate termination, such as the client's failure to benefit from treatment, services no longer required, services that no longer serve the client's needs or interests, client's failure to pay the fees charged, or agency or institution limits against provision of further counseling services. Make sure the appropriateness of the termination is fully documented.

Summary

A carefully drafted intake and consent form (perhaps lawyer-drafted to protect the therapist) sets out the steps and procedures for termination and will authorize the mental health professional to contact the client should termination occur by any means other than a mutual agreement and exit interview. Then, as the final notation in the file, the clinical case notes must reflect the circumstances of termination, the termination process, the fact that therapy has been successfully concluded and the file closed.

After the participatory therapist-client relationship has been terminated, the file must still be properly stored and preserved for the length of time required by both statute and ethical canons for adults and minors, for future therapy may be appropriate and the current clinical file will be of tremendous value and a treasure trove of information when offering future treatment by either this or a subsequent therapist. Thus termination does not really mean termination; it means abatement. The client is on therapeutic hold. The file will be preserved in a safe, secure, and confidential manner for as long as required by law and as set forth in state ethical codes. Hard copies are easy to preserve. Common sense, good practice, and the Health Insurance Portability and Accountability Act (HIPAA) Security Rules require that electronic files be periodically tested to ensure that they have not eroded or been corrupted. A file must be available for retrieval during its mandatory retention period.

Suggested Research Assignments

1. Locate and discuss any rules promulgated by licensing boards in your state dealing with termination and its documentation.
2. Locate and discuss any state and national professional association ethical guidelines that deal with termination. In reviewing ethical guidelines, do you notice any glaring inconsistencies?
3. Compare and contrast these state licensing board rules with the ethical rules promulgated by the state professional associations.
4. Compare and contrast state licensing board and professional association guidelines with the guidelines of national professional associations.
5. Research the decisions of your state licensing boards and state and national professional association ethics committees for termination violation sanctions.
6. Research legal case decisions for your state that involve improper termination by mental health professionals.
7. Talk to practicing mental health professionals in your area and ask them how they handle termination of clients. Do they have a termination protocol?
8. Develop a protocol for dealing with an angry client who abruptly terminates therapy with you.
9. Put together a referral list for use when a decision is made to terminate a client or the client elects to terminate with you.

Discussion Questions

1. A client you have been treating for several months calls to cancel an appointment, and when you ask why, he says because "It's not working." What do you say and do? What do you document?

2. A client misses an appointment without calling to cancel. What do you do? What do you document?

3. A client wants to terminate with you during a difficult session and demands a refund of all the money he has paid for "this worthless therapy." What do you say and do? What do you document?

4. The husband of a female adult client calls you, accuses you of having an affair with his wife, and threatens to kill you if you ever see his wife again for any reason. What do you say and do? What do you document? Do you tell the wife (your client) about the call?

PART II

ETHICS CODES AND LICENSING

14

Areas of Ethical Complaints

Joseph, a licensed professional counselor, accepted a dinner invitation from Karen, a former group therapy client. Karen was attractive and only attended two of the group sessions before deciding she did not enjoy the group and did not need further participation. After several bottles of wine, Joseph accompanied Karen to her high-rise apartment to take in the spectacular view of the city's skyline. Joseph eventually followed her into her bedroom and they made love. On leaving the apartment the next morning, he became appropriately and legitimately fearful about the consequences of what he had just done.

Wilma, a clinical social worker with a private practice devoted almost exclusively to geriatric patients, was having a difficult time getting timely payments remitted to her by a particular "reluctant to pay" insurance company. In financial frustration, she began billing for visits that did not occur, rationalizing that the clients' mental condition would not allow them to recall when or if they came to the office for the session and the insurance company's slowness in paying her justified the deception.

Joseph and Wilma both knowingly committed ethical violations. The difficult question to answer is why would they take such risks?

We are repeatedly asked for facts, statistics, and opinions about which kinds of ethical misconduct are most often reported to licensing boards and other disciplinary committees. What infractions should be carefully monitored in the daily life of the practicing professional? What red warning flags indicate a violation that is bound to come to the attention of the disciplinary authority? At what point does the hint of an ethical or legal impropriety deserve immediate attention and instant risk management?

We regularly review reports of mental health licensing boards' sanctions in our home state of Texas as well as those reported by other states and national organizations where available, and we are familiar with the offenses for which therapists are being sanctioned. In addition, having been in private law practice consulting with and working with mental health professionals for many years, we are aware of many wrongful actions by therapists that, although unethical, were never reported to a licensing board. Perhaps after consulting with us, the client never filed a formal complaint or the therapist who consulted with us revealed problems or unethical activities that, although revealed to an attorney, remained protected by the attorney-client privilege and continued to be strictly confidential. Not every ethical infraction or violation is reported by either a client or a therapist to the board. Not every client with a complaint chooses, after mature consideration, to become involved in the grievance process. For some clients, sharing a legitimate complaint with a lawyer or with another professional is sufficient airing of the situation and further pursuit is unnecessary and undesirable. The client discussed the grievance and feels better about it.

It has proven difficult to verify whether our Texas experience was representative and consistent throughout the United States. A few state licensing boards that we contacted shared limited complaint data that confirmed the information and opinions set out in this chapter. In many states, sanctions assessed against a mental health professional are available online. Insurance trusts and most licensing boards chose not to respond to our requests or declined to provide us with statistics. There is a need for better sharing and compiling of ethical violation information on a national level. An issue facing mental health disciplines investigating or considering portability of licenses is the lack of reporting of disciplinary actions. A national reporting system needs to be established to ensure availability and accuracy of complaint histories before a mental health professional is allowed to practice in another state. The establishment of a database for ethical infractions would make information available to clients, other professionals, and the credentialing organizations of sister states. Certainly, licensing authorities cannot rely on the veracity of sanctioned mental health professionals for reliable information of their complaint histories.

The good news is that very few therapists have complaints filed against them, and even fewer are sanctioned by their respective boards. It is difficult to even get a definitive idea of the number of mental health professionals in the United States, but consider the statistics in Tables 14.1, 14.2, and 14.3.

With the growing awareness possessed by educated and sophisticated consumers relating to ethical mental health services and the

Table 14.1   U.S. Mental Health-Care Professionals

Occupation	Number of Professionals
Clinical, counseling, and school psychologists	97,330
Industrial-organizational psychologists	1,140
Psychologists (all others)	7,960
Mental health counselors	91,830
Substance abuse and behavioral disorder counselors	75,940
Counselors (all others)	24,260
Marriage and family therapists	21,330
Educational, vocational, and school counselors	226,720
Child, family, and school social workers	262,830
Mental health and substance abuse social workers	116,750
Social workers (all others)	61,270
Psychiatrists	24,730
Total	1,118,520*

*Does not include psychiatric nurses.
Source: U.S. Department of Labor, Bureau of Labor Statistics, "Occupational Employment Statistics: May 2006," www.bls.gov/oes (accessed December 24, 2007).

Table 14.2   Mental Health Professional Association Membership
             Statistics

Professional Association	Approximate Number of Members
American Association for Marriage and Family Therapy	24,000
American Association of Pastoral Counselors	3,000
American Counseling Association	42,000
American Psychiatric Association	36,000
American Psychiatric Nurses Association	5,000
American Psychological Association	148,000
American School Counselor Association	20,000
National Association of Social Workers	150,000

Note: Compiled from information taken from each association's web page.

It appears that in any given year less than 2 percent of all mental health professionals are the subjects of an ethical complaint.

zealousness of our licensing boards and national organizations in policing the professions, the possibility of an ethical complaint is greater today than ever before.

The number of complaints filed each year is increasing. A therapist can ill afford a relaxed attitude about ethical issues and practice. Constant vigilance is the price of professional practice, and mental health professionals should be ever mindful of the constantly changing

Table 14.3   U.S. Licensed Mental Health Professionals

Profession	Number of Licensees
Professional counselors	103,865
Marriage and family therapists	51,116
Social workers	156,982
Total	311,963

Notes: Information is for the highest level of licensure for counselors and licensed marriage and family therapists (LMFTs). Includes social workers at all levels of licensure. Currently there is no counseling licensure in California. Currently there is no LMFT licensure in Montana and West Virginia.
Source: 2007 Mental Health Professions Statistics, American Counseling Association, www.counseling.org/Counselors/LicensureAndCert.aspx? (accessed December 24, 2007).

plethora of codes, statutes, and professional responsibilities that govern their profession. Mental health professionals should also be aware
of the ease of filing a complaint. One call to the board to obtain a form
or directions, a typewriter or computer, a one-page narrative indicating the alleged complaint or a statement of what the client perceives
as an inappropriate act, and an investigation begins. There is no expense to the theoretically injured client. However, to the provider,
this complaint begins a long journey of defensive activities, soul
searching, and angst, which causes untold hours of uneasiness. A licensing board or national organization complaint can cause years of
defensive activities that permeate each day of continuing practice.
Keep in mind that we live in a litigious, blame-seeking society, and
the licensing boards are a consumer-oriented, often politically appointed group. Boards are a serious and powerful critical entity to be
reckoned with. They do not have quick timetables for making decisions. Some have taken well over a year to ponder, and then the action results in a dismissal. Meanwhile the clinician must indicate
"case pending" in every application for insurance, hospital privileges,
or other application required by any entity with whom the clinician
wishes to associate.

So what unethical acts are therapists committing? The following
list ranks unethical behavior in order of frequency as illustrated by the
data and our personal experience:

- Sexual exploitation
- Dual relationships
- Boundary violations
- Breach of confidentiality/refusal to provide records
- Fraudulent billing
- Financial exploitation of a client
- Provision of services while impaired
- Violations of reporting statutes
- Miscellaneous acts

An example of a miscellaneous act is continuing to practice the
profession after a license has been revoked, suspended, or limited.

This usually occurs when a registration or renewal check is returned for insufficient funds, when a renewal is lost in the mail or some negligence in the office results in a failure to timely file, when continuing education hours are not timely reported, or when a disciplinary order by a board prevents the continuation of a practice.

Sexual exploitation leads the way in frequency. To make matters worse, we know from firsthand experience that many sexual exploitation complaints go unreported. The exploited person may not want to go public by making the complaint a matter of community gossip and placing a sordid affair in the public domain. Often married or committed individuals do not want their spouses or significant others to know about the liaison. Interestingly, many complaints are filed, yet by the time the case works its way through the investigative mill, the importance of the situation has retreated, life's circumstances have changed, or the complainant no longer wishes to proceed. We have also learned that although most complaints in this category are filed against male therapists, female therapists sexually exploit their clients in greater numbers than are being reported. Our practice has shown that male clients are not as likely to report their therapists for a sexual relationship, as female clients are likely to report male therapists.

Sexual exploitation leads the way in frequency.

We have grown weary of preaching that sex with clients, former clients, and any person in a close relationship with a client is prohibited (see Chapter 12, "Sexual Misconduct"). There is not a therapist in the country who does not know this ethical restriction and prohibition, yet it still happens with alarming frequency. On many occasions, a therapist who has attended one of our ethics workshops and did not heed the message has been forced to contact us for representation. It is very frustrating to lecture, observe the participants dutifully taking notes, and then realize when legal assistance is sought that some attendees at the seminar did not think that the lecture applied to them under their current circumstances. They somehow concluded that sex with a particular former client was the legitimate exception to the rule. Nothing could be further from the truth. There is zero tolerance by licensing boards and national organizations for sex with clients.

Avoiding dual relationships is a lesson preached in every educational program in the country as well. Many therapists cross this line for personal benefit or out of a misguided desire to help a client. Only one relationship is tolerated: the professional arm's-length therapeutic relationship. Entering into a business deal with a client or trading services with a client may seem harmless in a particular instance, but the risk of exploitation is too great to tolerate such arrangements under any circumstances.

Boundary violations occur in much the same way as dual relationships, and sometimes the terms are used interchangeably. Therapists are being sanctioned for their failure to maintain therapeutic boundaries, for personally violating them, and for allowing a client to do so. The therapist is responsible for establishing and maintaining the high protective wall between the client and the therapist. Continuing to provide services to a client who refuses to respect boundaries has resulted in sanctions against many therapists. We recommend that in the very first intake interview, when all contact is above board and before any relationship is established, the therapist determine the nature of the relationship and firmly set all the inflexible rules and boundaries. The therapist should impress on the client that boundaries are serious, that they provide for no exceptions, and that any violation will lead to immediate termination of the relationship.

Despite being well aware of the need to preserve client confidentiality, many therapists directly and sometimes inadvertently disclose confidential information about their clients. Failure to provide security for client thoughts and statements as well as files has resulted in sanctions against therapists who did not directly disclose the information (e.g., a snooping husband entered a therapist's office at night with a cleaning crew and perused his wife's clinical file). On the flip side of this issue, therapists who failed to disclose information or provide copies of records when legally required to do so have been sanctioned. This seems to occur most often in family law cases when a parent wants to review a child's records and the presenting parent does not want the information disclosed to the other parent.

Economic crimes and unethical acts are as old as humankind, and the mental health profession has seen its fair share. With managed care driving fees downward and competition for clients increasing, fraudulent billing activity probably will increase. Greed motivates

Therapists are being sanctioned for their failure to maintain therapeutic boundaries, for personally violating them, and for allowing a client to do so.

There is zero tolerance for sex with clients by either licensing boards or national organizations.

Greed motivates some therapists to bill fraudulently but we have learned that simple economic survival has pushed several mental health professionals to cross the line of honesty.

You can only bill for sessions that actually take place and that are substantiated by clinical notes.

some therapists to bill fraudulently, but we have learned that simple economic survival has pushed several mental health professionals to cross the line of honesty. No matter how disturbing one might find managed care or a particular payer of benefits, the risk in this area is too great. Civil, administrative, and criminal penalties are being leveled against the guilty and those who wish to stretch the truth to its limits. You can only bill for sessions that actually take place and that are substantiated by clinical notes.

Occasionally, a mental health professional takes advantage of the professional relationship to financially exploit a client, although the frequency is not as great as with sexual exploitation. Greed is usually the motivating factor and is inexcusable. It seems to be more prevalent among professionals providing services to elderly clients in nursing homes and assisted living settings.

Many therapists continue to provide services while they are impaired, most often due to substance abuse or addiction. We are aware of cases, however, where a therapist continued to practice when a physical disability impaired the therapist's ability to provide services (e.g., deafness) or after a license has been revoked, suspended, or canceled. Alcohol and illegal drug use occurs in all mental health disciplines as it does in all walks of life. Every mental health organization makes assistance available to impaired professionals, who recognize their impairment and seek help. Assistance cannot be imposed on providers.

Failure to report child abuse, threats by a client, elder abuse, or ethical violations by another mental health professional are actionable ethical violations for which therapists are sanctioned not just by licensing boards but often by the criminal justice system. Therapists have a general ethical duty to follow the law at all times with respect to their professional activities. Mandatory reporting statutes make this obligation much more specific under certain circumstances and cannot be ignored.

Under miscellaneous acts, we see such things as falsifying educational records, academic documentation, supervision records, and licensing applications; assisting the evasion of board rules; keeping sloppy records; practicing outside the scope of a license; poorly preparing expert testimony; and having felony convictions unrelated to the practice. Somewhere, sometime, somehow some mental health professionals have violated one or more of the ethical canons. It is our hope that better education of ethical issues through research, symposia, readings, and correct reporting of disobedience of ethical canons will keep future violations to a minimum.

Ethical Flash Points

- The number of complaints filed each year appears to be increasing. Therapists must be constantly vigilant in our increasingly litigious society.

- Having a casual attitude about ethics is almost sure to lead to an ethical violation.

- Most therapists who violate ethical canons know the rules.

- Sexual exploitation is the most frequently filed complaint, and everyone knows it is improper.

- Education and knowledge are not enough. Self-discipline and self-control are equally important to remain ethically compliant.

- Which category of violation is most often violated matters little. What really matters is that no violations occur.

Summary

Knowing the ethics canons of the national organizations and the licensing board rules in your state is just the first step in becoming ethically compliant. Educating mental health professionals about their ethics is the goal of this book, but we have learned that even therapists who know the rules violate them. Self-control and discipline are necessary to resist the temptation to bend or break the rules that will surely confront every mental health professional at some point. Be knowledgeable, be strong, and don't become a statistic.

Suggested Research Assignments

1. Research the ethical violations reported by the licensing boards for the mental health professions in your state, and develop a list of violations ranked by frequency.
2. Research the ethical violations reported by the state professional organizations for your state, and develop a list of violations ranked by frequency.
3. Research the ethical violations reported by the national professional organizations for your state, and develop a list of violations ranked by frequency.
4. Compare and contrast the three lists you have developed and discuss any patterns or inconsistencies.
5. Research the psychology behind sexual exploitation of clients by mental health professionals.
6. Talk to practicing mental health professionals in your area and ask them their view of the most common ethical violations.

Discussion Questions

1. Why do you think sexual exploitation complaints against mental health professionals occur with such frequency?
2. What can mental health professionals do for themselves and coprofessionals to prevent the most frequent ethical violations?
3. What would you tell a potential client about boundaries, and how would you document this?
4. What would you do if a client disrobed, sat on your lap, or touched you inappropriately during, before, or after a session? (*Note:* This has happened to several of our clients; it is not fiction.)
5. What would you do if you thought you were guilty of a serious ethical violation? A less serious obligation?

15

Ethics Codes as Evidence

Jane, a White, married, elected city council member living in a small southern community has carried on a two-year affair with a Black school principal. Racked by guilt because of her perception of community standards, Jane sought treatment for depression with a local psychologist, Dr. Kindheart. Aware of the sensitivity of the information received from Jane, Dr. Kindheart does not record any specific information in Jane's file. Session notes are limited to entries such as "explored pressures impacting client's depression." After several months of therapy, Dr. Kindheart leaves on a well-deserved European vacation after arranging for a colleague to cover for her. While Dr. Kindheart is on vacation, Jane's husband sues her for divorce, schedules a temporary custody hearing, and issues a subpoena for Dr. Kindheart to testify and produce Jane's records on her return. Jane, extremely distraught by the pending litigation, contacts Dr. Kindheart's office and schedules a session with the colleague. When she presents herself for the therapy session, Jane is unable to advise the colleague about her affair with the principal but does indicate she is upset over the custody hearing and the subpoena issued for Dr. Kindheart. The colleague, who knows nothing about the affair, tells Jane she has nothing to worry about and to get a good lawyer and relax. Later that evening, Jane commits suicide by running her automobile in the enclosed garage of her family home. She leaves a note apologizing to her husband and children. Her 12-year-old daughter discovers the body when she opens the garage door. The husband then sues the psychologist for malpractice due to negligent record keeping and failing to include significant and vital information in the clinical file. Can the ethics code provisions be used as evidence to support his case? On judicial scrutiny, will Dr. Kindheart's records be found deficient of significant facts and statements and inconsistent with minimum ethics requirements? Will the race of the principal be a significant fact, or would its inclusion in the progress notes indicate the treating therapist had some prejudice or tendency toward discrimination? Can community bias cloud clinical objectivity? In trying to protect Jane, did Dr. Kindheart make herself vulnerable?

Proving Malpractice

Malpractice has been defined as the unreasonable lack of skill or misconduct by a health-care provider.

Malpractice has been defined as the unreasonable lack of skill or misconduct by a health-care provider. The plaintiff in a malpractice lawsuit must show that the defendant had the duty to conform to a certain standard of conduct and failed to do so, and this failure caused the injury (*Watts v. Cumberland County Hosp.*, 75 N.C. App. 1, 300 S.E. 2d 242, 1985).

Generally, the plaintiff must prove four elements in a malpractice case: (1) that the health-care provider had a duty to conform to a certain standard of care, (2) that the health-care provider in question breached the standard of care in serving this particular client, (3) that the plaintiff suffered an injury, and (4) that there is a causal connection between the breach of the standard of care and the injuries suffered (*Pennington v. Brock*, 841 S.W. 2d 127, 129 [Tex. App.-Houston (14th District) 1992, *no writ*]). Further, the plaintiff must prove the standard of care in the locality where the treatment occurred, breach of the standard of care, and proximate cause by expert testimony (*Duff v. Yelin*, 721 S.W. 2d 365, 373 [Tex. App.-Houston (1st District) 1986], *aff'd*, 751 S.W. 2d 175, Tex. 1988).

Of these four elements, the easiest to establish is the standard of care, thanks in part to ethics codes. In a malpractice case, the ethics codes promulgated by a therapist's national and state organizations and by state statute or licensing board regulations can be used to help establish the standard of care that will be applied to the therapist, who is now the defendant in a malpractice suit. When presented to the court, the judge may admit them into evidence as indicating a standard of care. The weight to be given to the ethical codes depends on the judgment of the judge or the jury.

National Guidelines for Using Ethics Codes in Malpractice Litigation

American Association for Marriage and Family Therapy (AAMFT) Code of Ethics (2001)

Preamble

The ethical standards define professional expectations and are enforced by the AAMFT Ethics Committee. . . . Both law and ethics govern the practice of marriage and family therapy. When making decisions regarding professional behavior, marriage and family therapists must consider the *AAMFT Code of Ethics* and applicable laws and regulations. If the *AAMFT Code of Ethics* prescribes a standard higher than that required by law, marriage and family therapists must meet the higher standard of the *AAMFT Code of Ethics*. Marriage and family therapists comply with the mandates of law, but make known their commitment to the *AAMFT Code of Ethics* and take steps to resolve the conflict in a responsible manner.

American Counseling Association (ACA) Code of Ethics (2005)

The *ACA Code of Ethics* serves five main purposes:

1. The *Code* enables the association to clarify to current and future members, and to those served by members, the

(continued)

(*Continued*)

nature of the ethical responsibilities held in common by its members. . . .

2. The *Code* establishes principles that define ethical behavior and best practices of association members.

3. The *Code* serves as an ethical guide designed to assist members in constructing a professional course of action that best serves those utilizing counseling services and best promotes the values of the counseling profession. . . .

American Psychological Association (APA) Ethical Principles of Psychologists and Code of Conduct (2002)

Introduction and Applicability

The Ethics Code is intended to provide guidance for psychologists and standards of professional conduct that can be applied by the APA and by other bodies that choose to adopt them. The Ethics Code is not intended to be a basis of civil liability. Whether a psychologist has violated the Ethics Code standards does not by itself determine whether the psychologist is legally liable in a court action, whether a contract is enforceable, or whether other legal consequences occur. . . .

Preamble

The Ethics Code provides a common set of principles and standards upon which psychologists build their professional and scientific work. . . . This Ethics Code is intended to provide specific standards to cover most situations encountered by psychologists.

National Association of Social Workers (NASW) Code of Ethics (1999)

The *NASW Code of Ethics* is to be used by NASW and by individuals, agencies, organizations, and bodies (such as licensing and regulatory boards, professional liability insurance providers, courts of law, agency boards of directors, government agencies, and other professional groups) that choose to adopt or use it as a frame of reference. Violation of standards in this Code does not automatically imply legal liability or violation of the law. Such determination can only be made in the context of legal and judicial proceedings. . . .

Establishing Compliance with Standard of Care

Once the plaintiff establishes that the defendant owed a duty to the plaintiff to comport with the applicable standard of care, the plaintiff must then introduce evidence as to the applicable standard of care. The duty is proved by the relationship between the plaintiff and the defendant. If Jane's husband proves that Jane entered into a therapeutic relationship with Dr. Kindheart, her duty to provide services consistent with the applicable standard of care arises.

In examining the facts in Dr. Kindheart's case, the obvious question presented is whether Dr. Kindheart had a duty to record the information regarding Jane's affair with the Black school principal. Was race an issue at all? Should race, religion, national origin, or sexual orientation, and so forth be entered into a clinical record because of community bias and the feelings of the client or the therapist toward that bias? Section 6.01 of the APA Ethics Code (2002) states:

> Psychologists create, and to the extent the records are under their control, maintain, disseminate, store, retain, and dispose of records and data relating to their professional and scientific work in order to (1) facilitate provision of services later by them or by other professionals, (2) allow for replication of research design and analyses, (3) meet institutional requirements, (4) ensure accuracy of billing and payments, and (5) ensure compliance with law.

Did Dr. Kindheart appropriately document Jane's file to facilitate her colleague's provision of services while she was on vacation? This is the standard of care to which Dr. Kindheart should have complied. Arguably she did not. Her colleague probably would have taken the events of the divorce and subpoena much more seriously had she known all the information Jane shared with Dr. Kindheart. She may have perceived that Jane might contemplate suicide over these events if the consequences and nature of the affair were made public. On the other hand, a colleague may have considered race to be a nonissue.

The law requires Dr. Kindheart to possess and exercise the degree of skill and learning ordinarily possessed and exercised under similar circumstances by other psychologists in good standing, and to use ordinary and reasonable care and diligence, and her best judgment, in applying her skill to the case (70 CJS *Physicians and Surgeons* Sec. 41 [1951]). Ordinary and reasonable skill, learning, and care involve knowing and complying with the ethical provisions of the psychological organizations of which Dr. Kindheart is a member and those state boards that have issued her the licenses to practice. Pursuant to the APA Ethics Code, ordinary care requires Dr. Kindheart to appropriately document her file to facilitate the provision of mental health services later by her colleague or any subsequent professional who assumes responsibility for the file and for the continued treatment of the client. Dr. Kindheart failed to do this. Arguably, however, the affair could be considered the issue and race a nonissue. This is why there are judges and juries in civil trials and grievance committees and complaints committees for licensing boards to make these hard decisions regarding the appropriate documentation in clinical notations. Appropriate documentation is not a science, and no universal rules apply in all cases.

Having used the APA Ethics Code to establish the standard of care (that psychologists properly document their cases), Jane's husband could establish that she breached the standard of care by introducing into evidence Dr. Kindheart's inappropriately documented file. The husband has therefore satisfied two of the four elements of proof necessary to recover a money judgment against Dr. Kindheart. Keep in mind that the average jury is not composed of mental health professionals. Rather, judges are predominantly lawyers and juries are picked from a panel of citizens. Seldom, in a case such as this, will the jury include a psychologist, social worker, or counselor. Jurors are community people who happened to be on the list and who were not stricken or removed for cause. The issue of whether Dr. Kindheart's file is appropriately documented is determined by laypeople, possibly with only a passing knowledge or interest in mental health.

The average jury is not composed of mental health professionals.

Establishing the Connection between Breach of Standard of Care and Injury

In many malpractice cases brought against therapists, it is difficult to establish injury and the causal connection between the breach of the standard of care and the injury, particularly where there is no physical injury. Some courts still hold that absent physical injury there can be no recovery for mental suffering:

> Mental suffering is more difficult to estimate in financial terms, and no less a real injury. . . . Where the defendant's negligence causes only mental disturbance, without accompanying physical injury, illness or other physical consequence, and in the absence of some other independent basis for tort liability, the great majority of courts still hold that in the ordinary case there can be no recovery. . . . (W. Keeton, *Prosser and Keeton on Torts*, Sec. 54, at 361)

In Dr. Kindheart's case, there was a suicide and therefore physical injury as well as mental injury to Jane's family. It is conceivable that Dr. Kindheart's colleague would bridge the causal connection between Dr. Kindheart's failure to appropriately document Jane's case file and Jane's suicide. The colleague could testify that had she known about the details of the affair she might have better judged Jane's possible reaction to exposure, she would have appreciated the risk involved to Jane and possibly recommended inpatient care or immediately called in a psychiatrist who could have appropriately prescribed antidepressant medication.

Could Dr. Kindheart plead ignorance of the applicable APA ethics provisions? Would this be a defense to the malpractice action or limit the damages awarded in the case? Absolutely not.

Therapists are required to be familiar with their ethics codes. Ignorance will not excuse unethical conduct.

Therapists are required to be familiar with their ethics codes. Ignorance will not excuse unethical conduct. Section 8.02 of the APA Ethics Code states:

> Membership in the APA commits members and student affiliates to comply with the standards of the APA Ethics Code and to the rules and procedures used to enforce them. Lack of awareness or misunderstanding of an Ethical Standard is not itself a defense to a charge of unethical conduct.

We present workshops and seminars throughout the country stressing the importance of reading and understanding published ethical standards, canons, and codes and are amazed by how many seasoned professionals have not reviewed their associations' ethics codes since graduate school or their licensing examinations. Judging by the questions asked during the question-and-answer period following each presentation, therapists prefer to receive this knowledge through seminars rather than by making a careful examination of the codes. Don't wait to familiarize yourself with any applicable ethics codes. You need to know their provisions *before a problem arises, not after.* We are constantly amazed by how many mental health professionals call with ethical problems. Many have never read their ethical standards. Indeed, the norm is that many have not opened the envelope since it arrived, and when a problem arises, they have difficulty locating the envelope containing the ethics rules from the licensing board or national organization.

Ethical Flash Points

- Therapists are required to be familiar with their ethics codes. Ignorance of ethics code provisions is not a defense to unethical acts or omissions and will not lessen damages awarded.

- Ethics codes can be used to establish the minimum standard of care in a malpractice action. Their introduction into evidence in the litigation process is a significant event.

- Once a plaintiff establishes violation of an ethics code provision, the only real issue remaining is to decide the amount of monetary damages.

- Finding the appropriate provision in the canons of ethics is easy. Usually the canons are brief, to the point, and carefully thought out. Interpreting them and applying them to a detailed fact situation is often difficult, and the licensing boards and national organizations will offer general advice, but usually will not comment on specific questions. The therapist customarily determines what to document, as in the case used for illustration.

Summary

Ethical codes must be carefully reviewed and digested by every therapist. They are potent ammunition for a plaintiff in a malpractice case, and therefore knowledge and compliance are a strict necessity for every practicing therapist. Proving a departure from a published ethical requirement can relegate a malpractice case to a single issue: "How much money will compensate the client for the harm caused by the ethical violation?" Juries can be very generous with money belonging to someone else.

Suggested Research Assignments

1. Research malpractice cases against mental health professionals to ascertain the standard of care issue(s) presented in each case and whether an ethics code was cited.
2. Locate professional malpractice attorneys in your area and discuss with them the standard of care issue and how they prove breach or compliance in the cases that they handle.
3. Review the licensing rules and statutes that apply to the mental health professions in your state and explain how they could be used against a mental health professional in a malpractice case.
4. Identify resources you can consult with regarding standard of care issues or to resolve conflicts between standards or get clarification of standards.

5. Talk to practicing mental health professionals in your area and ask them whether they have ever experienced a conflict with state rules and law and professional association standards.
6. Develop a protocol that you will follow to resolve standard of care issues in your practice.

Discussion Questions

1. What will you do if you discover a conflict between licensing laws and rules in your state and professional association standards?
2. What steps can you take to fully document your compliance with the standards of care for your practice and in your community?
3. Should certified specialists be held to a higher standard of care than minimally licensed mental health professionals?
4. Do certain types of clients warrant a higher standard of care than others? If so, identify them and why a greater standard of care would be applicable.
5. What can be done to encourage mental health professionals to continue their education in the field of ethics?
6. Is "Don't do dumb stuff" a sufficient maxim that will avoid ethics complaints and malpractice litigation (see Chapter 33)?

16

Licensing Board Procedures

Albert, a licensed professional counselor in private practice for over 12 years, received a certified letter from his state licensing board. Although he had never before received a certified letter from the board, he instinctively knew it was not good news. As he suspected, it was not. For the first time in a stellar career as a helping professional, Albert was facing a complaint and investigation by his licensing board. Albert broke out in a cold sweat when he realized he did not know what to do. He had never been advised in graduate school or at any ethics continuing education seminar what action to take if an unhappy client filed a complaint with his licensing board. He was unsure whom he could call or wanted to call. After all, he really did not want to share information about the complaint. After a couple of days, he finally discussed the matter with a psychologist who practiced in the same building with whom he occasionally had lunch. The psychologist calmed his fears with a few stories from his own practice in which he had responded to complaints with long letters to his board, who then dropped the matter completely. Albert, following the psychologist's advice, dashed off a five-page letter to his licensing board letting them know about all the great things he had accomplished in the past 12 years. Basically, it amounted to a self-laudatory vitae.

Thinking the matter resolved, he put the original letter and the answer out of his mind until a second certified letter came three months later. This time, the licensing board advised him that based on their initial investigation, he had violated several sections of the state licensing act and they were pursuing revocation of his license. At this point, Albert contacted an attorney.

Dr. Sellers practiced for years. She was incensed when a client complained about not receiving a copy of her file in a timely fashion. She was so mad she refused to respond to a complaint notice from the licensing board. Big mistake. The board then proceeded with a complete investigation, discovered a number of discrepancies in billing practices and procedures, and followed with a revocation hearing. Only after engaging a lawyer did Dr. Sellers understand her precarious situation. Had she respectfully responded, perhaps with a half-hour attorney consultation, the matter might have been dropped.

A therapist responding to a complaint filed with his licensing board for having sex with a client ended his multipage self-laudatory biography noting: "Besides, I only did it once." Once was once too much. With zero tolerance sensitivity for sex with clients, the board revoked his license. A lawyer would have struck that remark from the letter had the therapist thought to have a legal review of his reply. Although the admission might have come out in future testimony had the case gone to trial, it would not have come from the therapist.

National Licensing Board Trends

The national trend is toward state licensing of all mental health disciplines. By their nature, licensing acts are an effort to regulate an industry or profession, protect the public at large, and create minimum standards of conduct and professional practice for a given profession. The mistake many mental health professionals make is to assume that the licensing board that bestowed their license is a "friend." A licensing board's mission is to regulate the mental health profession and to sanction mental health professionals when necessary. Simply put, licensing boards tell you what you can do, when you can do it, how you can practice, and what will happen if you violate their rules. Not only do therapists misperceive their licensing boards' attitudes and mission but frequently practitioners have little or no knowledge of complaint procedures and the administrative process. This chapter provides an overview of both actions. As stated in some places and implied in others, the licensing board is a consumer-oriented organization whose important and essential duty is to see that professionals practice ethically, and to punish those who do not. Their powers are awesome and deserve respect. Indeed, they demand deference.

The national trend is toward state licensing of all mental health disciplines.

Administrative Law

Most citizens are familiar with the civil and criminal justice systems either through personal interaction or what they acquire and assimilate through experience and the media. There is a third system or body of law known as *administrative law* that is not as well known nor understood even by most attorneys. Administrative law involves the law and rules of agencies, the decision-making parts of our government that are neither legislatures nor courts. We are familiar with numerous federal agencies, such as the Social Security Administration, the Food and Drug Administration, the Federal Communications Commission, and the Federal Trade Commission. Licensing boards are agencies. In the context of mental health, licensing boards are primarily state agencies, created by the states to regulate and police mental health providers. State licensing boards usually comprise individuals who are political appointees, one or more of whom are non-mental-health-professional members of the public. The professional members of the board consist of mental health professionals most of whom have the same license the board administers. All board members serve for a set number of years or at the pleasure of the state governor who appointed them. The actual appointment process and terms served varies with each state. Staff personnel, including an executive director who manages the day-to-day activities of the board, are salaried employees of the state.

Administrative law involves the study of agencies, the decision-making parts of our government that are neither legislatures nor courts.

Licensing Boards as State Agencies

Agencies are legislative creations enacted through statutes that are often referred to as their *enabling acts*. These enabling acts do not always establish the agency's precise procedures but do set forth the agency's mission or reason for existence. Procedure is dictated in part by a more general set of laws governing all agencies known as an *administrative procedure act*. The federal government's version is entitled the Administrative Procedure Act, 5 U.S.C. Sections 551-808. State administrative procedure acts can differ greatly but a model State Administrative Procedure Act has been promulgated. Many states have adopted this act totally or substantially follow it in enacting state laws.

An agency generally has wide discretion when creating the policies and procedures to fulfill its legislative mission. First, they make numerous rules designed to fulfill the purpose of the legislation. In addition to rule making, agencies have an adjudicative function by which they enforce the rules they adopt or promulgate. Courts have a very small role in supervising agency conduct. If a licensee is disciplined at the agency level, generally very little help is available through the courts. To appeal an administrative hearing (i.e., a determination lost at the hearing level) is difficult, cumbersome, and expensive, and an uphill process.

A state mental health licensing board is an agency governed by administrative law. It is created by the state legislature and given the mission of regulating mental health professionals through the licensing of those who practice. It passes rules, issues licenses based on qualifications it establishes, and enforces punishment if a licensee violates the licensing act or its ethics codes and board rules. Each state's administrative procedure act provides some procedural guidelines, and each board generally has wide discretion when creating detailed and specific procedures. Boards establish their own complaint and informal resolution procedures, but formal resolution, involving a hearing before an administrative law judge, is usually controlled by the state's administrative procedure act. Although it is not possible in one chapter to set out the complaint procedures for each state, we discuss a representative procedure. Every state has written rules and regulations, in addition to informal "understandings," that can guide both the boards and the licensee.

Knowing about these "understandings" is helpful when developing a defense to a complaint. It is worth noting that when engaging an attorney, some effort must be made to ensure that the lawyer has some experience with administrative law in the mental health field. A general legal education might not offer courses in the ramifications of mental health law. Generally, experience in this area is acquired by familiarity and know-how in the field, hopefully at the elbow of an experienced mental health expert. There are profound differences between criminal law, civil law, and administrative law. Each has its own practices and procedures.

Every state has written rules and regulations, in addition to informal "understandings" that can guide both the boards and the licensee.

The Complaint Procedure

The first step of a complaint procedure involves the receipt and an initial review of a complaint filed with the board by a client, another professional, any member of the public, or the board itself. Most state licensing boards require their licensees to provide information to each client on how and where to file a complaint against them with the licensing board. Some boards require the provider to post prominently the address and a toll-free number to contact the licensing board.

Either an individual or a committee may make the initial complaint review, but the introductory inquiry concerns whether the board has jurisdiction over the matter or parties complained of and, if so, whether the complaint states a violation of the licensing act, the ethics code, or a board rule. If the board does not find it has jurisdiction, it usually dismisses the matter and forwards information regarding the allegation and its findings (e.g., the board lacks jurisdiction over the matter or the complaint does not state a specific violation) to the licensed mental health provider and the complaining party. Numerous complaints are filed with licensing boards from clients who are dissatisfied with the results of therapy. Mental health professionals do not guarantee results. A valid complaint must indicate that a law or rule was violated. Clients filing a complaint state the facts as they

Most state licensing boards require their licensees to provide information to each client on how and where to file a complaint against them with the licensing board.

A valid complaint must indicate that a law or rule was violated.

perceive them; the board then determines whether a violation has occurred.

Finding a Violation

If the board finds that the provider has violated a rule, he or she will receive notice of the complaint and will be asked to respond to the allegations within a prescribed period. The initial time for responding is usually short but most boards are willing to extend the time for filing the response if they receive a timely and reasonable request. If the reviewer or committee that studies the therapist's response still perceives a likelihood that a violation has occurred, they may move directly to their adjudicative stage. If there is still doubt, the board may continue the investigation. An investigator may interview the parties or other witnesses and possibly check public records for relevant documentary evidence. Some investigations are open to the public; others are conducted behind closed doors. If the board concludes either (1) no jurisdiction or (2) no violation after the investigation is concluded, they will dismiss the matter and notify each party. Otherwise, the board moves on to the adjudicative stage.

Adjudicative Stage

The adjudicative stage is the time when the licensing board attempts to enforce the licensing act, ethics code, or its rules either through informal resolution or formal adjudication. The board thus fulfills its mission to protect the public from inappropriate, unfit, negligent, or fraudulent practitioners and harmful practices. Informal adjudication could be likened to plea bargaining in a criminal case. Here the board determines that although an ethical, licensing act, or board rule violation has occurred, the matter can best be resolved informally by agreement with the therapist. This is the usual procedure for less serious violations, such as failure to promptly forward copies of a client's file on request, maintaining incomplete records, or other minor infractions. Informal adjudication may be handled over the phone, by correspondence, or in a face-to-face settlement conference. Letters of instruction, public or private reprimands, requirements for continuing or continued education, and additional supervision are all techniques implemented for informal resolution. If an agreement cannot be achieved, the board will move on to formal adjudication.

It generally is in the best interest of the professional therapist to utilize an option to settle the matter informally, without a formalized record being transcribed and without a technical, adversary adjudication. Informal adjudication is quicker, more flexible, and less expensive and can be handled in a nonadversary hearing. When using this less formal approach, the board representatives are usually more amenable to the therapist suggesting alternatives and options to resolve the differing positions. A win-win solution can be the outcome.

The adjudicative stage is the time when the licensing board attempts to enforce the licensing act, ethics code, or its rules either through informal resolution or formal adjudication.

Formal Adjudication

Formal adjudication customarily means seeking revocation of a license through an administrative hearing governed by the rules and procedures of the state's administrative procedure act. An administrative procedure act requires the affected person to be given specific notice of the hearing time, date, place, nature of the hearing, the legal authority for convening the hearing, and information on the issues presented (see Federal Administrative Procedure Act, Sec. 554[b]). These matters are usually set forth in the original complaint. Since agency proceedings are civil cases (the defendant can't be sentenced to jail), the charged therapist need only be given reasonable notice of the violation (*Savina Home Industries v. Secretary of Labor*, 594 F.2d 1358 [10th Cir. 1979]). In criminal cases, the complaint against an individual must be very specific regarding the crime and the charge. A civil case does not require the same specificity. The therapist should always file a carefully documented, reasoned, and logical written response to the complaint with the licensing board prior to the hearing to set the tone for the defense. Providers should always consult a lawyer prior to filing their response to a complaint. It is easier for an attorney to create an effective defense in a letter than it is to explain away an admission once an unwitting and naive provider reduces it to writing.

Formal adjudication customarily means seeking revocation of a license through an administrative hearing.

The therapist should always file a written response to the complaint with the licensing board prior to the hearing to set the tone for the defense.

The Hearing

An administrative law judge conducts the hearing and takes testimony under oath through direct and cross-examination, allows documentary information into evidence, makes evidentiary rulings, and enters an order (Federal Administrative Procedure Act, Sec. 556). The hearing closely resembles a civil trial without a jury. The licensing board has the burden of proof (Federal Administrative Procedure Act, Sec. 556[d]), which means it is up to the board to introduce evidence of a violation.

An active, partici-
patory, but nonab-
rasive defense is
essential.

Because the board's original complaint may be general, how can a mental health professional prepare for the hearing? Most administrative procedure acts, including the federal act, make little mention of discovery except for subpoenas. Many states allow depositions with either the administrative law judge or the agency itself having the power to compel appearance. Record disclosure laws (Open Records Acts) may mandate that the board provide the therapist with copies of its file prior to the hearing. These tools should be actively employed in preparing for the hearing. An active, participatory, but nonabrasive defense is essential.

Burden of Proof

The law provides for three levels or "burdens" of proof depending on the issue or case involved:

1. Preponderance of the evidence
2. Clear and convincing evidence
3. Beyond a reasonable doubt

As a result of the media coverage of the O. J. Simpson murder trial and the popularity of *Court TV*, Americans have become well acquainted with the burden of proof in a criminal case: beyond a reasonable doubt. In civil cases, there are two burdens of proof: clear and convincing evidence and preponderance of the evidence. The Federal Administrative Procedure Act and many state acts fail to include a standard of proof to be applied by the administrative law judge in an administrative law hearing. In *Steadman v. S.E.C.* (450 U.S. 91, 1981), the Supreme Court held that absent a statutory requirement or an agency rule or practice, the burden of proof to be applied in agency proceedings is preponderance of the evidence. This is obviously the easiest of the three legal burdens to employ, which may be a chilling thought for a therapist accused of an ethical or licensing act violation.

Taking the Fifth

When facing a licensing board complaint, can a therapist claim his or her Fifth Amendment right against self-incrimination and refuse to release copies of records or to give testimony if called to do so? Professor K. C. Davis (1977), in his book *Administrative Law*, sets out five situations in which the Fifth Amendment cannot be used in response to a request for records including "(4) records that are required to be kept by statute or agency regulation" (p. 567). A therapist is unable to withhold records by asserting the Fifth Amendment for two reasons.

First, a therapist is generally required by the licensing act or the ethics code adopted by the licensing board to keep client records and notes. Because the board has this requirement, therapists *must* turn over the records to the board if ordered.

Second, if the complaining client consents and directs the therapist to turn over copies of his or her files, the therapist is obligated to surrender them usually pursuant to state statute or ethics code. A therapist may invoke the Fifth Amendment and preclude oral testimony; nevertheless, in all but the rarest cases, refusing to testify will make defending the complainant's allegations extremely difficult. Failing to testify will make it hard to rebut the complainant's statements, which will be taken as true if there is no contradicting evidence. The board must prove a violation of its licensing act, and they can meet the preponderance of evidence burden of proof with just the complainant's testimony. A therapist who holds his or her tongue may not be holding on to his or her license very much longer.

A therapist may invoke the Fifth Amendment and preclude oral testimony.

A therapist who holds his or her tongue may not be holding on to his or her license very much longer.

Sometimes, however, the therapist also faces a criminal prosecution in which a long-term jail sentence is a possible outcome, such as when a therapist sexually exploits a client. If criminal prosecution is likely or certain, asserting a Fifth Amendment right and losing a license could be a necessity. In determining whether to assert the Fifth Amendment privilege against self-incrimination, the risk-reward ratio must be considered. This is a carefully thought-out decision consciously made by clients with the advice and consent of their attorneys.

Prehearing Settlement Conference

Most licensing boards and administrative procedure acts favor informal resolution even after a hearing has been requested. Often referred to as a *prehearing settlement conference*, it can be an opportunity to persuade a licensing board to rescind its request for the formal hearing. In practical terms, this means the therapist attempts to persuade the board not to revoke the license and either dismiss the complaint or agree to a lesser, more agreeable, and less onerous sanction.

It is usually a mistake to fail to meet with the board in person after seeking the advice of a knowledgeable and informed attorney. Often, there is an opportunity to appear before an ethics panel or committee prior to the board making its final decision to proceed with sanctioning. Making a good appearance as early in the complaint process as possible can go a long way in convincing the committee to either close an investigation with no recommended sanction or to at least recommend the least draconian measure available to the board. Human nature makes it much easier to deal harshly with someone who is not in front of you. Preparing well for the face-to-face encounter and presenting the board with mitigating circumstances if a violation has occurred is well worth the time and expense involved.

It is best to be represented by an attorney who is familiar with the licensing act for your profession and the board's makeup and procedures. The attorney can best assist the therapist in putting the best case forward and can serve as a sounding board for arguments and theories to be presented to the committee. The general idea is that the provider's appearance should have the appearance of spontaneity while being thoroughly prepared and rehearsed. Engaging an attorney also lets the board know that you take the matter very seriously and may be willing to take the complaint all the way through the process to an administrative law hearing. Like most governmental entities today, cost and budget constraints are a reality for state licensing boards. It costs the board money allocated for its use to pursue administrative law hearings that it may need to devote to other operational needs.

Judicial Review

Once the administrative law judge has entered an order, there are few grounds on which to base a request for a court hearing or judicial review. Such grounds set out in administrative procedure acts include a decision that was arbitrary and capricious or unsupported by the great weight of the evidence, or an abuse of discretion (Federal Administrative Procedure Act, Sec. 706). The opportunity for a *de novo* (new) hearing on the merits before a civil or appellate judge after agency adjudication is available in very few states. Convincing a court to undo an agency result is possible but not very probable. It is critical for therapists to be aware of the board's complaint procedure and to put on the best possible case throughout its proceedings.

Ethical Flash Points

- When a complaint is received, seek peer and legal advice before finalizing any response. Prepare a rough draft response and have your lawyer review it prior to sending it to the board. Be cautious about talking with your peers. Colleagues may have some obligation to report infractions to the board. Any consultation with a board or a colleague should be theoretical, hypothetical, and about "another" person.

- Many lawyers are unfamiliar with administrative law, and even fewer mental health professionals are familiar with board rules and regulations. Consult with colleagues on

(continued)

(*Continued*)

practice issues, but engage an attorney familiar with board procedures and mental health law to defend you or represent you before the board.

- Responses to complaint letters should be succinct, addressing only the issues raised by the complaint or the board. Attorney review prior to submission is earnestly recommended.

- Don't wait for the board to seek revocation through a formal hearing before retaining competent legal assistance. There is an old saying in law that a lawyer who represents himself has a fool for a client.

- Be sure your malpractice insurance policy provides benefits for licensing board representation and costs. Defending against a complaint by a licensing board can cost thousands of dollars.

- Notify your malpractice insurance carrier the minute a complaint is filed; don't wait until a revocation hearing is requested. Policies contain specific notice provisions that, if not followed, can cause the loss of coverage.

- Vigorously pursue whatever discovery is available (e.g., depositions, letters, or other documents sent to the board) and take advantage of all statutes allowing access to the board's file, especially intraboard communications and memoranda.

- Mount a good defense but be courteous and respectful of the board and its staff at all times. Even if the result is favorable, those people will monitor your activities for a long time. A hearing before the board or an administrative judge is not the same as a full adversary hearing before a court. It is less dramatic and more conversational and conciliatory. Mount an effective defense, but do it with tact, finesse, and collegiality.

- Utilize every opportunity for informal resolution of the complaint even after a formal revocation hearing has been requested.

- Take the earliest opportunity to meet face-to-face with the board or a panel or committee of board members to present your side of the case.

- Even though the board has the burden of proving a violation by a preponderance of the evidence, approach the case as if the burden is shifted and prove innocence or compliance beyond all reasonable doubt. This will help ensure high energy and a strong defense.

- Assert the Fifth Amendment right against self-incrimination only if absolutely necessary when faced with possible criminal punishment.

- Familiarize yourself with the board's complaint procedure before a complaint is filed and develop a response plan to implement a defense the minute notification of a complaint is received.

- Don't rely on the fact that you have never had a complaint filed against you. Many complaints that are filed are without merit. Even the most consciously ethical practitioner has the risk that an unhappy client may file a complaint.

- There is no risk to a client when filing a frivolous complaint. Only the practitioner is at risk.

- Whenever there is the hint of a complaint or an unsatisfied client, stop, look at the circumstances, and listen to all the client's gripes. Often all the client wants is immediate attention and satisfaction. Frequently a free session satisfies this need to be heard. Be sure to listen intently.

Summary

With the increasing number of complaints filed against mental health professionals and the increased knowledge of consumers with respect to mental health practice issues, no therapist is immune from an ethical or licensing act violation allegation. Board complaint procedures involve administrative law with which most therapists are totally unfamiliar. Competent legal assistance and direction is critical. Life and liberty may not be at risk before the licensing board, but a license revocation could certainly impact a therapist's pursuit of happiness. Total revocation of a license to practice can make a person unemployable. Remember, competent representation may not result in a dismissal, but it may diminish or reduce the punishment. Practice ethically, but be informed and prepared to defend against a specious and fabricated allegation. Take every complaint seriously.

Take every complaint seriously.

Suggested Research Assignments

1. Research the complaint procedures for the licensing boards for the mental health professions in your state. What are the similarities and differences?

2. Research the licensing act requirements for the mental health professions in your state with respect to advising clients about complaint procedures.

3. Locate attorneys in your area who represent mental health professionals in connection with ethics complaints and discuss with them their experiences with the state boards.

4. Review the complaint procedures for the state and national professional organizations and compare them with the complaint system for your state licensing boards.

5. Research the sanctioning options of the licensing boards for the mental health professions in your state and any published criteria or mitigating circumstances.

6. Develop a protocol you will use in your practice if a complaint is ever filed against you.

7. Develop a protocol for dealing with upset clients who you believe may be considering the filing of a complaint against you.

8. Research available insurance coverage for licensing board complaints and compare and contrast them.

Discussion Questions

1. What action would you take if a client advised you that she believes you have violated an ethical canon or licensing act provision? What do you document?

2. What do you recommend a colleague do if he receives notice from a licensing board of a complaint filing?

3. What steps would you take if a former client filed a complaint against you?

4. Is it appropriate to obtain "testimonials" from satisfied clients and submit them to a licensing board as part of your response to the complaint?

5. Do your state law and the HIPAA Privacy Rule preclude you from discussing the complaint with any third parties? Does it make a difference if the complaint was filed by the former spouse of your former client?

17

Office of Civil Rights

Bethany, a licensed marriage and family therapist, spent several months counseling a couple and who seemed to be successfully reconciling their marriage. Over a weekend, things unraveled and the couple ended up pursuing a divorce. During the divorce proceedings, the wife accused the therapist of breaching confidentiality by relating information to the husband that was shared with the therapist in a private session. When a complaint was filed with the state licensing board, the husband provided an affidavit that stated he had learned the information allegedly disclosed by the therapist by reading his wife's diary that she kept hidden in the glove compartment of her car. The therapist breathed a long sigh of relief when the state board found no violation. The next day, however, the therapist received a notice of complaint filed by the wife with the Office of Civil Rights.

Herb, employed at a local hospital as a social worker, worked with patients who suffered catastrophic injuries and their families. The mother of a recently paralyzed 18-year-old man filed a complaint with the Office of Civil Rights accusing the hospital and its staff, including Herb, of violating the young man's privacy rights by providing protected health information to the

*young man's father. The parents had divorced when the young man was
4 years old, and the father had not had any contact with his son after the
divorce. He owed the mother a substantial sum for unpaid child support.
Three months after the accident occurred, the father learned of the accident
from a newspaper article. The newspaper reported that government investigators found that a negligent driver of a tractor-trailer rig owned by a major
corporation caused the accident. Two other motorists had been killed in the
crash. The next day the father came to the hospital with a lawyer, and they
identified themselves to hospital staff as the boy's father and uncle. While the
young man slept, the father and his lawyer peppered staff, including Herb,
with questions about his son's condition and prognosis. When the mother
came to the hospital, she overheard one of the nurses talking to the father
and his lawyer about the young man's physical therapy. She was instantly
incensed and demanded the two men leave. When the young man awoke,
he backed his mother and ordered them to leave. Hospital security was eventually called to escort the father and his lawyer out of the hospital. Rereading
a copy of the hospital's notice of privacy practices prompted the mother to file
the complaint with the Office of Civil Rights.*

Federal Oversight

The Health Insurance Portability and Accountability Act (HIPAA)
created a new level of oversight and regulation for mental health providers across the country. The HIPAA Privacy Rule allows for complaints of violations to be filed against a covered entity with the U.S.
Department of Health and Human Services (HHS) Office of Civil
Rights (OCR), which is charged with compliance and enforcement
responsibility. A covered entity is a health plan, health-care clearinghouse, and any health-care provider who conducts certain health-care
transactions electronically.

OCR has stated that enforcement will be primarily complaint-
driven. OCR will investigate complaints and work to make sure that
consumers receive the privacy rights and protections that HIPAA requires. When appropriate, OCR can impose civil monetary penalties
for violations of the privacy rule provisions. Potential criminal

violations of the law are referred to the U.S. Department of Justice for further investigation and appropriate action.

Penalties

Congress provided civil and criminal penalties for covered entities that misuse personal health information. For civil violations of the standards, OCR may impose monetary penalties up to $100 per violation, up to $25,000 per year, for each requirement or prohibition violated. Criminal penalties apply for certain actions such as knowingly obtaining protected health information in violation of the law. Criminal penalties can range up to $50,000 and one year in prison for certain offenses; up to $100,000 and up to five years in prison if the offenses are committed under false pretenses; and up to $250,000 and up to 10 years in prison if the offenses are committed with the intent to sell, transfer, or use protected health information for commercial advantage, personal gain, or malicious harm.

Congress provided civil and criminal penalties for covered entities that misuse personal health information.

Complaints

Complaints to the Office for Civil Rights must:

- Be filed in writing, either on paper or electronically;
- Name the entity that is the subject of the complaint and describe the acts or omissions believed to be in violation of the applicable requirements of the HIPAA Privacy Rule; and
- Be filed within 180 days of when you knew that the act or omission complained of occurred. OCR may extend the 180-day period upon a showing of good cause.

Anyone can file written complaints with OCR by mail, fax, or e-mail. A person needing help filing a complaint or having a question about the complaint form can call the OCR toll-free number: (800) 368-1019. OCR has 10 regional offices, and each regional office covers certain states. Complaints should be filed with the appropriate OCR regional office, based on the region where the alleged violation took place. Complaints should be sent to the attention of the appropriate OCR regional manager.

The complaint may be submitted in any written format. An OCR Health Information Privacy Complaint Form can be found on the OCR web site (www.hhs.gov/ocr/hipaa) or at an OCR regional office. A complainant may submit a written complaint in his or her own format, but it should include the following information:

- Complainant's name, full address, home and work telephone numbers, e-mail address.
- If the complaint is filed on someone's behalf, the name of the person on whose behalf the complaint is filed.
- Name, full address and phone of the person, agency, or organization the complainant believes violated the complainant's (or someone else's) health information privacy rights or committed another violation of the HIPAA Privacy Rule.
- A brief description of what happened. How, why, and when the complainant believes his or her (or someone else's) health information privacy rights were violated, or the HIPAA Privacy Rule otherwise was violated.
- Any other relevant information.
- The complaint should be signed and dated.

The following information is optional:

- Whether special accommodations are necessary for OCR to communicate with the complaint about the complaint and if so what type. The identity of another person for OCR to contact if they cannot reach the complainant directly.
- Whether the complaint has been filed somewhere else.

HIPAA requires health-care professionals to advise clients how to contact OCR in the event they wish to file a complaint. It also prohibits the alleged violating party from taking retaliatory action against anyone for filing a complaint with OCR. An OCR complaint can be e-mailed to OCRComplaint@hhs.gov or reported by telephone at at: (866) 627-7748 (toll-free).

OCR Regional Addresses

Region I: CT, ME, MA, NH, RI, VT
Office for Civil Rights
U.S. Department of Health & Human Services
JFK Federal Building, Room 1875
Boston, MA 02203
(617) 565-1340; (617) 565-1343 (TDD)
(617) 565-3809 FAX

Region II: NJ, NY, PR, VI
Office for Civil Rights
U.S. Department of Health & Human Services
26 Federal Plaza, Suite 3313
New York, NY 10278
(212) 264-3313; (212) 264-2355 (TDD)
(212) 264-3039 FAX

Region III: DE, DC, MD, PA, VA, WV
Office for Civil Rights
U.S. Department of Health & Human Services
150 S. Independence Mall West, Suite 372
Philadelphia, PA 19106-3499
(215) 861-4441; (215) 861-4440 (TDD)
(215) 861-4431 FAX

Region IV: AL, FL, GA, KY, MS, NC, SC, TN
Office for Civil Rights
U.S. Department of Health & Human Services
61 Forsyth Street, SW, Suite 3B70
Atlanta, GA 30323
(404) 562-7886; (404) 331-2867 (TDD)
(404) 562-7881 FAX

Region V: IL, IN, MI, MN, OH, WI
Office for Civil Rights
U.S. Department of Health & Human Services
233 N. Michigan Ave., Suite 240
Chicago, IL 60601
(312) 886-2359; (312) 353-5693 (TDD)
(312) 886-1807 FAX

Region VI: AR, LA, NM, OK, TX
Office for Civil Rights
U.S. Department of Health & Human Services
1301 Young Street, Suite 1169
Dallas, TX 75202
(214) 767-4056; (214) 767-8940 (TDD)
(214) 767-0432 FAX

(continued)

OCR Regional Addresses (Continued)

Region VII: IA, KS, MO, NE
Office for Civil Rights
U.S. Department of Health &
Human Services
601 East 12th Street, Room 248
Kansas City, MO 64106
(816) 426-7278; (816) 426-7065
(TDD)
(816) 426-3686 FAX

**Region VIII: CO, MT, ND, SD,
UT, WY**
Office for Civil Rights
U.S. Department of Health &
Human Services
1961 Stout Street, Room 1426
Denver, CO 80294
(303) 844-2024; (303) 844-3439
(TDD)
(303) 844-2025 FAX

**Region IX: AZ, CA, HI, NV, AS,
GU, The U.S. Affiliated Pacific
Island Jurisdictions**
Office for Civil Rights
U.S. Department of Health &
Human Services
50 United Nations Plaza, Room 322
San Francisco, CA 94102
(415) 437-8310; (415) 437-8311
(TDD)
(415) 437-8329 FAX

Region X: AK, ID, OR, WA
Office for Civil Rights
U.S. Department of Health &
Human Services
2201 Sixth Avenue, Mail Stop
RX-11
Seattle, WA 98121
(206) 615-2290; (206) 615-2296
(TDD)
(206) 615-2297 FAX

OCR's policy is to resolve a covered entity's noncompliance through "informal means," before resorting to monetary penalties. Informal means can include demonstrating compliance to OCR, completing a corrective action plan (i.e., a plan to remedy the noncompliance), or entering into some other type of agreement with OCR.

If informal means do not work, the proposed rule provides that HHS must give the covered entity an opportunity to submit written evidence of any mitigating factors or affirmative defenses, as it proceeds to the civil monetary penalty phase.

The Enforcement Rule identifies three specific affirmative defenses that would bar the imposition of civil money penalties:

1. The violation is a criminal offense;
2. The covered entity did not have actual or constructive knowledge of the violation; and

3. The failure to comply was due to reasonable cause and not to willful neglect, and the failure to comply was corrected during a 30-day period beginning on the first date the person liable for the penalty knew, or by exercising reasonable diligence would have known, that the failure to comply occurred.

The covered entity has 30 days to respond and raise any of these affirmative defenses. The proposed rule describes the specific manner in which investigational inquires will be conducted, how testimony will be given, and how evidence obtained during an investigation may be used.

Finally, the proposed rule includes a provision that prohibits covered entities from threatening, intimidating, coercing, discriminating against, or taking any other retaliatory action against anyone who complains to HHS or otherwise assists or cooperates in the HIPAA enforcement process.

Imposition of Civil Monetary Penalties

The maximum civil money penalty (i.e., the fine) for a HIPAA breach is $100 per violation and up to $25,000 for all violations of an identical requirement or prohibition during a calendar year. The Enforcement Rule identifies the following three variables to be used singly or collectively, at the discretion of HHS, in calculating the number of violations: (1) actions—the number of times a covered entity takes a prohibited action or fails to take a required action; (2) persons—the number of persons involved or affected; and (3) time—the duration of a violation in terms of days.

The proposed rule also provides that HHS may consider the following factors, as either aggravating or mitigating the violation, when determining the amount of the penalty: the nature of the violation; the circumstances under which the violation occurred; the degree of culpability; any history of prior offenses; the financial condition of the covered entity; and such "other matters as justice may require."

Importantly, while a monetary penalty can potentially be imposed on a covered entity based on the conduct of a business associate, if the covered entity complies with HIPAA business associate rules, a penalty *will not* be assessed.

Conversely, if it fails to comply with those rules, such as by failing to enter into a Business Associate Agreement or failing to take steps to cure a breach or end a violation that it knows about, the covered entity could be held liable for the actions of its business associate and be penalized.

Procedures for Hearings

The HIPAA Privacy Rule sets out procedures for the prehearing and hearing phases of the enforcement process, including the establishment of prehearing conferences, exchange of witness lists, subpoenas for attendance at the hearing, the burden of proof at the hearing, and the nature of the administrative record. It also provides for initial review by an administrative law judge, and appeal of the administrative law judge's decision to the HHS Department Appeals Board.

Ethical Flash Points

- Mental health professionals need to be fully compliant with HIPAA's Privacy Rule.

- The Office of Civil Rights has the authority to investigate complaints and compliance with the Privacy Rule.

- Even small technical violations could lead to bigger problems if OCR exercises its authority to investigate possible noncompliance of other sections of the Privacy Rule.

- Complaints must be filed with OCR within 180 days of learning of the violation.

- Remember that state law that is more protective of privacy will supersede the federal Privacy Rule.

- A state licensing board could take action against a mental health professional even when OCR finds no violation if there is a state rule in effect that is more protective of a client's privacy rights.

Summary

No mental health professional should overlook the power, jurisdiction, and authority the federal government has over his or her practice and services. In the opening scenario, you could assume that Bethany would be able to achieve the same result with the OCR (no action on the complaint) by providing the same information that she provided to the state licensing board. However, she will incur the time, expense, and anxiety a second time.

Herb's case poses an interesting situation in that the HIPAA Privacy Rule allows for health-care providers to share protected health information with family members, friends, or others the patient identifies who are involved with the patient's health care unless the patient objects. Herb, the hospital, and other staff members who were named in the complaint would probably defend on the basis of this provision. OCR could find, however, that the 18-year-old son had not identified the father as a person involved in his care.

Clearly there was no intentional or malevolent disclosure of the patient's private health-care information, so criminal sanctions are highly unlikely. A civil penalty could be considered, however. Taking into account the factors—the nature of the violation; the circumstances under which the violation occurred; the degree of culpability; any history of prior offenses; the financial condition of the covered entity; and such "other matters as justice may require"—could result in the $100 fine being imposed. Not a serious consequence? Well, what if OCR now decides to exercise its compliance investigatory authority and begins to look at all the privacy issues and how they are handled at the hospital? Multiple violations could be uncovered, leading to more serious consequences.

One of the unique features of the HIPAA Privacy Rule is that where it conflicts with state law the rule that is most protective of a patient's right to privacy will prevail. For example, if state law does not allow for identified victims to be contacted if a client threatens them with physical harm but the Privacy Rule does, then the state law provision will supersede the federal rule. This is not typical in that federal law most often will trump state law. It is possible then for the

OCR to find no violation while a state licensing board could sanction a mental health professional on the same set of facts.

It is possible that a state licensing board could treat Herb with greater severity even if the OCR declines to take any action.

Compliance with the HIPAA Privacy Rule is critical for all healthcare professionals. Taking the time to educate yourself on its requirements and to periodically review policies and procedures for compliance is the best way to avoid a complaint. See *The Portable Lawyer for Mental Health Professionals* (Bernstein and Hartsell, 2004), chapters 37 through 45 for a more in-depth discussion of the Privacy Rule. Where applicable, relevant provisions of the Privacy Rule have been incorporated into the discussion in other chapters of this book. Knowing the complaint process and how OCR approaches complaints can help guide the mental health professional in responding to a complaint if notice of one is received.

Treat a complaint filed with OCR just as seriously as a state licensing board complaint, and follow the suggestions set out in Chapter 16 for responding to and defending against the complaint.

Suggested Research Assignments

1. Compare and contrast the ethical rules for your discipline and/or license with the HIPAA Privacy Rule and cite similarities and differences.
2. Compare and contrast the differences in sanctions available to OCR and your state licensing board.
3. Write out a plan of action you would follow if a complaint were filed against you with OCR.
4. Identify resources/persons you would consult with if a complaint were filed against you with OCR.
5. Interview mental health professionals in your area about their experiences with the Privacy Rule and OCR compliance enforcement.

Discussion Questions

1. A complaint has been filed against you with OCR, and you wish to consult with a colleague. What concerns if any should you have about talking to the colleague about the matter?
2. How might a sanction issued by OCR against you impact your ability to practice?
3. An investigator enters your office and indicates a complaint has been filed. How do you ensure that the presenting person is, in fact, an investigator, and what steps do you take to protect yourself, your employer, and your client's privacy rights?
4. How will your approach or method of doing business change now that you are aware of the Privacy Rule and its enforcement provisions?

18

Centers for Medicare and Medicaid Services

Penny, a licensed clinical social worker, recently resigned from a state agency where she had worked as a child abuse investigator. She rented a small office with a waiting room and began a private practice to provide therapy to children and families. Her former colleagues at the state agency represented a steady source of client referrals. Her first two months were a success. Then she received a subpoena to testify in a divorce trial and to provide a copy of her client's record. Her client signed a written consent for the release, but when Penny attempted to print a copy of the client's records from the personal computer she used to store client records, the computer failed. After frantically working to restore the system, she was forced to call in an expert. The expert advised Penny her hard drive was defective and it was unlikely she could recover her lost data. Penny had an external backup drive, but when the expert attached it to another computer, he discovered that Penny must have incorrectly installed or used the software or backup drive because no files were found on the external drive. When Penny appeared in court the next day in response to the subpoena, she was forced to testify why she was unable to produce the client's records. The client *received an unfavorable ruling in the case and upon advice from her lawyer filed a complaint against Penny with the Centers for Medicare and Medicaid Services alleging violations of the HIPAA Security Rule.*

Phillip is a licensed psychologist who was in private practice for 22 years when he received notice that a disgruntled client had filed a complaint against him with the Centers for Medicare and Medicaid Services. Phillip had refused to provide the client with an affidavit supporting the client's claim for disability benefits from his employer because he did not believe the client's mental condition prohibited him from working. The client alleged that Phillip had failed to provide him with notice of the identity of the practice's security officer and, further, that Phillip had not taken any action required of health-care providers with respect to the electronic personal health information dictated by the HIPAA Security Rule. This in fact was true. Phillip had brought his practice current and compliant with the HIPAA Privacy Rule but had not gotten around to tackling the requirements of the Security Rule.

Federal Oversight

The Health Insurance Portability and Accountability Act (HIPAA) Security Rule allows for complaints for violations to be filed against a covered entity with the U.S. Department of Health and Human Services Centers for Medicare and Medicaid Services (CMS), which is charged with compliance and enforcement responsibility. Just like with the Privacy Rule, a covered entity is a health plan, health-care clearinghouse, and any health-care provider who conducts certain health-care transactions electronically.

The rule applies to electronic protected health information (EPHI), which is individually identifiable health information (IIHI) in electronic form. IIHI relates to (1) an individual's past, present, or future physical or mental health or condition; (2) an individual's provision of health care; or (3) past, present, or future payment for provision of health care to an individual. The principal purpose of the Security Rule is to protect the confidentiality, integrity, and availability of EPHI when it is stored, maintained, or transmitted.

Electronic transmission includes the Internet, extranets (using Internet technology to link a business with information only accessible to its employees), dial-up lines, computer-generated faxes (not traditional paper-to-paper faxes), private networks, and EPHI that is physically moved from one location to another using magnetic tape, disk, or compact disc media.

The following standard electronic transactions are specified by the Security Rule and trigger the need to be HIPAA-compliant:

- Health-care claims
- Health-care payment and remittance advice
- Coordination of benefits
- Health-care claim status, enrollment, or disenrollment from a health plan
- Eligibility for a health plan
- Health plan premium payments
- Referral certification and authorization
- First report of injury
- Health claims attachments

Complying with the Security Rule is a process that begins with a risk analysis. The risk analysis is a careful and thorough documented evaluation of whether a practice's administrative activities, physical environment, and computer systems are secure, and whether EPHI is accessible only to appropriate and authorized individuals.

The risk analysis will help the mental health professional to determine and document any security threats or vulnerabilities (e.g., computer viruses or break-ins) in the practice by comparing current activities with the administrative, physical, and technological requirements of the Security Rule. The risk analysis should assess the likelihood and impact of identified threats and vulnerabilities and lead to any necessary preventive and corrective actions to bring the practice into compliance in the event of a breach of security.

Each stage of the risk analysis must be documented and the completed risk analysis document added to the practice's HIPAA compliance records. Policies and procedures should be updated to reflect any administrative, physical, or technical safeguards that have been implemented as a result of the risk analysis.

CMS's approach to Security Rule Enforcement is to rely on complaints to learn of violations, seek voluntary compliance using informal means, and to provide technical assistance and information to help covered entities come into compliance. If the complaint is not resolved informally, then CMS can initiate the process that could lead to the imposition of administrative fines and penalties. CMS also has been given the authority to initiate compliance reviews.

Civil Penalties

CMS can assess a penalty of up to $100 per day for each violation up to a maximum of $25,000 per calendar year for identical violations.

On February 16, 2006, the Department of Health and Human Services (DHHS) published a final rule that details the bases and procedures for imposing civil monetary penalties on covered entities that violate the HIPAA Security Rule. CMS can assess a penalty of up to $100 per day for each violation up to a maximum of $25,000 per calendar year for identical violations. Factors that may affect the amount of the proposed penalty are the type of the violation, the surrounding circumstance and consequences of the violation, the extent of the covered entity's blame, the covered entity's record of compliance or lack of compliance, and the size and financial condition of the covered entity.

A covered entity has the right to request a formal hearing before an administrative law judge. This proceeding allows for prehearing discovery, presentation of evidence, witnesses, and oral arguments. The decision of the administrative law judge may be appealed to the Health and Human Services Department of Appeals Board. The Board's decision is then reviewable in court.

Complaints

Complaints may be filed with CMS by:

1. Internet using the Administrative Simplification Enforcement Tool at http://htct.hhs.gov. The complaint form can be found at:

www.cms.hhs.gov/Enforcement/Downloads/HIPAANon-Privacy
ComplaintForm.pdf.
2. Mail at: The Centers for Medicare and Medicaid Services, HIPAA
   TCS Enforcement Activities, P.O. Box 8030, Baltimore, MD
   21244-8030.

Complaints must meet all of the following requirements:

- Be filed in writing, either on paper or electronically. CMS will not
  accept faxed complaints.
- Describe the acts or omissions believed to be in violation of the applicable administrative simplification provisions.
- Provide contact information, including name, address, and telephone number, for the complainant and the covered entity that are
  the subject of the complaint.
- Be filed within 180 days of when the complainant knew or should
  have known that the act or omission that is the subject of the complaint occurred, unless this time limit is waived by CMS for good
  cause shown. Complainants may, but are not required to, use the
  CMS complaint form referenced earlier.

Procedures for Initial Processing of Complaints

On receipt of a complaint, CMS will review the complaint to determine if CMS will accept it for processing. CMS reserves the right to
reject complaints. CMS will acknowledge its receipt of a complaint
filed within 14 calendar days of receipt. That acknowledgment may be
either electronic or on paper. After CMS receives the complaint,
CMS will make a preliminary review of the complaint to determine
whether it is complete and appears to allege a failure to comply with
an administrative simplification provision.

The review will typically proceed as follows:

1. If the complaint is complete and appears to allege a failure to comply with the applicable administrative simplification provisions,
   CMS will notify the complainant that the complaint is accepted

for processing and further review. Acceptance of a complaint for processing and further review does not represent a determination that a compliance failure has occurred.

2. If additional information is required to make the preliminary determination, CMS will ask the complainant to provide the additional information within a reasonable time, and the complaint will be held in abeyance until that information is received. Failure to provide the requested additional information when requested by CMS may lead to closure of the complaint, without prejudice to the complainant's right to refile the complaint.

3. CMS will close a complaint if it does not state a claim on which CMS may act. A complaint may be withdrawn at any time, upon notice to CMS in such form and manner as CMS may require. Even if a complaint is withdrawn, CMS may nonetheless determine to continue its investigation of the alleged noncompliance complaint. In general, a complaint that has been withdrawn before investigation may be refiled. Complainants are, however, cautioned that they must refile their complaint within 180 days of the date on which the complainant knew or should have known that the act or omission that is the subject of the complaint occurred, and should not assume that this time limit will be waived by CMS.

CMS will close a complaint if it does not state a claim on which CMS may act.

Complaint Processing and Review

If after initial processing, as outlined in the previous section, a complaint is accepted for processing and review, CMS will begin an investigation of the complaint. CMS may request from the complainant such additional information and materials as it may require in order to evaluate whether a compliance failure may have occurred, as alleged in the complaint. Failure to provide the information when requested may result in closure of the complaint. If based on the preliminary review and any additional information gathering CMS ascertains that a compliance failure by a covered entity may have occurred, CMS will advise the covered entity that a complaint has been filed and will inform the covered entity of the alleged compliance failure.

CMS will work with covered entities to obtain voluntary compliance. CMS will ask the covered entity to respond to the alleged compliance failure by submitting in writing: (1) A statement demonstrating compliance, or (2) a statement setting forth with particularity the basis for its disagreement with the allegations, or (3) a corrective action plan. CMS will afford the covered entity a reasonable time to respond to CMS's request for information, generally 30 days. Extensions may be granted, on a case-by-case basis, at CMS's sole discretion, and for good cause shown. It is expected that, in most cases, no more than one extension, of an additional 30 days, will be granted.

A covered entity that disagrees with the allegations made should set forth and document, where possible: (1) Compliance, (2) in what respect it believes the allegations to be factually incorrect or incomplete, and/or (3) why it disagrees that its alleged actions or failures to act constitute a failure to comply. On receipt of this response from the covered entity, CMS may communicate further with the covered entity and request the opportunity to interview knowledgeable persons or to review additional documents or materials. CMS expects that additional information or access to witnesses will be provided in a timely manner. CMS may also seek additional information from the complainant.

A covered entity may amend or supplement its response at any time and may propose voluntary compliance through a corrective action plan at any time. CMS may require modifications in the terms of a proposed corrective action plan as a prerequisite to accepting the corrective action plan. If a corrective action plan is accepted, CMS will actively monitor the plan, and the covered entity will be required to periodically report to CMS its progress toward compliance. If the covered entity comes into voluntary compliance, CMS will notify the complainant by mail or electronically. The parties to the complaint will be notified, as appropriate, when the complaint is closed.

A covered entity may amend or supplement its response at any time and may propose voluntary compliance through a corrective action plan at any time.

CMS states that it will make reasonable efforts to secure a timely response from the covered entity. If the covered entity fails or refuses to provide the information sought, an investigational subpoena may be issued in accordance with 45 C.F.R. 160.504 to require the attendance and testimony of witnesses and/or the production of any other evidence sought in furtherance of the investigation.

After finding that a violation exists, CMS will pursue other options, such as, but not limited to, civil money penalties.

Ethical Flashpoints

- Mental health professionals need to be fully compliant with HIPAA's Security Rule.

- The security rule is more complicated and requires greater effort to become compliant and to document compliance.

- The Centers for Medicare and Medicaid Services has the authority to investigate complaints and compliance with the Security Rule.

- Complaints must be filed with CMS within 180 days of learning of the violation.

- Bringing oneself quickly into compliance will be critical if a complaint is filed with CMS if noncompliance is a fact.

Summary

In many ways, the HIPAA Security Rule is more complicated and more difficult to implement than the Privacy Rule. However, if the mental health professional is transmitting patient health-care information electronically, even if the only transmitting is carrying home a portable back up drive each night, he or she must comply with its provisions. The authors refer readers to *The Portable Lawyer for Mental Health Professionals* (Bernstein and Hartsell 2004), Chapter 46, "HIPAA Security Rule," for a more in-depth discussion of the Security Rule. Where applicable, relevant provisions of the security rule have been incorporated into the discussion in other chapters of this book.

Knowing and understanding the complaint process that CMS will impose will be helpful in responding to a complaint if one is filed. Penny and Phillip, the mental health professionals who each failed to be compliant with the Security Rule in the opening scenarios, face being sanctioned at the rate of $100 per day for noncompliance. It is possible that CMS will allow them each a period of time to bring themselves into compliance before considering sanctions. There is no guarantee of this especially when you consider that little or no effort was made to be compliant.

Take any complaint filed with CMS seriously and react to it promptly, especially if noncompliance is a fact. The quicker one is able to become fully compliant the better the outcome that can be expected.

Suggested Research Assignments

1. Compare and contrast the ethical rules for your discipline and/or license with the HIPAA Security Rule and cite similarities and differences.
2. Compare and contrast the differences in sanctions available to CMS and your state licensing board.
3. Write out a plan of action you would follow if a complaint were filed against you with CMS. Should this plan include an attorney?
4. Identify resources/persons you would consult with if a complaint were filed against you with CMS.
5. Interview mental health professionals and/or attorneys in your area about their experiences with the Security Rule and CMS compliance enforcement.

Discussion Questions

1. A complaint has been filed against you with CMS and you wish to consult with a colleague. What concerns if any should you have about talking to the colleague about the matter?
2. How might a sanction issued by CMS against you impact your ability to practice?
3. An investigator enters your office and indicates a complaint has been filed. How do you ensure that the presenting person is, in fact, an investigator and what steps do you take to protect yourself, your employer, and your clients privacy rights?
4. How will your approach or method of doing business change now that you are aware of the Security Rule and its enforcement provisions?

19

Reporting Statutes and Obligations

Cheryl scheduled an afternoon counseling session with Dr. Kindheart, a child psychologist, after receiving a referral from a school counselor. Cheryl suspected her second husband had sexually molested her 12-year-old daughter, Susan. After the initial session with Susan, Dr. Kindheart told her mother there was a strong probability Susan was sexually or physically abused. Cheryl assured him she would contact the child welfare authorities and make a report. Cheryl wrote down the telephone number on the back of Dr. Kindheart's business card. Dr. Kindheart practiced in a state that requires reporting suspected child abuse. Relying on Cheryl's assurance that she would file a report, Dr. Kindheart scheduled a second appointment for Susan three days later. Cheryl went home and, fearful of the unpredictable outcome of a report, did not call child welfare. The night before the second appointment, Susan's stepfather sexually assaulted her again. When the police investigated the case, they found out that neither Cheryl nor Dr. Kindheart had reported the suspected prior abuse. Criminal charges were filed against each of them for failure to comply with the reporting statute. They each pleaded guilty to the misdemeanor offense, paid fines, and performed community service. The lead detective on the assault case against the stepfather also filed a complaint with the state board responsible for disciplining and licensing psychologists. Dr. Kindheart received a public reprimand that was published in the board's newsletter.

After becoming romantically and sexually involved with a recently terminated client, Kevin, a licensed social worker, confided in Jerome, also a licensed social worker, and a longtime friend. Jerome counseled Kevin regarding the obvious inappropriateness of the relationship and strongly urged Kevin to discontinue dating the client. Kevin decided to do just that and told the client about his conversation with Jerome and the advice he received. The client was devastated about the breakup, but later became incensed at the rejection and filed a complaint with the social work licensing board. When she spoke with the board's investigator, she told him about Kevin's conversation with Jerome that precipitated the breakup. The licensing board sought and secured the revocation of Kevin's license and simultaneously sanctioned Jerome for failing to report sexual exploitation under a state reporting statute and ethics code provision. Jerome was placed on two years' probation, a fact he was required to disclose to each client and on every malpractice renewal application along with the ethics code provision he had violated.

John, Richard, and Carolyn, licensed professional counselors, shared office space together for over 10 years. They maintained separate practices but contributed equally to common office expenses, referring clients to one another and covering for each other during absences. After experiencing a difficult marital breakup, Carolyn began to drink excessively. Her alcohol abuse became evident to John and Richard, and they became concerned for her. They made excuses for her with clients and suggested repeatedly that she take some time off. Richard even tried to convince her that she needed help for substance abuse. Carolyn politely thanked them each time they tried to help her but kept insisting she was going to be all right. She was not impaired. She just needed some time. Late one afternoon, Carolyn screamed obscenities at a client and physically pushed her out of her office and out the front door of the building. The client immediately called the state licensing board. When an investigator interviewed John and Richard, they honestly shared how they had been concerned for some time regarding Carolyn's drinking and erratic behavior. They indicated this was not the first time she had been abusive to a client when she was under the influence of alcohol. To their surprise, the board sanctioned them for failing to report unethical conduct by another licensed counselor. Most state ethical canons provide procedures concerning impaired colleagues. At a minimum, call the licensing board anonymously and seek guidance.

What Is a Reporting Statute?

Every state has laws that will circumvent or supersede general principles of confidentiality. The general perception of U.S. consumers—that information shared between a client and a therapist is sacrosanct and absolutely privileged—is erroneous. The belief in this myth must be dispelled by a therapist as part of informed consent (i.e., informing a client about the numerous exceptions to confidentiality). The HIPAA Privacy Rule purports to protect disclosure of protected healthcare information but specifically provides that covered entities may disclose such information in certain situations. The difference between the Privacy Rule and state reporting statutes is that state laws usually mandate a report. The Privacy Rule uses the word "may." For example C.F.R. 164.512 (b)(1)(ii) provides that covered entities may disclose protected health information to report child abuse or neglect if the report is made to a public health authority or other appropriate government authority that is authorized by law to receive such reports.

Reporting statutes include some of the exceptions to confidentiality that must be disclosed to a client prior to the commencement of therapy. The typical matters that most often fall within a statutory obligation to report are child abuse and neglect, elder abuse, abuse of the physically or mentally impaired, sexual exploitation by a mental health professional, and imminent danger to a client or a third party. The mechanics of each statute and the authorities to whom a report should be made vary with each state and statute. Therapists are sometimes compelled by their professional duties and obligations to disclose

The typical matters that most often fall within a statutory obligation to report are child abuse and neglect, elder abuse, abuse of the physically or mentally impaired, sexual exploitation by a mental health professional, and imminent danger to a client or a third party.

confidential information that ordinarily would be protected by the mental health privilege and ethical concepts of confidentiality. The law has determined that in these instances society's right to protection outweighs a client's right to confidentiality.

National Guidelines for Breaching Confidentiality

American Association for Marriage and Family Therapy (AAMFT) Code of Ethics (2001)

2.2 Marriage and family therapists do not disclose client confidences except by written authorization or waiver, or where mandated or permitted by law.

American Counseling Association (ACA) Code of Ethics (2005)

B.1.c. Respect for Confidentiality

Counselors do not share confidential information without client consent or without sound legal or ethical justification.

B.2.a. Danger and Legal Requirements

The general requirement that counselors keep information confidential does not apply when disclosure is required to protect clients or identified others from serious and foreseeable harm or when legal requirements demand that confidential information must be revealed.

American Psychological Association (APA) Ethical Principles of Psychologists and Code of Conduct (2002)

4.05 Disclosures

(a) Psychologists may disclose confidential information with the appropriate consent of the organizational client, the individual client/patient, or another legally authorized person on behalf of the client/patient unless prohibited by law.

(b) Psychologists disclose confidential information without the consent of the individual only as mandated by law, or where permitted by law for a valid purpose such as to (1) provide needed professional services; (2) obtain appropriate professional consultations; (3) protect the client/patient, psychologist, or others from harm; or (4) obtain payment for services from a client/patient, in which instance disclosure is limited to the minimum that is necessary to achieve the purpose.

National Association of Social Workers (NASW) Code of Ethics (1999)

1.07 Privacy and Confidentiality . . .

(c) Social workers should protect the confidentiality of all information obtained in the course of professional service, except for compelling professional reasons. The general exception that social workers will keep information confidential does not apply when disclosure is necessary to prevent serious, foreseeable, and imminent harm to a client or other identifiable person. In all instances, social workers should disclose the least amount of confidential information necessary to achieve the desired purpose; only information that is directly relevant to the purpose for which the disclosure is made should be revealed.

Know the Codes

Mental health professionals are obligated to know all exceptions to confidentiality, including mandatory reporting statutes. Ignorance of

Mental health professionals are obligated to know all exceptions to confidentiality, including mandatory reporting statutes. Ignorance of the law or ethical rules is not an excuse and will not provide a defense.

the law or ethical rules is not an excuse and will not provide a defense. When legally required to disclose confidential information, a mental health professional is under a legal and ethical obligation to do so. Too many times, mental health professionals are reluctant to make reports because of uncertainty or a reluctance to get involved in what may turn out to be a very messy or nasty legal matter. In most instances, the therapist cannot rely on a client or a third party to make the report. Ethically and legally, it is the provider's primary responsibility to report such behavior. Just as importantly, the therapist should document the report to prove compliance with the statute and ethics code.

In the first vignette, Dr. Kindheart relied on her client to report the child abuse to the proper authorities. Cheryl failed to do so, and it was easily argued that had Dr. Kindheart fulfilled her legal and ethical duty to report the suspected abuse, Susan's stepfather would not have had an opportunity to continue the abuse. An investigation would have commenced immediately. The liability under these facts is threefold. First, we are unaware of any state that does not impose criminal penalties for failure to report child abuse. Second, the damages suffered by the child make a civil lawsuit highly probable. Third, failing to report as required by law is an ethical violation that could lead to licensing board sanctioning. It is foolish to fail to report when one considers the potential consequences as well as that most statutes provide for civil and criminal immunity from prosecution for reports made in good faith.

In the second vignette, Jerome failed in his legal duty as well as his ethical obligation to report Kevin's sexual relationship to the state licensing board as required by the statute dealing with a mental health professional's sexual exploitation of a client. A sanction against Jerome was entirely appropriate. A mental health professional cannot afford to protect friends and colleagues by ignoring ethical obligations.

Ethics codes require reporting ethical violations to state or national organization ethics committees and to state licensing boards.

Ethics codes require reporting ethical violations to state or national organization ethics committees and to state licensing boards. In the third vignette, when Richard and John knew Carolyn was seeing clients while intoxicated and therefore impaired clinically, they had an ethical duty to report her after they had confronted her and she refused to take steps to correct her problem.

National Guidelines for Reporting Ethical Violations

American Association for Marriage and Family Therapy (AAMFT) Code of Ethics (2001)

Principle I: Responsibility to Clients . . .

1.6 Marriage and family therapists comply with applicable laws regarding the reporting of alleged unethical conduct.

American Counseling Association (ACA) Code of Ethics (2005)

H.2 Suspected Violations . . .

H.2.b. Informal Resolution

When counselors have reason to believe that another counselor is violating or has violated an ethical standard, they attempt first to resolve the issue informally with the other counselor if feasible, provided such action does not violate confidentiality rights that may be involved.

H.2.c. Reporting Ethical Violations

If an apparent violation has substantially harmed, or is likely to substantially harm a person and is not appropriate for informal resolution or is not resolved properly, counselors take further action appropriate to the situation. Such action might include referral to state or national committees on professional ethics, voluntary national certification bodies, state licensing boards, or to the appropriate institutional authorities. This standard does not apply when an intervention would violate confidentiality rights or when counselors have been retained to review the work of another counselor whose professional conduct is in question.

(*continued*)

(*Continued*)

American Psychological Association (APA) Ethical Principles of Psychologists and Code of Conduct (2002)

1.04 Informal Resolution of Ethical Violations

When psychologists believe that there may have been an ethical violation by another psychologist, they attempt to resolve the issue by bringing it to the attention of that individual, if an informal resolution appears appropriate and the intervention does not violate any confidentiality rights that may be involved.

1.05 Reporting Ethical Violations

If an apparent ethical violation has substantially harmed or is likely to substantially harm a person or organization and is not appropriate for informal resolution under Standard 1.04, Informal Resolution of Ethical Violations, or is not resolved properly in that fashion, psychologists take further action appropriate to the situation. Such action might include referral to state or national committees on professional ethics, to state licensing boards, or to the appropriate institutional authorities. This standard does not apply when an intervention would violate confidentiality rights or when psychologists have been retained to review the work of another psychologist whose professional conduct is in question.

National Association of Social Workers (NASW) Code of Ethics (1999)

2.11 Unethical Conduct of Colleagues

(a) Social workers should take adequate measures to discourage, prevent, expose and correct the unethical conduct of colleagues.

(b) Social workers should be knowledgeable about established policies and procedures for handling concerns about colleagues' unethical behavior. Social workers should be familiar with national, state, and local procedures for handling ethics complaints. These include policies and procedures created by NASW, licensing and regulatory bodies, employers, agencies, and other professional organizations.

(c) Social workers who believe that a colleague has acted unethically should seek resolution by discussing their concerns with the colleague when feasible and when such discussion is likely to be productive.

(d) When necessary, social workers who believe that a colleague has acted unethically should take action through appropriate formal channels (such as contacting a state licensing board or regulatory body, an NASW committee on inquiry, or other professional ethics committees).

Interpreting the Ethics Codes

These provisions impose an affirmative duty on mental health professionals to informally take action and if necessary formally report and prevent unethical conduct by other mental health professionals. Mental health professionals must report inappropriate dual relationships, unethical sexual relationships, substance abuse, billing fraud, exceeding competence levels, and so forth even if the offender is a close friend or colleague. Providers are obligated to self-police the profession and failing to take action as required is itself an ethical violation.

Providers are obligated to self-police the profession and failing to take action as required is itself an ethical violation.

These cited provisions should cause every practicing professional to be careful when consulting with colleagues about ethical concerns or violations. To do so may impose an ethical dilemma on the friend and colleague concerning whether to report you. A better course would be to consult with a knowledgeable attorney or a person outside the profession who is not under an ethical duty to report a therapist's misconduct. If providers do consult other colleagues about an ethical concern, they should ensure the conversation is agreed to be an academic, hypothetical, or theoretical situation regarding a theoretical case, which "might" present itself. In that way, real circumstances are not discussed, and no one would feel obligated to report questionable behavior.

Ethical Flash Points

- Confidentiality must be breached when legally required by law (i.e., there is a legal duty for the sharing of the information).

- A mental health professional must be knowledgeable regarding all exceptions to confidentiality including mandatory reporting statutes, and these exceptions must be explained to the client before therapy begins. It is an ethical part of informed consent.

- Ignorance is not an excuse or defense, and mandatory reporting statutes must be strictly observed. Mandatory means do it.

- Document all reports to prove compliance.

- It is the therapist's obligation to report abuse or possible harm to the client or a third party.

- Many states have statutes that specifically provide that reporting to a third party (a school principal or supervisor) is not adequate.

- Criminal, civil, and administrative penalties can be imposed for failing to strictly comply with reporting statutes.

- Ethics codes impose a duty on practitioners to self-police and report unethical conduct by other members of the discipline.

- Failure to report a close friend's or colleague's unethical conduct is itself an ethical violation.

- Consulting with a knowledgeable attorney or another person outside the profession regarding unethical conduct may be safer than talking to colleagues since the outsider generally does not have an obligation to report you.

Summary

Although confidentiality is the backbone of therapy, there are numerous times when confidential information must be disclosed. It is absolutely essential for a mental health professional to be thoroughly knowledgeable about all reporting statutes and ethics code provisions that mandate a report of client information or unethical conduct by another mental health professional. Reporting statutes and provisions are designed to protect societal interests, whether it be to protect a child from abuse by a parent or stepparent or to protect an unsuspecting client from misconduct by a therapist.

Strict mandatory compliance is ethically demanded and failure to do so will lead to serious criminal, civil, and administrative (disciplinary) penalties.

Suggested Research Assignments

1. Locate and discuss the reporting obligations required by licensing boards and the law in your state. Which mandatory reporting obligations are most likely to affect your practice?
2. Locate and discuss any state and national professional association reporting obligations. What are their similarities and differences?
3. Compare and contrast the obligations imposed by the state licensing boards in your state with the rules promulgated by the state professional associations.
4. Compare and contrast state licensing board and professional association obligations with the guidelines of national professional associations.
5. Research the decisions of your state licensing boards and state and national professional association ethics committees for reporting obligation violation sanctions.
6. Research the specific reporting statutes in your state applicable to mental health professionals and ascertain the consequences of a failure to comply.
7. Research legal case decisions (criminal and civil) for your state that involve a failure to report by mental health professionals.
8. Talk to practicing mental health professionals in your area and ask them how they handle reporting obligations. Do they have a protocol?
9. Develop a protocol for identifying issues that may require a report and your compliance with that duty.
10. Identify resources that you would consult if you were in doubt regarding a reporting obligation.

11. Locate knowledgeable lawyers in your community whom you can call for immediate advice should a mental health practice–related legal problem occur.

12. Research and determine what information you need to disseminate to potential clients regarding your reporting obligations and the best way to provide them this information.

Discussion Questions

1. A client you have been treating for several months advises you that her husband has been physically abusing her son. What do you do? What do you document?

2. This same client instructs you not to tell anyone because her husband will kill her and her son. What do you do? What do you document?

3. What advice do you give a colleague who thinks the daughter of her 85-year-old client is neglecting the physical needs of the client, is spending the client's money on trips for herself, and is paying her gambling debts?

4. A licensed professional counselor and suite mate with whom you share office space and expenses is coming in to the office in an inebriated state several days per week. What do you do? What, if anything, do you document?

5. A new client asks you to review his therapy records from a previous therapist to see what the therapist might have done wrong. The new client believes that since the therapy did not achieve any appreciable improvement in the client's problems that this previous therapist must be negligent and the licensing board should be notified. What do you do?

6. You see a psychologist whom you know using cocaine in a bathroom during a Christmas party sponsored by a large mental health organization. What do you do?

PART III

PRACTICE CONSIDERATIONS

20

Billing

Susan, a recently retired licensed professional counselor, was unexpectedly subpoenaed to appear at an attorney's office and give a deposition in a divorce case involving a couple she had seen for marriage counseling three years earlier. After reading the subpoena, she immediately contacted her attorney to represent her in a fruitless effort to quash the subpoena. After a court hearing in which she was ordered to appear for the deposition and give testimony, she became inordinately anxious. When her attorney asked her why she was so upset, she advised him that the subpoena required her to produce her case file for this couple, including her billing records. The billing records were her main concern. Although she saw the couple for marital therapy, she billed the husband's insurance company as if she were providing the husband individual counseling for depression because his employer-provided insurance did not pay for marriage counseling. At the time, both husband and wife were happy with the arrangement because it meant they would not have to pay for their marital or family therapy. Now that the couple was in the midst of a custody fight, the husband might not want to have a billing record that suggested he was being treated for depression. Susan was justifiably frightened about the consequences of her billing practices and her questionable creativity in receiving third-party payments. She had documented comments concerning depression, but not enough to justify the diagnosis. Any qualified professional reviewing the case notes would discover fudging in the records and could substantiate this conclusion by interviewing the clients.

When Carol missed her third scheduled therapy appointment without calling to cancel, Robert, her licensed psychologist, sent her a billing statement charging her for the three missed appointments. On receiving the invoice, Carol became incensed and called Robert demanding an explanation. When Robert advised her he felt justified in billing her, she swore she would never pay him. Several months, several invoices, and several disparaging notes from Carol later, Robert filed suit against Carol in small claims court for $300. Carol immediately filed a complaint with the state licensing board accusing Robert of failing to inform her that she would be billed for skipped appointments, for not advising her on a procedure for canceling appointments, and for causing her stress and aggravation that only exacerbated the mental and emotional condition for which she was being treated. Robert brought a lot of grief on himself for $300 that he was unable to collect anyway.

Jane, a suburban housewife, had an affair with her next-door neighbor, the husband of her close friend, for over a year. Overwhelmed with grief, shame, and depression, she contacted Sarah, a licensed professional counselor, for help. Jane didn't want anyone to know she was seeking counseling and told Sarah she wouldn't be in a position to pay her until the end of the month without her husband finding out. They agreed to five sessions over the next 30 days, at the end of which Sarah would bill Jane and Jane would come in and pay cash.

Thirty days later, Sarah sent Jane a bill for her services. The return address on the envelope contained an address without any name or description identifying Sarah. By chance, Jane's husband, George, came home early and removed the mail from the family mailbox. Glancing at the envelope from Sarah, he became curious but did not open it. Instead, he wrote down the return address and the next day on the way to his attorney's office found the address and learned it was the office of Sarah, LPC. He was meeting with his lawyer to finalize divorce pleadings and strategy. When he mentioned Sarah and the envelope, his attorney had a subpoena issued for Sarah, together with Jane's records, for the temporary hearing scheduled to decide temporary custody and exclusive use and possession of the family home.

Sarah was served with the subpoena the night before the hearing, and when she attempted to call Jane at home, her husband answered each time and Sarah hung up without identifying herself. When Sarah walked into the courtroom the next morning, Jane shrieked. Sarah was ordered to testify and turn over her file to the opposing attorney for examination. This file contained information about Jane's affair. Jane lost temporary custody and was ordered to move out of the family home.

Jane was furious with Sarah and filed a complaint with the licensing board alleging breach of confidentiality and failure to obtain written consent to forward billing or any other information to Jane's home. Sarah did not lose her license over this matter, but was publicly reprimanded by the board for the careless practice of contacting a client without the authorization to do so. She was told that she must have permission to write or call a client at any specific number or address. Failure to obtain that permission was a breach of confidentiality.

Billing Practices

It may be hard to believe that billing clients for services can create ethical issues and lead to ethical violations, but it is true. Mental health professionals practice in a climate of consumer protectionism. As consumers, clients must be adequately advised about how they will be charged and billed for services provided, as well as their obligation to pay. Informed consent must be obtained to bill for services rendered, as well as for appropriate billing of missed appointments that were not canceled, sometimes called "no shows."

It is not improper to bill a client for a missed appointment that was not canceled within a proscribed period of time. It is only inappropriate if the client was not previously informed of the cancellation policy and procedure or if a contract with a managed care entity precludes such charges. Likewise, late fees can be billed to a client for payments

Informed consent must be obtained to bill for services rendered, as well as for appropriate billing of missed appointments that were not canceled, sometimes called "no shows."

not received within a set period as long as the practice is disclosed before providing the services. Ethical charges include no-show fees, late fees, interest on past-due accounts, and even attorney's fees and court costs if the account is placed in the hands of an attorney for collection, as long as these charges are disclosed in advance and are part of the signed informed consent in the intake contract.

A therapist providing services to a client pursuant to a provider contract with a managed care entity or insurance company must be aware, however, of any contractual restrictions or limitations. Some provider contracts prohibit the provider from charging and billing the client for any fee except a copay. Under those circumstances, the therapist is not free to bill for skipped or noncanceled appointments. There is no "standard" or "uniform" managed care contract. Each contract is unique, carefully drafted by and for the protection of the managed care entity and must be read carefully.

Protecting Client Confidentiality

The client's right to confidentiality also poses an ethical concern for the therapist with regard to billing. Billing for services requires at a minimum a description of the service provided (i.e., a treatment plan), the date of service, and if submitted to a third-party payer, a diagnosis together with an ongoing and updated prognosis. When the billing is submitted to a third-party payer, it will be reviewed by someone other than the therapist and the client. Consent to submit the information required by the third party should be obtained from the client on intake and when treatment begins, and should be documented before a bill is ever submitted for payment.

The HIPAA Privacy Rule CFR §164.506 (c)(1) provides that a covered entity may use or disclose protected health information for its own treatment, payment, or health-care operations. Even though consent from the client is not mandated for billing purposes, it is permitted by the Privacy Rule and we strongly recommend doing this. The goal should be to leave a consumer without doubt as to the mental health professional's intended uses and disclosures of the consumer's confidential information and to obtain written consent. This will eliminate any potential risk of a sanction or malpractice suit if a client subsequently complains to a licensing board or alleges lack of informed consent. Therapists should obtain a specific address, phone number, e-mail, address, fax number, and other information so that they can contact clients. Therapists should be able to forward billing and other information to them using these contact methods with the client's advance permission. Billing records contain confidential information that therapists usually can share only with client consent. Informing a third party that a person is a client is a breach of confidentiality. Such information must be carefully guarded and protected.

Billing records contain confidential information that therapists usually can share only with client consent.

Confidential information includes all information concerning a client, including whether a person is a client. Allowing a third party to learn an individual is a client through a return address or caller ID on the telephone can be a breach of confidentiality. If the client consents to contact by mail at a particular address or at a specific telephone number, he or she bears the risk and the sole blame and responsibility if a breach of confidentiality occurs. All authority for disclosure can easily be included in an intake and consent form. The consequences for a client of an improperly viewed billing invoice may seldom be as severe as Jane experienced in the second opening scenario, but the result for the mental health professional will still usually be a sanction by the licensing board.

Informing a third party that a person is a client is a breach of confidentiality.

Allowing a third party to learn an individual is a client through a return address or caller ID on the telephone can be a breach of confidentiality.

This might be an appropriate time to review the intake and consent form. It is not sufficient to simply have the client complete or provide an address, but it is important to include specific consent to contact the client at the addresses provided. There can often be a good reason a client does not want to receive e-mails, letters, calls, or bills at any given address. Just because the therapist has this information does not indicate the therapist has a right to use it. A bill from a mental health professional is often more than the spouse needs to know.

Misrepresenting Treatment for Billing Purposes

It is improper to intentionally misstate or miscode a diagnosis on billing statements. Such misrepresentations are considered ethical violations and are punishable offenses. Accuracy and truth in connection

It is improper to intentionally misstate or miscode a diagnosis on billing statements. Such misrepresentations are considered ethical violations and are punishable offenses.

with billing records are absolutely required. Failing to be accurate and truthful not only can lead to ethical violations and licensing concerns but also may lead to criminal charges for fraud or theft. Governmental and private insurance payers are not hesitant to seek criminal prosecution for fraudulent billing practices. The right to audit the provider's accounts, billing records, and procedures is usually included in every managed care contract. Many managed care companies routinely spot-check providers to ensure that billing practices meet company standards.

Susan, the LPC who thought she was doing her clients a favor and helping her cash flow at the same time by miscoding her billing invoices, risked serious consequences for her actions in billing for depression and, in fact, providing marital therapy. She advised her attorney that she had done this with many clients and could name at least 10 colleagues who had submitted similar bills in the past. Susan was lucky because her billing records, although subpoenaed, were not specifically requested by either attorney when she gave her deposition. Her ethical violation in providing one treatment and billing for another did not come to light, and she undoubtedly is still having sleepless nights hoping no one else decides to subpoena, audit, examine, or review her records. More than one unlucky health-care provider has been caught billing for services not actually provided. Accuracy dictates that only services actually performed can be billed and collected. Criminal prosecution is a real probability for this kind of billing practice (e.g., substituting clients or including skipped appointments as if services were rendered).

Collection Agencies/Lawsuits to Collect Fees

The use of third-party debt collection agents to assist mental health professionals is permitted by ethical codes but prior notice to clients is required. The HIPAA Privacy Rule requires the collection agent to execute a Business Associate Agreement (C.F.R. §164.502(e)(2)) to document the agent's adequate assurance to safeguard the protected health information received. Likewise an exception to confidentiality and the mental health privilege usually exists for suits to collect fees for services. (See Chapter 3, "Confidentiality.") The problem with these options is that they may anger a client who already may harbor ill feelings toward the therapist. An angry client is more likely to file a complaint against a therapist with a regulatory authority, and even if the complaint lacks merit it will cause the therapist angst, distress, and expense to defend against it. A lawsuit against the client to collect fees will usually result in the client contacting an attorney who will immediately begin to strategize on counterclaims and suits that will include allegations of malpractice. No professional liability insurance carrier would advocate for aggressive collection practices by an insured party. Walking away from the unpaid fee will almost always be the most prudent option. The occasional unpaid fee is a routine business expense. Good practice would indicate that once a few sessions are unpaid, the therapist should recognize a "collection" problem and termination and a referral should be considered.

Walking away from the unpaid fee will almost always be the most prudent option.

This is often the time when a client suggests a trade-out or bartering arrangement. This, too, is to be avoided, although technically it may be ethical as long as it is completely fair. Figure out a method to terminate the treatment with the consent of the client. Do not be maneuvered into a bartering arrangement, which will ultimately lead to a disastrous future conflict of interest. (See Chapter 23, "Kickbacks, Bartering, Fees, and Gifts")

National Guidelines for Billing Practices

American Association for Marriage and Family Therapy (AAMFT) Code of Ethics (2001)

Principle VII: Financial Arrangements . . .

7.2 Prior to entering into the therapeutic or supervisory relationship, marriage and family therapists clearly disclose and explain to clients and supervisees: (a) all financial arrangements and fees related to professional services, including charges for canceled or missed appointments; (b) the use of collection agencies or legal measures for nonpayment; and

(*continued*)

(Continued)

(c) the procedure for obtaining payment from the client, to the extent allowed by law, if payment is denied by the third-party payer. Once services have begun, therapists provide reasonable notice of any changes in fees or other charges.

7.3 Marriage and family therapists give reasonable notice to clients with unpaid balances of their intent to seek collection by agency or legal recourse. When such action is taken, therapists will not disclose clinical information.

7.4 Marriage and family therapists represent facts truthfully to clients, third-party payors, and supervisees regarding services rendered.

American Counseling Association (ACA) Code of Ethics (2005)

A.10.b. Establishing Fees

In establishing fees for professional counseling services, counselors consider the financial status of clients and locality. In the event that the established fee structure is inappropriate for a client, counselors assist clients in attempting to find comparable services of acceptable cost.

A.10.c. Nonpayment of Fees

If counselors intend to use collection agencies or take legal measures to collect fees from clients who do not pay for services as agreed upon, they first inform clients of intended actions and offer clients the opportunity to make payment.

American Psychological Association (APA) Ethical Principles of Psychologists and Code of Conduct (2002)

6.04 Fees and Financial Arrangements

(a) As early as is feasible in a professional or scientific relationship, psychologists and recipients of psychological services reach an agreement specifying compensation and billing arrangements.

(b) Psychologists' fee practices are consistent with law.

(c) Psychologists do not misrepresent their fees.

(d) If limitations to services can be anticipated because of limitations in financing, this is discussed with the recipient of services as early as is feasible.

(e) If the recipient of services does not pay for services as agreed, and if psychologists intend to use collection agencies or legal measures to collect the fees, psychologists first inform the person that such measures will be taken and provide that person an opportunity to make prompt payment.

National Association of Social Workers (NASW) Code of Ethics (1999)

3.05 Billing

Social workers should establish and maintain billing practices that accurately reflect the nature and extent of services provided and that identify who provided the service in the practice setting.

Ethical Flash Points

- Accuracy and honesty are essential ethical requirements when billing a client.

- This applies to billing, diagnosis, treatment, and prognosis.

- Intentionally miscoding a diagnosis to secure payment for services by a third-party payer can lead to criminal prosecution for fraud or theft.

- Billing for services not actually provided is also unethical and can lead to criminal prosecution.

(continued)

(*Continued*)

- Confidentiality should be a concern for every therapist each time mail or e-mail is sent or calls are placed directly to the client. (Beware of messages delivered to answering machines or call notes.)

- Forward billing to a client only at an authorized address. Follow the same procedures with mail, e-mail, telephone, or other communication.

- Remember, even a casual "You can call me any time," or "Just send the bill to my home (office)" should be noted in the file. Written consent is best. Note the sage words: An oral contract is not worth the paper it is written on. This is true now more than ever.

- Document the client's contact authorization in writing. Include it in your intake and informed consent form, and have the client sign a copy for you to insert in the client file.

- Using third-party collectors or filing a lawsuit to collect unpaid fees is almost always a bad decision because they invite aggressive responses from the client including malpractice counterclaims and licensing board complaints.

An oral contract is not worth the paper it is written on.

Summary

As with sexual exploitation, most billing sins are obvious and blatant ethical violations that may lead to criminal prosecution if committed with intent to defraud a third-party payer. Good judgment and honest behavior will ensure ethical billing practices. Inadvertent breaches of confidentiality may be more innocent but certainly can cause a lot of trouble for a mental health professional. Aggressive collection actions such as the use of third-party debt collectors or filing a lawsuit usually pose an unacceptable risk and should be avoided. Thoughtful and accurate billing procedures will contribute to a healthy and long-term mental health practice and career. One caveat is that when the mental health professional is doing the collecting, the mental health professional has complete control over the collection system—what is said, implied, and represented. However, once a claim is referred to a third party, especially if a third party is receiving a percentage of the amount collected, the therapist loses control over the lines of communication. Thus, while it makes legal sense to be a tough collector, it defies common sense. The rule: Don't let accounts increase to significant amounts. Manage debt sensibly, and, if it gets out of control, stop treatment and make a referral.

Don't let accounts increase to significant amounts. Manage debt sensibly.

Suggested Research Assignments

1. Locate and discuss the billing provisions of the ethical codes promulgated by the mental health profession licensing boards and the law in your state. What limitations do they impose on billing practices?
2. Locate and discuss any state and national professional association billing rules. What are their similarities and differences?
3. Compare and contrast the obligations imposed by the state licensing boards in your state with the rules promulgated by the state professional associations.
4. Compare and contrast state licensing board and professional association obligations with the guidelines of national professional associations.
5. Research the decisions of your state licensing boards and state and national professional association ethics committees for billing violation sanctions.
6. Research state and federal criminal law with respect to health-care billing. Start with your state insurance code and federal fraud and abuse statutes. What are the consequences for a failure to comply?
7. Research legal case decisions (criminal and civil) for your state that involve improper health-care billing by mental health professionals.
8. Talk to practicing mental health professionals in your area and ask them how they handle client billing and the typical billing issues they encounter in their practices.
9. Research and determine what information you need to disseminate to potential clients regarding your billing and collection practices.
10. Develop a protocol for dealing with a client who fails to pay your bill.
11. Identify resources that you would consult if you were having problems collecting an unpaid bill from a client or former client.

12. Contact your professional liability insurance carrier and ask its representatives for advice on billing and collecting from clients.

Discussion Questions

1. A client you have been treating for several months advises you that her husband has lost his job and she can't afford to pay you right now. She asks you if it is okay to keep coming and for the fees to be paid after he goes back to work. What do you do? What do you document?

2. A colleague calls to discuss a matter with you. She had agreed to five sessions with a client over 30 days and to bill the client after the last session when the client anticipated receiving a bonus from his employer. Three bills and 90 days after the last session, the bill is still unpaid. What advice do you give the colleague?

3. A family friend and a church pastor asks you as a favor to him to see a couple who need marriage counseling and are having financial problems. He has referred you much business over the years. When the couple comes to the first session, they advise you that they still have coverage for 30 days under the husband's insurance policy through his former employer. They ask you to schedule as many sessions over the next 30 days as possible and for you to bill the insurance company. What do you say? What do you do? What, if anything, do you document?

4. A client who has turned out to be suffering from borderline personality disorder calls and demands you refund the fees she has paid you for seven sessions she now views as worthless and incompetent therapy sessions. What do you say? What do you do? What, if anything, do you document?

5. A significant rise in the costs of operating your office necessitates an increase in your fees. How will you raise your fees? What steps should you take? Can you prospectively begin billing your existing clients at the higher rate?

21

Establishing a Practice

Albert, a licensed social worker, toiled for many years in a state agency providing social work services. When he got fed up, he abruptly resigned, took a 2-week vacation, and went to the mountains. He then opened his own office when he returned to town. His immediate supervisor at the agency was incensed by the fact that Albert quit without notice while he was servicing and responsible for a large caseload. After shuffling Albert's clients to other social workers, the supervisor filed a complaint with the state licensing board. He charged Albert with patient abandonment and unprofessional conduct. Albert was sanctioned by the licensing board and put under supervision for a 12-month period.

Carolyn spent 2 years working for a local counseling center as an LPC intern and employee accumulating the necessary supervised hours for full licensure. When she became a fully licensed counselor, she resigned from the counseling center and opened her own office. Shortly thereafter, the counseling center learned that Carolyn, without their knowledge, consent, or approval, had sent out a notice to all clients and former clients of the counseling center announcing her departure, providing the address and phone number for her new practice location and inviting clients to contact her if they were in need of services. She had also removed the files for each client with whom she had direct client contact while employed at the center. The counseling center director sent a letter demanding return of the files and threatening legal action. Who had the right to possession of the files?

Karen and Susan attended graduate school together and remained in close contact with one another as they completed the licensing process for marriage and family therapists in their state. When each secured a state license, they decided to open a therapy office together. They rented space and began promoting their practice. Their brochures indicated they offered services for all emotional and psychological conditions on a sliding-fee scale. The pastor of a large local church approached them about referring members of his congregation who had substance abuse problems. Although Karen and Susan had never personally worked with substance abusers in the past, they indicated to the pastor that they would gratefully work with anyone the pastor referred to their practice. Are they heading for trouble?

Transitioning to an Independent Practice

Many people choose to become licensed professional service providers with the specific goal of having an independent practice. Being one's own boss and controlling one's destiny appeals to many people. Starting a professional therapy practice can be an exciting and career-fulfilling dream. It can also be a time when the practitioner is confronted with the increased risks of an ethical dilemma and violation. Most practitioners do not experience instant financial success when opening a new practice, and start-up and operational costs can be overwhelming. The temptation to take on more than the therapist is competent or prepared to handle can be great. Careful and deliberate consideration and planning must precede the opening of an independent practice prior to welcoming the first patient into the office.

Careful and deliberate consideration and planning must precede the opening of an independent practice prior to welcoming the first patient into the office.

With the requirement of provisional licensing by virtually all mental health licensing boards, practitioners will first have to consider how and when they transition to an independent practice. They will be employed or practicing under supervision at the time they become fully licensed. Even if they have been fully licensed for some time, therapists wishing to open an independent practice have duties and obligations to their existing clients and employers. In the opening scenario, Albert inappropriately handled his transition to an independent practice and was appropriately sanctioned. His actions were both unfair and unprofessional to his employer and constituted unethical abandonment of his clients. Good practice would dictate appropriate notice to the agency, a review of current and past files, and the arranging of an orderly transition that supports the procedures of the agency, together with compliance with ethical and legal guidelines and the needs of the clients.

National Guidelines for Termination of Practice

American Association for Marriage and Family Therapy (AAMFT) Code of Ethics (2001)

Principle I: Responsibility to Clients . . .

1.10 Marriage and family therapists assist persons in obtaining other therapeutic services if the therapist is unable or unwilling, for appropriate reasons, to provide professional help.

1.11 Marriage and family therapists do not abandon or neglect clients in treatment without making reasonable arrangements for the continuation of such treatment.

American Counseling Association (ACA) Code of Ethics (2005)

A.11. Termination and Referral

A.11.a. Abandonment Prohibited

Counselors do not abandon or neglect clients in counseling. Counselors assist in making appropriate arrangements for the continuation of treatment, when necessary, during interruptions such as vacations, illness, and following termination.

(continued)

(Continued)

National Association of Social Workers (NASW) Code of Ethics (1999)

1.16 Termination of Services

(b) Social workers should take reasonable steps to avoid abandoning clients who are still in need of services. Social workers should withdraw services precipitously only under unusual circumstances, giving careful consideration to all factors in the situation and taking care to minimize possible adverse effects. Social workers should assist in making appropriate arrangements for continuation of services when necessary. . . .

(e) Social workers who anticipate the termination or interruption of services to clients should notify clients promptly and seek the transfer, referral, or continuation of services in relation to the clients' needs and preferences.

(f) Social workers who are leaving an employment setting should inform clients of appropriate options for the continuation of services and of the benefits and risks of the options.

Before a therapist can step out into an independent practice, existing clients receiving services must be effectively provided for. Until such provision can be made, a therapist would have to delay plans to leave in order to open his or her own office (see Chapter 13, "Terminating Therapy").

Is it appropriate for withdrawing therapists to take clients with them into an independent practice? Generally speaking, clients choose the provider from whom they secure services. A client would be free to follow the therapist into that therapist's private practice. However, the therapist must not exploit clients by soliciting them when establishing the independent practice. It may be that the client will be better served by continuing to receive services from the entity the therapist has withdrawn from. If so, the therapist establishing the independent practice has a duty to discuss this with the client.

National Guidelines for Client Transfer

American Psychological Association (APA) Ethical Principles of Psychologists and Code of Conduct (2002)

10.04 Providing Therapy to Those Served by Others

In deciding whether to offer or provide services to those already receiving mental health services elsewhere, psychologists carefully consider the treatment issues and the potential client's/patient's welfare. Psychologists discuss these issues with the client/patient or another legally authorized person on behalf of the client/patient in order to minimize the risk of confusion and conflict, consult with the other service providers when appropriate, and proceed with caution and sensitivity to the therapeutic issues.

National Association of Social Workers (NASW) Code of Ethics (1999)

3.06 Client Transfer

(a) When an individual who is receiving services from another agency or colleague contacts a social worker for services, the social worker should carefully consider the client's needs before agreeing to provide services. To minimize possible confusion and conflict, social workers should discuss with potential clients the nature of the clients' current relationship with other service providers and the implications, including possible benefits or risks, of entering into a relationship with a new service provider.

Sometimes therapists enter into contractual agreements with employers when they begin working for that employer. These contracts may limit the options upon withdrawal from employment with respect to contact and future treatment with current and former clients and those clients of the entity that the therapist did not treat. The entity and its officers will have a duty to work with the departing therapist to best provide continuing care for clients being treated by that therapist. Unilateral action as taken by Carolyn in the second opening scenario may be prohibited. Absent such an agreement, Carolyn still may have acted unethically in sending promotional material to her own clients and those clients of her former employer that she did not provide services to. This could be considered inappropriate solicitation. It is hard to imagine Carolyn being referred any clients from her former employer as a result of her actions. If there is an employment contract with the agency, the terms of that contract are controlling. An employed therapist who wishes to enter private practice or other employment would be wise to have an attorney review the current contract in order to determine if the transition will be trouble free or if the change will be the beginning of an ethical violation or continuing litigation.

If there is an employment contract with the agency, the terms of that contract are controlling.

National Guidelines for Recruiting Clients and Staff

American Counseling Association (ACA) Code of Ethics (2005)

Section C, Professional Responsibility

C.3.d. Recruiting through Employment

Counselors do not use their places of employment or institutional affiliation to recruit or gain clients, supervisees, or consultees for their private practices.

National Association of Social Workers (NASW) Code of Ethics (1999)

2.04 Disputes Involving Colleagues

(a) Social workers should not take advantage of a dispute between a colleague and an employer to obtain a position or otherwise advance the social workers' own interests.

> (b) Social workers should not exploit clients in disputes with colleagues or engage clients in any inappropriate discussion of conflicts between social workers and their colleagues.

Mental health professionals have a duty to uphold the integrity of their disciplines and attempting to lure clients away from a previous employer or another therapist can be unseemly, undignified, and unethical. It does not serve the best interests of the profession or the client and should be avoided. The departing therapist should strive to take the high ground at all times. Former employers and colleagues can be great referral sources if the departure is handled openly, amiably, and cooperatively.

In withdrawing from employment, consideration should be given to client records. Mental health professionals and employers often get crosswise concerning who has a right to possess client records. A withdrawing therapist may wish to take records for the clients treated and will assert an ethical obligation to maintain client records for the requisite retention period (see Chapter 25, "Record Keeping"). The entity will assert that the clients treated by the withdrawing therapist are in fact entity clients and the entity has the obligation to create, maintain, and secure the records. An important motivation behind the dispute is the future business (income) represented by the clients. The departing therapist should defer to the entity's claim. The entity may own the file (have the right and duty to maintain and secure the information), but the client has the right to the information in the file. If clients choose to follow a therapist into a new or independent practice, then these clients can request a copy of their files and present the copy to the withdrawing therapist. Alternatively, the withdrawing therapist, with the client's authorization, can also request a copy directly.

The transition requires thoughtful planning and processing on client care, notification of clients, and maintenance and security of client records. Until each of these areas is appropriately managed and provided for, with the client's best interest at the forefront, actual opening of the independent practice should not occur.

Former employers and colleagues can be great referral sources if the departure is handled openly, amiably, and cooperatively.

Opening the Practice

Opening the independent practice involves many practical, legal, and ethical considerations. Unfortunately, therapists cannot turn to their professional guidelines for a precise and recommended course of action to follow in establishing a practice. Their graduate school education may have provided them with little insight on how to go about setting up an independent office. Taking business and accounting classes is not the norm for students pursuing a master's degree in a mental health discipline. Even if the therapeutic services are of the highest quality, a practice can fail due to poor business practices. Business relationships and contracts are a necessity; poorly negotiated agreements can doom the practice to failure before the first client ever walks in the door. Getting good, competent professional advice from attorneys, real estate or leasing agents, accountants, insurance agents, bankers, financial planners, and other colleagues is critical in successfully establishing a practice.

Ethical overtones are found in just about every decision made in establishing a practice, including legal, contractual, or business matters. These decisions must be made well in advance of opening the practice. Some of the more obvious areas of ethical concern that must be thought out prior to opening the practice are discussed next.

Practice Forms

Before a client is seen in the practice, the appropriate forms should be prepared and reviewed by the therapist and a knowledgeable attorney. These would include, but are not limited to, intake and consent forms, history forms, authorizations, HIPAA Notice of Privacy Practices, and business associate agreements. These forms should ensure compliance with the therapist's ethical duty to secure informed consent for treatment and disclosure of information to third parties when required (see Chapter 7, "Informed Consent").

Privacy

Therapy must be provided in an environment that ensures client confidentiality and privacy. Consideration must be given to the physical location in which services will be provided. Will the conversations between the therapist and the client be private, or is there a possibility for a third party to overhear what is being said? Consideration must also be given to the privacy, physical maintenance, preservation, and security of client records. What medium will be used to create and store records? How will the records be maintained and secured (see Chapter 25, "Record Keeping")?

Competency

It would be a very unusual and gifted therapist who could rightly conclude that he or she was competent to treat every client and every psychological condition or problem that came into the office. Determining your competence and confidence level and then matching them to clients and problems you accept into your practice is key to avoiding an ethical or malpractice mistake. Each therapist has to be aware of his or her own limitations and restrictions. Knowing who and what you will treat and being firm in the application of this knowledge can preclude taking on a client when financial necessity tempts you. Exceeding your level of competence is ethically prohibited (see Chapter 4, "Dangerous Clients"; Chapter 5, "Discrimination"; Chapter 9, "Prohibited Clients"; and Chapter 13, "Terminating Therapy," for discussions on competency). Knowing who and what problems you wish to treat will be helpful if you intend to do any promotion or advertising for your practice.

Karen and Susan in the third opening scenario are probably making a huge mistake in trying to assist clients with substance abuse issues when they have never worked with these problems. They should at least consider engaging a colleague with substance abuse treatment experience who can offer supervision.

Consultation and Referral

At some point, sooner rather than later, a therapist opening a new practice will need to consult with a colleague on a treatment issue or refer a client to another therapist. Creating a list of licensed, competent colleagues to call on when and as the need arises will benefit not only the therapist but the client as well. Mental health professionals have an ethical duty to consult and refer when necessary and must be prepared for this eventuality (see Chapter 13, "Terminating Therapy," and Chapter 22, "Closing or Interrupting a Practice," for discussions on referrals).

Practice Interruption or Cessation

All practitioners have a duty to prepare, and have ready for implementation, procedures in the event they die, become incapacitated, or simply wish to take a vacation. These procedures must be in place before any clients are treated. It is a wise practice to secure client consent to the proposed procedures at the time informed consent to treatment is obtained (see Chapter 22, "Closing or Interrupting a Practice"). Determine if clients will have the option of reaching you outside of normal business hours and, if so, how this will be accomplished. Note that if you offer to be available, you will need to respond to any late-night client contacts you receive.

Staff Training and Supervision

If the hiring of full- or part-time employees will occur, planning for their training, especially with respect to client privacy, HIPAA regulations, and confidentiality, is critical. Therapists who hire employees are responsible for the actions of their employees committed in the course and scope of their employment. Ethical guidelines require appropriate training and supervision of employees and the services they provide. There is a duty to hire competent staff and to assign duties that are compatible with an employee's ability and experience. Clients need to be made aware of the function of employees and the confidential information that the employees will be accessing to do their jobs. HIPAA Privacy and Security Rules require documentation of employee training in the areas of privacy and security of protected health-care information. Before an employee can begin work and before the first client presents at the office, the employee must be thoroughly trained and commit to respecting the privacy of patient identities and information (see Chapter 3, "Confidentiality").

Therapists who hire employees are responsible for the actions of their employees committed in the course and scope of their employment.

Fees

Pricing is a key factor in just about every business. This is usually determined by the cost of operations and the desire to make a profit. Mental health professionals, however, have an ethical duty to charge reasonable fees. Extravagant office expenses may not justify a fee significantly out of the norm for practitioners in the same area. The fee policy must be disseminated to clients before treatment begins. In opening a practice, a therapist will have to decide how much to charge and whether the practice will accept third-party payments or only direct payments from clients. Imbedded in this decision will be the question of making application for inclusion in managed care programs that necessitate accepting third-party payments (see Chapter 23, "Kickbacks, Bartering, Fees and Gifts").

Advertising and Promotion

If "you build it, they will come" is not going to be true 99 percent (or more) of the time. It will be essential to get the word out about your new practice. Truthful advertising is ethically permissible, but deceitful or misleading information is never permitted. In addition, direct one-on-one client solicitation, no matter how accurate, may not be allowed. Advertising consultants need to be advised of the special ethical considerations that a mental health professional has in promoting the practice (see Chapter 6, "False and Misleading Statements").

National Guidelines for Ethical Issues in Establishing a Practice

American Association for Marriage and Family Therapy (AAMFT) Code of Ethics (2001)

Principle II: Confidentiality . . .

2.4 Marriage and family therapists store, safeguard, and dispose of client records in ways that maintain confidentiality

(continued)

(Continued)

and in accord with applicable laws and professional standards.

Principle VII: Financial Arrangements

Marriage and family therapists make financial arrangements with clients, third-party payors, and supervisees that are reasonably understandable and conform to accepted professional practices.

7.2 Prior to entering into the therapeutic or supervisory relationship, marriage and family therapists clearly disclose and explain to clients and supervisees: (a) all financial arrangements and fees related to professional services, including charges for canceled or missed appointments; (b) the use of collection agencies or legal measures for nonpayment; and (c) the procedure for obtaining payment from the client, to the extent allowed by law, if payment is denied by the third-party payor. Once services have begun, therapists provide reasonable notice of any changes in fees or other charges.

American Counseling Association (ACA) Code of Ethics (2005)

Section C Professional Responsibility . . .

C.2.a. Boundaries of Competence

Counselors practice only within the boundaries of their competence, based on their education, training, supervised experience, state and national professional credentials, and appropriate professional experience. Counselors gain knowledge, personal awareness, sensitivity, and skills pertinent to working with a diverse client population.

Section D Relationships with Other Professionals . . .

D.1.f. Personnel Selection and Assignment

Counselors select competent staff and assign responsibilities compatible with their skills and experiences.

American Psychological Association (APA) Ethical Principles of Psychologists and Code of Conduct (2002)

5.06 In-Person Solicitation

Psychologists do not engage, directly or through agents, in uninvited in-person solicitation of business from actual or potential therapy clients/patients or other persons who because of their particular circumstances are vulnerable to undue influence. However, this prohibition does not preclude (1) attempting to implement appropriate collateral contacts for the purpose of benefiting an already engaged therapy client/patient or (2) providing disaster or community outreach services.

National Association of Social Workers (NASW) Code of Ethics (1999)

1.07 Privacy and Confidentiality

(c) Social workers should protect the confidentiality of all information obtained in the course of professional service, except for compelling professional reasons. . . .

(i) Social workers should not discuss confidential information in any setting unless privacy can be ensured. Social workers should not discuss confidential information in public or semipublic areas such as hallways, waiting rooms, elevators, and restaurants.

2.05 Consultation

(a) Social workers should seek the advice and counsel of colleagues whenever such consultation is in the best interests of clients. . . .

(continued)

(Continued)

2.06 Referral for Services

(a) Social workers should refer clients to other professionals when the other professionals' specialized knowledge or expertise is needed to serve clients fully or when social workers believe that they are not being effective or making reasonable progress with clients and that additional service is required.

Ethical Flash Points

- Transition obligations:

  - Inform employers and existing clients as soon as practicable of your intention to withdraw and open an independent practice.

  - Work with the employer and clients in the systematic and smooth transfer of clients and client care responsibilities to other professionals. If time and circumstances permit, conduct an exit interview with each client.

  - Prepare transfer summaries where needed and, with client permission, call the therapist taking over the file to discuss the case in more detail. Make sure the client and subsequent therapist know you will be available for a limited period of time. Document this offer to cooperate with subsequent providers.

  - All case notes, client files, and progress notes must be up-to-date. All correspondence that pertains to a file should be answered.

  - Discuss with the employer the issue of client files. Seek an agreement to remove the client files for any clients that will be moving with you to your new practice. If the employer is reluctant to allow the files to be moved, attempt to reach agreement on obtaining a photocopy of the file.

  - Be sure that the files for the clients you treated will be adequately maintained and secured by the employer for the requisite retention period if you do not take these files with you.

- Work out the details with the employer on how clients and former clients will be notified of your departure and what information should be provided to them. Cooperating with the employer may be critical to letting clients and former clients know how to find you.

- The best approach is to be open, straightforward, fair, and reasonable with the employer. Remember the entity and its professionals can be a good referral source for you in the future.

- Business contracts:

- Contracts with managed care companies, hospitals, insurance companies, and businesses must be analyzed and when possible, negotiated. Ethical obligations of the therapist must be kept in mind. For example, if a managed care contract requires that all clients be referred back to the managed care company if the treating therapist is unable to assist the client and the therapist knows there is not a therapist on the company's panel qualified to treat the client, there is an ethical dilemma. The therapist has a duty to refer the client to a source that can help that client. Special language may be required in the contracts to protect the therapist's ethical obligations and options. Seek competent legal and professional assistance early.

- Real property leases or purchase contracts must be entered into. Most mental health professionals starting a practice lease office space. Should you lock in a favorable rent for a longer period of time or negotiate a short-term lease at a higher rent, possibly with options? Consideration must be given to all financial terms, and, as with other contracts, special concern must be given to the therapist's ethical duties. Most commercial leases allow for the landlord to lock out the tenant in the event of default by the tenant. Because a mental health professional has a duty to maintain, secure, and make available client files, an exception for access to or removal of client files must be provided for in the lease. The office space must be adequate for the practice and provide for the maximum amount of client privacy. Work with your own leasing agent when possible.

- Rental agreements and contracts for telephone, Internet and fax, Yellow Pages advertisements, Web pages, and other services must be viewed from a financial and ethical perspective. Price shopping and product and service comparisons will result in more prudent selections. When working with advertising agents, make sure they are acquainted with your ethical obligations as a mental health professional.

(continued)

(Continued)
- Make sure you have adequate insurance, including professional liability (malpractice), general liability (premises), content insurance, business interruption insurance, and document protection insurance. Engage a reputable independent insurance agent to assist you in obtaining the best coverage at the best price. Usually, securing multiple kinds of coverage from the same company will result in the best overall pricing.

- You will have a choice of entities to choose from in establishing your practice. These will include a sole proprietorship, a partnership, a corporation, a limited liability company, and a professional limited liability company. You should consult with a knowledgeable business attorney and tax advisor in making this decision. The type of entity chosen does matter.

- Practice matters:

  - Practice forms that are tailored for your practice, including a detailed client consent form, should be drafted, reviewed, and revised before the first client arrives. Get competent legal assistance and ask colleagues to review your forms as well.

  - Determine the medium in which client information will be created and stored. Develop policies and procedures for the creation, retention, and dissemination of client information. If records are created, stored, and transferred electronically, be sure the policies and procedures are compliant with the HIPAA Security Rule.

  - Develop and be prepared to implement a practice cessation or interruption plan. Ask colleagues to review your proposed plan for completion and effectiveness.

  - Determine your level of competency, and make a conscious decision on what types of clients and problems you will treat and which ones you will not treat. Talk to colleagues who know you best to see if they agree with your self-assessment.

  - Put together a list of competent therapists you can consult with and refer to when necessary.

  - If full- or part-time employees are to be hired, seek the most capable candidates possible and then plan and implement an internal training program that will thoroughly acquaint them with privacy and security issues. Document the training and ask employees to commit in writing to protecting client privacy and confidentiality. If possible, arrange for employees to take continuing education courses to increase their knowledge and to polish and improve their skills.

(Continued)

- Determine your fee policy and reduce it to writing and include it in your intake and consent forms. Talk to other practitioners in your area to determine the reasonableness of your fees.

- Memberships, licenses, and subscriptions:

  - Be sure you have a copy of your current professional license to display as well as all other information your licensing board requires you to display in your office. This will usually include a sign with information on how clients can contact the licensing board to file a complaint.

  - Take a look at the options you have for membership in professional organizations, especially local chapters. They can provide good networking opportunities, support, and sometimes access to insurance programs. Each of these organizations has annual dues, so it is important to prioritize the organizations that offer the most advantages.

  - Consider local chambers of commerce or other business or professional organizations to provide you with networking and promotional opportunities.

Summary

Establishing an independent practice can be the culmination of a life-long dream. It can result in tremendous satisfaction and reward. It also brings greater financial obligation and risk. It is often the financial pressures that tempt a therapist into an ethical violation or just poor judgment. Taking the time to plan, research, and develop policies and procedures for the practice well in advance of opening the doors to clients will give the practice the greatest chance of success and limit the risk of an ethical miscue. If the competency level and confidence of the therapist are low, opening an independent practice should be a last resort. If there is no other option for gaining experience, the therapist should consider engaging a seasoned therapist to consult with on a regular basis as the therapist and practice develop.

Assemble a team of competent and knowledgeable professionals to work with you on establishing and then operating the practice. These will include attorneys, accountants, bankers, financial experts, and in-surance specialists. Look for individuals who can be with you for the long term and with whom you would be comfortable providing and receiving referrals.

Suggested Research Assignments

1. Locate and discuss the provisions of the ethical codes promulgated by the mental health profession licensing boards and the law in your state that impact on the establishment of an independent practice. What obligations to they impose? What guidance do they offer?

2. Locate and discuss any state and national professional association rules impacting on the establishment of an independent practice. What are their similarities and differences?

3. Compare and contrast the obligations imposed by the state licens-ing boards in your state with the rules promulgated by the state professional associations.

4. Compare and contrast state licensing board and professional associ-ation obligations with the guidelines of national professional associations.

5. Research the decisions of your state licensing boards and state and national professional association ethics committees for violation sanctions related to practice establishment.

6. Talk to practicing mental health professionals in your area and ask them how they went about establishing their practices. What ad-vice do they have for you?

7. Identify resources that you would consult to assist you in establish-ing an independent practice.

8. Contact your professional liability insurance carrier and ask its representatives for advice on establishing an independent practice.

9. Apply the state licensing board rules for your discipline to the sce-narios at the beginning of the chapter. What would you advise? What are the possible outcomes?

Discussion Questions

1. A colleague calls and asks you to consider opening a counseling office with her. She has just been fired by her employer but wanted to go into business for herself anyway. What concerns would you have? What questions would you ask?

2. What documents and forms would you want to prepare in advance of establishing your independent practice? How would you go about preparing them?

3. You have made the decision to leave your employment with a counseling center to open your own practice. What steps do you take, when do you take them, and why?

4. What considerations would you expect from a mental health professional whom you employed for five years if this person was about to withdraw from your company?

5. How would you promote your new independent practice?

6. What would you do if an employee resigned from your counseling practice without notice and took all the files for each client this person was currently treating and had treated during her years of employment?

22

Closing or Interrupting a Practice

With a busy practice, Penny, a licensed professional counselor, enjoyed a good income and lifestyle. One day on her way to the office, she was involved in an automobile accident. Weeks later, she was still in a coma. Her distraught husband had no idea what he should do about her practice so he just ignored it and concentrated on Penny and her ongoing medical care. A client became angry because she had taken off work to come to a scheduled therapy session and then was unable to reach Penny by phone. She had no knowledge of the car accident and filed a complaint against Penny with the state licensing board. Months later when Penny recovered, she was sanctioned by the board for her lack of a plan for her practice should death or incapacity occur.

Dr. Stern has been in practice for 35 years and is ready to retire. His office lease, Yellow Pages ad, and managed care contracts are all terminating at the end of the year. His malpractice insurance will also run out on December 31. All his client files are in order and he has maintained them for 10 years, although he also kept his first client's file for sentimental reasons. Now that he has decided to retire, Dr. Stern is unsure what to do first. The decision to retire was difficult. The steps to a successful retirement are even more complex and require more detailed concentration and implementation.

Alice Gump is a play therapist. Over the past few years, she has had an active practice treating children and young adolescents using the latest techniques and some advanced theories she has developed herself. Because of her cutting-edge therapy, several clients whose children she treated have filed complaints with the licensing board, others have written to the national organization of play therapists, and one has retained a lawyer to file a malpractice suit. Alice has ample insurance, but she feels she can do better financially and live a happier and more carefree life if she changes professions. "Dealing with unhappy clients makes the practice not worth the effort," she said. She decides to close her office and focus on a very successful family business.

Drs. Tom, Dick, and Harry have leased office space together, use the same stationery, share a sign on the door, and use the same general telephone number with individual extensions. To some extent, they cooperate when managed care and insurance are concerned, and they have a lawyer-drafted contract that provides that any unhappy professional can withdraw from the group at any time on 60-days' notice. It also provides that the person leaving is fully accountable for all personal therapy contracts that extend beyond the withdrawal date. Dick becomes ill, and his physician insists he retire. Can he simply shake hands with Tom and Harry, wish them well, and retire on his income disability insurance? What must he do?

The Puentes are a husband-and-wife therapy team both licensed by the state and operating a thriving business consisting primarily of private pay clients. He deals principally with marriage and family problems, whereas she is a highly regarded play therapist. After a routine physical and additional testing, Dr. Puente's physicians discover he has Alzheimer's, a debilitating disease that will become progressively worse with time. His wife is not able to incorporate her husband's clients into her practice. What do the Puentes do now?

Deciding to Close a Practice

There are many reasons for closing a practice. In two-career families, the mental health professional's spouse might be transferred or
offered a position in another city that is "too good to resist." Or,
after years of practice, the therapist may feel burned out and ready
to establish a new career. Some practitioners have attended risk
management workshops and concluded that, in the age of consum-
erism, the risk of continuing in a private practice is not worth the
income or rewards received. Some entrepreneurial therapists have
sold their practices to large organizations for significant profit and
closed their therapeutic doors. Then there are the fortunate ones
who over the years have accumulated a substantial nest egg, built a
thriving practice, and are ready now to retire and bask in the good
memories of thousands of satisfied and paying clients. Whichever
way it comes about, a mental health professional with client files;
former and current clients; listings and memberships in local, state,
and national organizations; and state-issued licenses cannot simply
wait until a lease is up, buy a sign that says "gone fishing" or "retired" or "call 123-4567 if you need assistance," insert a new message on the answering machine, and disappear. A therapist, social
worker, counselor, psychologist, addictions specialist, or mental
health professional who leaves a practice for any reason—personal
or business, expressed or implied, forced or voluntary—must follow
correct procedures. There are ethical provisions for terminating a
professional practice and handling a temporary practice interruption, and therapist-client relationships can become legal problems
(i.e., a malpractice suit) if ignored or followed incorrectly. Lawyers
may introduce an ethics violation into evidence to demonstrate
that a provider breached his or her duty to the client and damaged
the client by not following the ethic provisions for closing a practice (see Chapter 15, "Ethics Codes as Evidence"). Ethics and law
are intertwined to a significant degree when it comes to malpractice
allegations. In our litigious society, technical rules for closing a
practice must be followed meticulously.

There are ethical provisions for terminating a professional practice and handling a temporary practice interruption, and therapist-client relationships can become legal problems if ignored or followed incorrectly.

Covering All the Bases

For some therapists, closing their practice is the result of a carefully conceived, orchestrated, and thought-out plan in which the practitioner has consulted the licensing board, national organizations, the attorney, accountant, professional colleagues, and malpractice carrier. Armed with the knowledge and input from all these sources, the therapist gradually and systematically implements the agreed-on plan and shuts down the practice. These therapists have made all preparations, met all deadlines, and considered the termination dates of all agreements. They have appropriately referred all clients, made arrangements for the security and confidentiality of the files, and taken steps to retrieve the files on a selective basis if needed. No client is abandoned or neglected.

On other occasions, the end of the road is not predictable. Therapists sometimes cannot predict when they will retire. Sickness or sudden mental or physical disability may impair therapists to a degree that prevents them from continuing their practice on a temporary or permanent basis. To continue would be inappropriate and unethical in itself and might lead to negligence and malpractice actions.

Sometimes a practice is closed because a licensing board has revoked the therapist's license to practice. Numerous board complaints may have accomplished the same result by inhibiting the therapist's ability to obtain malpractice insurance, attract or maintain clients, or gain hospital privileges. Complaints may also make it difficult to obtain referrals or associate with colleagues. Some professionals inadvertently lose their licenses because they fail to continue forwarding their Continuing Education Units or neglect to pay their licensing fees.

Still other mental health professionals simply find the paperwork, approval procedures, or complexities of dealing with insurance companies for third-party reimbursement too cumbersome. They decide they are no longer willing or able to confront and process the mountain of necessary forms and paperwork and opt instead to retire or pursue a different career—coaching or consulting, for example.

The reasons for retirement or withdrawal are not important. A practitioner who chooses to withdraw from the practice for any reason may do so, but to do so ethically, he or she must consider certain concerns and hazards.

Considerations When Closing a Practice

A therapeutic practice is not like a bookstore or grocery chain where the owner simply has to gather the remaining inventory, sell it to the public or donate it to charity, and then close the shop. Therapists have numerous long- and short-term obligations to colleagues, their profession, clients, and business associates. In addition, therapists must honor their contractual agreements with individuals, corporations, and partnerships. Therapists cannot turn to their professional guidelines for a precise and recommended course of action to follow in transitioning into retirement, or a new profession or a practice interruption. The ethics codes do not delineate a definitive retirement or interruption sequence or a critical path to retirement heaven or a well managed temporary break from the practice. Many graduate-level programs of an advanced rank do not focus on what happens when a practice is closed, and what the consequences are to a retiring or disabled professional.

Therapists cannot turn to their professional guidelines for a precise and recommended course of action to follow in transitioning into retirement, a new profession, or a practice interruption.

Ethical and Legal Obligations

When closing a mental health practice or planning for a practice interruption, therapists need to consider potential legal liabilities, contractual obligations, and ethical and moral dilemmas. They must also decide what to do with client files and how long to maintain them. Should they be stored in a closet or garage, put through a shredder, or sent to the dumpster? In the case of an interruption in services, who will be responsible for client records in the therapist's absence must also be considered. And, should the client file be required for legal or therapeutic reasons, who will be responsible for releasing and then re-preserving them further at a later time when they are no longer needed?

When closing a mental health practice, therapists need to consider potential legal liabilities, contractual obligations, and ethical and moral dilemmas.

Although some professional obligations are contractual and legal, they may also have ethical overtones:

- Leases are contractual obligations. If they continue after the projected date of retirement or interruption of the practice, they must be considered and negotiated either by paying an agreed amount or by fulfilling the balance of the lease term. Leases cannot be abandoned without legal consequences.
- Advertising and listing contracts with telephone companies, newspapers, magazines, and Yellow Pages are often for long terms that must be honored. Therapists must make arrangements for responding to potential clients who answer these print, radio, or other types of perpetual advertisements. Also, the printed matter or hard copy can survive long after the contractual obligation terminates. Individuals have a habit of preserving old phone books and advertising literature.
- Mental health professionals often belong to associations, partnerships, joint ventures, corporations, and limited partnerships. The precise terms of these organizational structures may contain the process and procedure for termination and withdrawal. Each contract and agreement must be reviewed and analyzed. The terms of the agreements voluntarily entered into years ago bind the retiring or withdrawing individuals.
- External contracts between the individual and organizations may be continuing and long term. Not only leases, but contracts with managed care entities, insurance companies, hospitals for in- or outpatient services, and contracts to provide mental health treatment to groups for extended periods have to be considered and honored. Failing to honor these and other long-term obligations can easily lead to licensing board complaints, as well as a breach of contract or malpractice suit. In general, malpractice policies will not cover contractual defaults.
- Review malpractice policies to ensure that acts of commission or omission covered during practice continue to be covered after retirement.
- For an interruption in your practice, make sure policies are renewed and maintained in force until you return to the practice and then reestablished.

- In some situations, professional guidelines are not specific concerning retirement, relocation, the total and complete closing of a practice, and future temporary or permanent unavailability of the therapist. When this occurs, the client's best interests should always be considered and reasonable steps taken to protect the client, client records, and the client's future needs.
- Retirement or practice interruption should be considered with the same thoughtfulness and consideration as establishment of a practice. Disestablishment has different legal and ethical considerations. Each individual should have his or her own critical checklist so no stone is left unturned.

Planning for Retirement

An ethical complaint can be filed after retirement as can a malpractice or breach of contract suit. Continuing insurance coverage is desirable in the event of either of these unpleasant events. Likewise, litigation, ethical complaints, and current contracts "in the mill" have to be legally, ethically, and contractually honored and concluded.

An ethical complaint can be filed after retirement as can a malpractice suit. Continuing insurance coverage is desirable in the event of either of these unpleasant events.

Planning for all obligations to terminate on a given date is impossible. Leases have different termination dates. Clients likewise recover at different times. Therapists planning to retire need to consider when to start declining additional clients. Group practices must be terminated in an orderly fashion, with consideration given to colleagues, clients, and business associates.

The perfect blend is a detailed retirement plan that considers the needs of the retiring professional, the requirements of the consumer or the client, and the general reputation of the profession. Retiring and closing a practice with dignity and risk free is achievable, although complex. It requires thorough and careful planning.

Planning for a Practice Interruption

An ethical complaint can be filed during an interruption in a therapist's practice, as Penny discovered in the opening scenario when she recovered from her car accident. A malpractice suit is also a real possibility. As with retirement, continuing insurance coverage is desirable in the event of a practice interruption. Likewise litigation, ethical complaints, and current contracts "in the mill" have to be legally, ethically, and contractually honored and concluded.

Many practice interruptions are planned. A sabbatical of sorts for the practitioner is one example. In those instances, the therapist faces very similar issues and should implement similar procedures that apply to retirement. Unexpected interruptions, however, pose different concerns and considerations. What should be done in the short term becomes critical. If the therapist is unable to resume practicing, then either the therapist or the therapist's legal representative should follow the steps necessary for closing the practice.

A death or incapacity plan must be in place before the unexpected occurs because ethical practice requires anticipation by the mental health professional of the unexpected.

There must be advance planning with respect to who initially can step in and access and maintain files, contact clients, transition clients to new treatment providers, and deal with the myriad contract obligations of the practice or practitioner. A death or incapacity plan must be in place before the unexpected occurs because ethical practice requires anticipation by the mental health professional of the unexpected. Ensuring the best possible outcome for clients when a therapist is permanently or temporarily unavailable is the achievable goal.

National Guidelines for Closing or Interrupting a Practice

American Association for Marriage and Family Therapy (AAMFT) Code of Ethics (2001)

Principle I: Responsibility to Clients

1.10 Marriage and family therapists assist persons in obtaining other therapeutic services if the therapist is unable or unwilling, for appropriate reasons, to provide professional help.

1.11 Marriage and family therapists do not abandon or neglect clients in treatment without making reasonable arrangements for the continuation of such treatment.

Principle II: Confidentiality

2.5 Subsequent to the therapist moving from the area, closing the practice, or upon the death of the therapist, a marriage and family therapist arranges for the storage, transfer, or disposal of client records in ways that maintain confidentiality and safeguard the welfare of clients.

American Counseling Association (ACA) Code of Ethics (2005)

A.11. Termination and Referral

A.11.a. Abandonment Prohibited

Counselors do not abandon or neglect clients in counseling. Counselors assist in making appropriate arrangements for the continuation of treatment, when necessary, during interruptions such as vacations, illness, and following termination.

C.2. Professional Competence

C.2.h. Counselor Incapacitation or Termination of Practice

When counselors leave a practice, they follow a prepared plan for transfer of clients and files. Counselors prepare and disseminate to an identified colleague or "records custodian" a plan for the transfer of clients and files in the case of their incapacitation, death, or termination of practice.

American Psychological Association (APA) Ethical Principles of Psychologists and Code of Conduct (2002)

3. Human Relations

3.12 Interruption of Psychological Services

Unless otherwise covered by contract, psychologists make reasonable efforts to plan for facilitating services in the event that psychological services are interrupted by factors such as

(continued)

(Continued)

the psychologist's illness, death, unavailability, relocation, or retirement or by the client's/patient's relocation or financial limitations.

6. Record Keeping and Fees

6.02 Maintenance, Dissemination, and Disposal of Confidential Records of Professional and Scientific Work

(a) Psychologists maintain confidentiality in creating, storing, accessing, transferring, and disposing of records under their control, whether these are written, automated, or in any other medium.

(b) Psychologists make plans in advance to facilitate the appropriate transfer and to protect the confidentiality of records and data in the event of psychologists' withdrawal from positions or practice.

National Association of Social Workers (NASW) Code of Ethics **(1999)**

1.07 Privacy and Confidentiality

(o) Social workers should take reasonable precautions to protect client confidentiality in the event of the social worker's termination of practice, incapacitation, or death.

1.15 Interruption of Services

Social workers should make reasonable efforts to ensure continuity of services in the event that services are interrupted by factors such as unavailability, relocation, illness, disability, or death.

3.04 Client Records

(d) Social workers should store records following the termination of services to ensure reasonable future access. Records should be maintained for the number of years required by state statutes or relevant contracts.

Ethical Flash Points

- Executory contracts (contracts to be performed in the future):

  - Contracts with managed care, hospitals, insurance companies, and businesses have to be terminated. Many can be terminated satisfactorily by negotiation, but they cannot be ignored. For example, many professionals have long-term contracts to provide mental health treatment to clients, employees, and staff. These must be terminated and other providers substituted, if possible.

  - Rental agreements and contracts for telephone and fax services, Yellow Pages advertisements, Web pages, and other services must be timed to end on the retirement date or negotiated so they do not carry postretirement obligations.

  - Cancel utilities, phone, and other services where appropriate.

- Client obligations:

  - Inform clients as soon as practicable of your intention to close your practice.

  - If not accomplished in the intake form, obtain authorization from the client to deliver the client record to another competent professional.

  - Prepare transfer summaries where needed and, with client permission, call the therapist taking over the file to discuss the case in more detail. Make sure the client and subsequent therapist know you will be available for a limited period of time.

  - All case notes, client files, and progress notes must be up-to-date. All correspondence that pertains to a file should be answered.

  - Check with your national and state organization, as well as the licensing board, and then call the malpractice carrier. Make sure you have scrupulously followed all the prerequisites for closing a practice.

  - Client files are confidential, and this obligation continues postretirement. Most state licensing laws as well as civil statutes indicate the number of years a file must be maintained, secured, and preserved. Clients have a right to view these files for the number of required years and afterward as long as they are in existence and in the possession of the therapist or a successor therapist. In case of any complaint, the preserved file is the first line of defense.

  - Even retired therapists can sue and be sued, and may be subpoenaed into court at any time, either with or without the file. Therefore, the file must be accessible as

(continued)

(Continued)

well as secure. The retained file protects both the provider and the consumer. A well-preserved, complete file that cannot be located is no file at all. This is also true for a computer record where disks or drives are no longer operable. The preservation of confidential files implies that the files are accessible in readable form.

- Although a therapist may terminate the therapeutic relationship and retire at any time without obtaining client permission, there remains an ethical obligation to cooperate with a subsequent therapist in a meaningful manner. An available file will ensure that the information offered will be accurate and helpful to a subsequent therapist as well as the client.

- Continuing clients normally are entitled to an exit interview. The client should be advised of additional community resources, other competent providers, and be provided with written posttreatment recommendations. A termination letter would be appropriate.

- Individual client needs or circumstances may require a therapist to provide therapy even after all other clients are terminated. As with any termination, careful consideration must be given to the client's emotional and psychological condition and to timing the termination properly.

- For former clients who are only now discovering the therapist has retired, a recorded message should direct them to a relief therapist who has not reviewed their file but has access. Confidentiality should be maintained.

- Client obligations continue for the statute of limitations period even after therapy has terminated. Confidentiality continues until the file is destroyed. The statute of limitations is extended for minors or individuals who are out of the country.

- Since death, disability, relocation, forced retirement, and other unforeseen circumstances are always a possibility, the intake form should contain a clause that permits the therapist to arrange for the transfer of the clinical record to another competent professional if any of these circumstances should occur. Thus, the client would give the provider or the professional permission in advance to store and preserve the file in a protected facility with a licensed professional in charge. Arrangements could then be made between professionals to make the files accessible.

- Clinical files:

  - Files should be summarized, indexed, and itemized so that they can be located.

  - If boxed, each box must be clearly marked and labeled.

- The storage facility must be secure, locked, dry, and free of mildew and rodents. Storing files after therapy has terminated and postretirement is a necessary expense.

- Access to client records must be limited to such individuals with a legal right to know the contents and a legal right of entry. All access should be on a "need-to-know" basis.

- Mail, phone, e-mail, and other correspondence:

  - Mail addressed to a retired therapist should be forwarded to the therapist for response, if possible. Otherwise, a designated responsible professional should send a prepared letter to the addressee explaining the therapist's retirement and nonavailability and suggesting alternative resources. Some arrangements have to be made to access the file if therapeutically warranted or if desired by the client.

  - A telephone message must notify callers of the therapist's retirement and list alternative sources for treatment.

  - If e-mail is used as a treatment option, it should be recognized in the intake and consent form, and an "all-points" e-mail should be sent announcing the retirement and outlining alternative treatment options. Confidentiality is as important with e-mail as it is for other addresses and phone numbers. Client information must be safeguarded regardless of the communication medium involved.

- Terminating business relationships:

  - Most business contracts have termination provisions and procedures established in the agreement. Before retirement, these must be reviewed to determine whether the parties have terminated in the prescribed manner. Litigation of any type should be avoided. Mediation, if needed, can be a big help to parting (soon to be former) associates. Consider including mandatory mediation and/or arbitration clauses into any contract before it is signed.

  - Many technical details must be taken care of to dissolve a partnership, corporation, limited partnership, professional association, and other created entities and relationships. Therapists should employ a lawyer and banker, as well as an accountant and financial planner to facilitate the dissolution.

  - Usually a lawyer-drafted written termination or dissolution agreement is appropriate.

  - A handshake, pat on the back, and mutual good wishes do not comprise a sound legal dissolution.

(continued)

(*Continued*)
- Memberships, licenses, and subscriptions:

  - Continuing professional memberships should be terminated. Send notices to professional groups and organizations as needed. It is better to have a termination letter in the professional association's file than for the provider to be finally dropped from the association because of delinquency or nonpayment of dues.

  - If your license is to lapse or terminate, make sure it is properly handled according to licensing board requirements.

  - Ongoing subscriptions can either lapse or be stopped if a refund is possible. Some subscription contracts for advertisements and magazines have automatic renewal clauses, so canceling such subscriptions in writing is preferred.

  - Malpractice insurance may terminate on the date of retirement; however, it is important to obtain continued coverage for claims made due to past actions. Check with the insurance professional and seek out all the options. Generally, it is a good idea to purchase a "tail," a continuing policy that offers the provider coverage for all the years of practice whether or not any claim is or has been made or threatened. Such a policy enables the mental health professional to sleep at night knowing that past activities are covered by insurance to the extent of the policy coverage and limits.

Summary

The list of retirement considerations contains many suggestions for the retiring therapist as well as the therapist planning a temporary leave from the practice. Many of these same ideas should be reviewed and incorporated into the active therapist's death or incapacity plan. In addition, the following suggestions should be addressed by a mental health professional long before something unexpected occurs:

- Arrange for a qualified mental health professional who can *immediately* step in and appropriately access confidential client information in order to alert clients of their treatment provider's death or incapacity, to safeguard client records and make them available to clients or subsequent treatment providers, make appropriate referrals to new treatment providers, inform the licensing boards, professional organizations

and malpractice insurance carrier of the therapist's condition and practice interruption.

- Secure written client consent for the selected qualified mental
  health professional to access the client's confidential information or
  at least secure written consent for the therapist to designate a competent mental health professional who can access the client's information in the event of an unexpected practice interruption.
- Have a will and guardian document prepared that designates a per-
  son(s) who can qualify for court appointment as the therapist's estate representative or legal guardian. This person will need to step
  in and make all the decisions necessary to keep the practice viable
  during the therapist's incapacity or to close it down if the therapist
  dies. This same person should be provided in advance with all relevant information about contractual obligations and insurance coverages of the therapist and practice. This person will be able to access
  bank accounts and make necessary payments and handle the business decisions that will need to be made.
- Create and maintain good client and up-to-date business records
  and make sure they can be located, accessed, and understood by the
  person(s) selected to step into the therapist's shoes.

Whatever the reason for the practice interruption or cessation,
the mental health professional must be prepared in advance so client harm is minimized. A review of ethical canons makes clear this
duty exists, but little specific direction is provided. This is one area
of practice that most health-care providers give too little thought to
because to do it correctly requires a great deal of advance planning
and preparation. Do yourselves and your clients a big favor: Plan and
prepare.

Suggested Research Assignments

1. Locate and discuss the practice closing and interruption provisions of the ethical codes promulgated by the mental health
   profession licensing boards and the law in your state. What obligations do they impose? What guidance do they offer?

2. Locate and discuss any state and national professional association practice closing and interruption rules. What are their similarities and differences?

3. Compare and contrast the obligations imposed by the state licensing boards in your state with the rules promulgated by the state professional associations.

4. Compare and contrast state licensing board and professional association obligations with the guidelines of national professional associations.

5. Research the decisions of your state licensing boards and state and national professional association ethics committees for practice closing and interruption violation sanctions.

6. Research legal civil case decisions for your state that involve improper practice closing or interruption by mental health professionals.

7. Talk to practicing mental health professionals in your area and ask them how they handle actual and anticipated practice interruptions. See if they take it seriously as recommended in this chapter.

8. What clauses might be inserted in your original intake and consent form that will protect both you and the client?

9. Research and determine what information you need to disseminate to potential clients regarding your practice interruption procedures.

10. Develop a protocol for dealing with an anticipated practice interruption (i.e., if you and your spouse take a 3-month sailing trip).

11. Develop an actual death or incapacity plan that you will implement in your practice.

12. Identify resources that you would consult with to assist you in developing a practice interruption plan.

13. Contact your professional liability insurance carrier and ask its representatives for advice on planning for retirement or a practice interruption.

14. Apply the state licensing board rules for your discipline to the scenarios at the beginning of the chapter. What would you advise? What are the possible outcomes?

Discussion Questions

1. A colleague calls and asks for your help. She has been diagnosed with cancer and will require extensive treatment that will necessitate her shutting down her practice at least temporarily. What do you advise her to do?

2. What characteristics would you want a person to have if you were going to designate him or her as the person who would step into your practice in the event of your death or incapacity?

3. What information would you want to have if a colleague indicated you were his choice to step into his practice if anything happened to him?

4. What is your responsibility if you take over the file of another professional?

5. What do you do if you take over a colleague's file and discover that the colleague was professionally negligent by acts of omission or commission?

6. Your wife has just been named dean of the social work program for a major university and you will be moving shortly. When you advise your clients that you will be terminating with them and will assist them in finding a new therapist, one of your most needy clients refuses to consider letting you terminate. This client indicates you will be abandoning her and you are the only person who can help her. What do you say? What do you do? What do you document?

7. Can you transition all your clients to Internet therapy in the event you are going to relocate to another state? What ethical and treatment implications does this idea present?

23

Kickbacks, Bartering, Fees, and Gifts

Over several years, Sharon, a school counselor and licensed professional counselor, referred more than 100 clients to Dr. Kindheart, a licensed marriage and family therapist and a member of Sharon's church. As an expression of gratitude, Dr. Kindheart bought two tickets to a series of musicals— a $300 value—and sent them with a card to Sharon. When Sharon shared her delight at having received the unexpected gift with another school counselor, she was surprised by her colleague's response. She was advised that accepting the gift was unethical and that it was unethical and perhaps illegal for Dr. Kindheart to send the gift.

When Carol, a recently licensed social worker, answered an advertisement regarding office space for lease, the psychiatrist who owned a small office building offered her a terrific deal. He offered her a corner office without a fixed rental payment. He suggested that Carol simply pay him 20 percent of all fees she collected from her clients and an additional 10 percent of any fees collected from clients referred to her by the psychiatrist. Without an established practice, Carol found the offer very appealing, moved in, and began faithfully paying the appropriate percentages to the psychiatrist. Two years later when the psychiatrist was investigated for insurance fraud, Carol came under investigation by state law enforcement officials for an illegal fee-sharing arrangement. She was also challenged by the state licensing board.

Cheryl, a discontented and separated housewife, offered a psychologist an old piano in payment for therapy. After much deliberation, the psychologist, a pianist of some accomplishment, agreed to provide 20 hours of therapy at the normal session rate of $120 per hour in exchange for the piano. Six months later, Cheryl and her husband reconciled thanks in part to improvements achieved through the therapy. When Cheryl's husband moved back into the marital residence, he was shocked to see the piano missing. He became furious when he learned Cheryl had traded it for $3,000 worth of therapy. The piano, when new 20 years ago, had been purchased for $15,000. He filed suit, and judgment was entered against the psychologist for the fair market value of the piano plus attorney fees. The husband also filed a complaint with the therapist's licensing board.

Dr. Mortale was spending a long overdue and well-deserved secluded summer vacation in Big Bucks Point, Florida, when a call came in on his cell phone. He had published widely in the field of suicide prevention and catered to a wealthy clientele of retired, but unhappy and bored, mature children of the "old money" generation. Mrs. Frantic was calling from the suspension bridge over the bay, where her husband (who had tried and conspicuously failed three times so far to commit suicide) was threatening to jump.

Dr. Mortale knew that a therapist should not treat a client without first negotiating a fee, and that the fee should be within the client's ability to pay. Knowing that this client (Mrs. Frantic) could pay just about any fee charged, he quoted, and she accepted, a $1 million fee to talk-by-cell-phone to Mr. Frantic, who would talk only to Dr. Mortale. Thirty minutes later, a more relaxed and relieved Mr. Frantic came down from the bridge, hugged his wife, and returned home. Can Dr. Mortale send the bill for $1 million, or is the transaction unreasonable? After all, the therapist saved Mr. Frantic's life, as well as avoiding incredible public exposure and embarrassment.

Referral Fees

Most therapists sense that paying someone for making referrals is wrong or at least questionable. Ethics codes leave little room for doubt. When a psychologist pays, receives payment from, or divides fees with another professional other than in an employer-employee relationship, the payment to each is based on the services (clinical, consultative, administrative, or other) provided and not on the referral itself.

The payment of referral fees is an acceptable practice in many other industries but is not tolerated in the delivery of mental health services. Why not? Why shouldn't we allow therapists to develop and cultivate referral sources to enhance income and increase a practice? Isn't that consistent with good American business principles? Isn't it appropriate and in good character to thank people appropriately for a kindness rendered? In the mental health field, it is not good business nor acceptable because the potential for abusing the client is too great. Mental health professionals have an obligation to make referrals to the best possible sources of care for their clients. If payment is made to a referring party, a question could arise concerning why the referral was made. Was it made so a referral fee could be collected or because it was the best possible source of care? This is another area in which the mental health profession strives to avoid even the hint or appearance of abuse or the risk of exploitation. Making a referral is a clinical decision, and a decision based even in small part on an actual or potential referral fee would have a difficult time passing muster against a challenge of clinical objectivity.

Are arrangements whereby a mental health professional pays a percentage of fees earned and collected in lieu of rent permissible? Fees can be split if the shared fee is reasonably and rationally related to the services actually provided by the nontreating person or entity. It may be difficult to establish the reasonable and rational relationship between the fees paid to a landlord and the value of the space provided to the treating therapist. The burden will be on the mental health professional to establish the relationship. Such arrangements, although not absolutely forbidden, should be avoided. Good

When a psychologist pays, receives payment from, or divides fees with another professional other than in an employer-employee relationship, the payment to each is based on the services (clinical, consultative, administrative, or other) provided and not on the referral itself.

Mental health professionals have an obligation to make referrals to the best possible sources of care for their clients.

bookkeeping over a protracted period of time can furnish evidence of a rational relationship.

National Guidelines Regarding Accepting Kickbacks

American Association for Marriage and Family Therapy (AAMFT) Code of Ethics (2001)

Principle VII: Financial Arrangements

7.1 Marriage and family therapists do not offer or accept kickbacks, rebates, bonuses, or other remuneration for referrals; fee-for-service arrangements are not prohibited.

American Psychological Association (APA) Ethical Principles of Psychologists and Code of Conduct (2002)

6. Record Keeping and Fees

6.07 Referrals and Fees

When psychologists pay, receive payment from, or divide fees with another professional, other than in an employer-employee relationship, the payment to each is based on the services provided (clinical, consultative, administrative, or other) and is not based on the referral itself.

National Association of Social Workers (NASW) Code of Ethics (1999)

2.06 Referral for Services

(c) Social workers are prohibited from giving or receiving payment for a referral when no professional service is provided by the referring social worker.

National and State Statutes

Federal and state statutes make kickback arrangements in connection with health-care criminal acts subject to fine and imprisonment. They are typically much broader in scope than just criminalizing fee-sharing or fee-splitting arrangements. According to national and state statutes, offering or accepting a seemingly innocent and thoughtful gesture such as musical tickets in connection with one or more referrals would be a criminal as well as an unethical act. Doing more than offering a verbal thank-you is prohibited. Receiving more than verbal appreciation from the professional to whom the referral was made is also prohibited. Anything more would constitute a reward and bring the act within the purview of criminal statutes.

Vernon's Texas Statutes Annotated Prohibition on Illegal Remuneration

A person commits an offense if the person intentionally or knowingly offers to pay or agrees to accept any remuneration directly or indirectly, overtly or covertly, in cash or in kind, to or from any person, firm, association of persons, partnership, or corporation for securing or soliciting patients or patronage for or from a person licensed, certified, or registered by a state health-care regulatory agency.

Bartering

Mental health professionals should also avoid bartering for services. A trade has potential for unfair advantage since the playing field is never level. Bartering leaves a mental health professional open to allegations of abuse and the risk of client exploitation. Bartering is an ancient and long-accepted method of exchanging goods and services. It was a necessity when there was no monetary system to drive and facilitate commerce. It is common today in many countries with devalued currency. However, due to the potential for exploitation, bartering is not a recommended practice by any of the mental health disciplines.

If bartering is accepted, it has to be at the client's suggestion, but also it must not be exploitative, must be documented by written

According to national and state statutes, offering or accepting a seemingly innocent and thoughtful gesture such as musical tickets in connection with one or more referrals would be a criminal as well as an unethical act.

Receiving more than verbal appreciation from the professional to whom the referral was made is also prohibited.

Bartering leaves a mental health professional open to allegations of abuse and the risk of exploitation.

informed consent, and must be an accepted practice among professionals where the therapist is providing services. It will be a very unusual and rare circumstance that can meet this burden. Even though bartering, just as fee sharing, is not absolutely prohibited, payment for services rendered in cash, by check, or by credit card appears to be the most ethically sound and defensible practice.

National Guidelines Regarding Bartering

American Association for Marriage and Family Therapy (AAMFT) Code of Ethics (2001)

Principle VII: Financial Arrangements

7.5 Marriage and family therapists ordinarily refrain from accepting goods and services from clients in return for services rendered. Bartering for professional services may be conducted only if: (a) the supervisee or client requests it, (b) the relationship is not exploitative, (c) the professional relationship is not distorted, and (d) a clear written contract is established.

American Counseling Association (ACA) Code of Ethics (2005)

A.10.d. Bartering

Counselors may barter only if the relationship is not exploitive or harmful and does not place the counselor in an unfair advantage, if the client requests it, and if such arrangements are an accepted practice among professionals in the community. Counselors consider the cultural implications of bartering and discuss relevant concerns with clients and document such agreements in a clear written contract.

American Psychological Association (APA) Ethical Principles of Psychologists and Code of Conduct (2002)

6. Record Keeping and Fees

6.05 Barter with Clients/Patients

Barter is the acceptance of goods, services, or other nonmonetary remuneration from clients/patients in return for psychological services. Psychologists may barter only if (1) it is not clinically contraindicated, and (1) the resulting arrangement is not exploitative.

National Association of Social Workers (NASW) Code of Ethics (1999)

(b) Payment for Services

Social workers should avoid accepting goods or services as payment for professional services. Bartering arrangements, particularly involving services, create the potential for conflicts of interest, exploitation, and inappropriate boundaries in social workers' relationships with clients. Social workers should explore and may participate in bartering only in very limited circumstances when it can be demonstrated that such arrangements are an accepted practice among professionals in the local community, considered to be essential for the provision of services, negotiated without coercion, and entered into at the client's initiative and with the client's informed consent. Social workers who accept goods or ser-vices from clients as payment for professional services assume the full burden of demonstrating that this arrangement will not be detrimental to the client or the professional relationship.

Fees

What can a mental health professional charge for professional services? In the United States and within its free enterprise system, is it

The Ethics Code requires fees to be reasonable and not excessive.

not what the market will bear? In these days of $100 million professional sports contracts, why shouldn't the therapist be able to charge whatever the client is willing to pay? Why? Because the Ethics Code requires fees to be reasonable and not excessive.

The sky is not the limit in setting fees even if the therapist by virtue of education, experience, and skill is considered to be the top practitioner in the community. A "reasonable fee" is dependent on the client's ability to pay and what other therapists in the community are charging. Therapists should avoid even the appearance of exploitation. Fees, including late charges, the use of collection agencies, and charges for responding to record requests or subpoenas to give testimony, must be disclosed prior to beginning therapy (see Chapter 7, "Informed Consent" and Chapter 20, "Billing"). Nevertheless, providing clients with all necessary information concerning fees and obtaining informed consent does not excuse an excessive or unreasonable fee. The unequal power positions of the mental health professional and the client in the therapeutic relationship necessitate special consideration and divergence from free-market concepts in the areas of setting fees and bartering.

A "reasonable fee" is dependent on the client's ability to pay and what other therapists in the community are charging.

The intent of the Ethics Code is to protect the client from monetary exploitation by mental health professionals. The ACA even expects its members to assist clients in finding affordable services if the counselor's reasonable fee is beyond the client's ability to pay. Charging an excessive fee even if the client agrees to it is an ethical violation subjecting mental health professionals to the full range of sanctions and consequences.

National Guidelines for Setting Fees

American Association for Marriage and Family Therapy (AAMFT) Code of Ethics (2001)

Principle VII: Financial Arrangements

Marriage and family therapists make financial arrangements with clients, third-party payors, and supervisees that are reasonably understandable and conform to accepted professional practices.

American Counseling Association (ACA) Code of Ethics (2005)

A.10. Fees and Bartering

A.10.B. Establishing Fees

In establishing fees for professional counseling services, counselors consider the financial status of clients and locality. In the event that the established fee structure is inappropriate for a client, counselors assist clients in attempting to find comparable services of acceptable cost.

American Psychological Association (APA) Ethical Principles of Psychologists and Code of Conduct (2002)

6. Record Keeping and Fees

6.04 Fees and Financial Arrangements

(a) As early as is feasible in a professional or scientific relationship, psychologists and recipients of psychological services reach an agreement specifying compensation and billing arrangements.

(b) Psychologists' fee practices are consistent with law.

(c) Psychologists do not misrepresent their fees.

National Association of Social Workers (NASW) Code of Ethics (1999)

1.13 Payment for Services

(a) When setting fees, social workers should ensure that the fees are fair, reasonable, and commensurate with the services performed. Consideration should be given to clients' ability to pay.

Gifts

As with bartering, gifts are not strictly prohibited by ethical codes. In Texas, the rule applicable to licensed professional counselors states: "The licensee shall not give or accept a gift from a client or a relative of a client valued at more than fifty dollars" (Title 22 Texas Administrative Code§681.41(k)(2)). There are two concerns regulatory authorities have with gifts. One is the possibility of client exploitation, which could be significant. The other issue is the erosion of therapeutic boundaries that could occur if a therapist accepts even nominal gifts from a client. Gifts are fraught with peril because of a therapist's inability to be 100 percent certain of the client's motivation in bestowing the gift. If the client has an ulterior motive and does not obtain the desired result from the gift, the therapist can expect problems including a complaint with a licensing board. Although gifts of small value under certain circumstances can be permitted, a wiser practice is to maintain and disseminate to clients prior to commencing treatment a rigid policy of not accepting or giving gifts.

We are often confronted with this question in ethics workshops: "What about the flowers or crayon drawings I am given by the children that I work with?" Our response is that we perceive young children as being pure in heart and we don't have the same concern for some improper underlying motivation behind the gift as we would with adolescents or adults.

National Guidelines Regarding Gifts

American Association for Marriage and Family Therapy (AAMFT) Code of Ethics (2001)

Principle III: Professional Competence

3.10 Marriage and family therapists do not give to or receive from clients (a) gifts of substantial value or (a) gifts that impair the integrity or efficacy of the therapeutic relationship.

American Counseling Association (ACA) Code of Ethics (2005)

A.10. Fees and Bartering

A.10.E. Receiving Gifts

Counselors understand the challenges of accepting gifts from clients and recognize that in some cultures, small gifts are a token of respect and showing gratitude. When determining whether or not to accept a gift from clients, counselors take into account the therapeutic relationship, the monetary value of the gift, a client's motivation for giving the gift, and the counselor's motivation for wanting or declining the gift.

Ethical Flash Points

- Paying or receiving referral fees is unethical and illegal.

- Never give or receive more than a hearty verbal thank-you (a cordial note is also acceptable) in connection with the referral of a client.

- Clients are to be referred to the best possible sources for care and treatment consistent with their ability to pay.

- Splitting fees in lieu of rent is problematic and could be construed as illegal fee sharing.

- Bartering, although not absolutely prohibited, should be avoided. The therapist has the burden of establishing that the transaction is ethical. The therapist will always have an obligation to show that the transaction was inherently "fair."

- Bartering must be requested by the client; must not be exploitative; must be documented in the form of written, informed consent; and must be practiced by professionals in the community.

- Only rarely is bartering considered ethical.

(continued)

(*Continued*)
- Fees must be reasonable and not excessive.

- The mental health professional cannot charge whatever the client will pay even after obtaining informed consent. The client's agreement to pay does not make the fee ethical.

- Reasonableness is a function of what is charged in the locality and the client's ability to pay.

- Accepting gifts from a client, although not absolutely prohibited, should be avoided as well. The therapist has the burden to establish that the client was not exploited and the gift was appropriate under the circumstances.

- A better policy will be an absolute prohibition on accepting gifts from clients or giving clients gifts.

- Occasional small gifts or artwork from children are not as problematic.

Summary

Regardless of the fee arrangement, the burden will always be on the mental health professional to establish that the fee was reasonable, appropriate in the community where the services were rendered, and adequately disclosed in advance of therapy to the client. Establishing that the client was not exploited becomes problematic when high fees are charged or bartering takes place in lieu of exchanging money for services. The same is true with gifts accepted from a client. The free-enterprise, whatever-the-market-will-bear mentality, is not acceptable in the delivery of mental health-care services. The relationship of therapist and client is not the same as that of the store clerk and customer.

Suggested Research Assignments

1. Locate and discuss the provisions of the ethical codes promulgated by the mental health profession licensing boards and the law in your state with regard to referral fees, bartering, fees, and gifts. What is prohibited and what obligations do they impose?

2. Locate and discuss any state and national professional association rules with regard to referral fees, bartering, fees, and gifts. What are their similarities and differences?

3. Compare and contrast the obligations imposed by the state licensing boards in your state with the rules promulgated by the state professional associations.

4. Compare and contrast state licensing board and professional association obligations with the guidelines of national professional associations.

5. Research the decisions of your state licensing boards and state and national professional association ethics committees for sanctions imposed for violations relating to referral fees, bartering, fees, and gifts.

6. Is bartering or the giving of gifts altered if the counseling entity is sponsored by a church or other religious organization?

7. Research legal civil case decisions for your state that involve improper referral fees, bartering, fees, or gifts by mental health professionals. Have they heard rumors about bartering or excessive fees?

8. Talk to practicing mental health professionals in your area and ask them about their fees and how they determine what fee to charge a client.

9. Research and determine what information you need to disseminate to potential clients regarding your fees.

10. Research state statutes and federal fraud and abuse statutes. What are the penalties they impose for violations?

11. Contact your professional liability insurance carrier and ask its representatives for advice on setting fees.

Discussion Questions

1. A physician who refers you a significant number of clients each year calls and asks if he and his family can use your lake house for the weekend. What do you say? What do you do?

2. The wife of a couple in family therapy creates Plexiglas works of art. Each time she comes to your office, she brings a small sample and moves around your personal collectables so she can fit the new object on the shelf. What do you do? What do you document? At this time it is of negligible value, but who knows what these creations will be worth in the future?

3. What would you consider a reasonable fee in your location for your services? Why?

4. What do you tell a client who presents you with an expensive art piece during the termination session? What do you say? What do you do? What do you document? Would your answers be different if the session was not the final termination session?

5. What would you do about a colleague who shows you a pearl necklace she says she just received from a recently terminated client?

6. The spouse of one of your clients sends you a pair of theater tickets with a note thanking you for the work you have done with his wife. What do you say? What do you do? What do you document?

7. Is it reasonable and permissible to charge a higher rate for giving testimony in a client's case than for your therapy sessions?

24

Malpractice Insurance

Allen, a licensed marriage and family therapist, became sexually involved with the 32-year-old daughter of a retired couple he saw for marital therapy. She lived with her parents and became acquainted with Allen when she provided transportation for her parents to and from therapy sessions after her father broke his hip and was unable to drive. It was several months before the parents noticed the way their daughter and Allen looked at each other when they met in the reception area of Allen's office. When they asked their daughter on the way home about these intimate glances, she laughed and told them she had been dating Allen and was in love with him. The parents were upset and immediately called Allen to confirm the news. The next day they filed a complaint with the state licensing board and consulted an attorney regarding a malpractice lawsuit. Should Allen be comforted by the fact that he faithfully paid all his malpractice insurance policy premiums?

Susan is a licensed social worker. She made a practice of miscoding billing statements to bring her services within the coverage scope of her clients' insurance policies. Her clients were delighted with this practice, and Susan made a decent living until an insurance provider investigated, discovered the deception, and reported Susan to the district attorney's office and the state licensing board. In addition, the insurance provider brought a civil action to recover thousands of dollars in payments made to Susan over the years. Can Susan relax, secure in the knowledge that her malpractice insurance carrier will take care of these problems for her?

Scott, a psychologist under investigation by his state licensing board for sexual misconduct, agreed to a license suspension. In need of income, he continued to see a few direct-pay clients during the board's investigation and during the period of his license suspension. One of the direct-pay clients filed a malpractice case against Scott in connection with his diagnosis and treatment for repressed memories. Eventually the licensing board cleared Scott of the sexual misconduct charges, but when he turned the malpractice complaint over to his malpractice insurance provider, was he assured of a defense? Scott assumed he was covered because he had kept his premiums current during the board's investigation.

Why Have Malpractice Insurance?

In today's litigious and consumer-oriented society, a mental health professional would be foolish to practice without obtaining and retaining professional liability (i.e., malpractice) insurance. Disgruntled clients can file claims with relative ease and impunity even if there is no merit to the allegations. The cost of defending these claims can run into thousands of dollars. (Lawyers' fees can range from $150 to $500 per hour, and are climbing.) A professional liability insurance policy provides benefits for defending claims asserted while the professional is practicing his or her licensed profession during the covered period in the policy and for the payment of damages.

What Is Malpractice Insurance?

The typical professional liability insurance policy provides benefits

The typical professional liability insurance policy provides benefits including the cost of defense, settlements, appeals, and judgments within the stated policy limits. Most policies provide a benefit for representation and defense before licensing boards. This is the good news. The bad news is that these same policies contain between 15 and 20 stated policy exclusions (see example policies in Appendixes B and C). Complaints regarding certain ethical violations are not covered by the policy, leaving the offending mental health professional exposed to damage awards that must be paid from personal assets or future earnings.

including the cost of defense, settlements, appeals, and judgments within the stated policy limits.

There are two major types of professional liability policies, claims-made and occurrence policies. An occurrence policy covers you for any incidents that happen while you are insured by the policy—regardless of when the claim may be filed. A claims-made policy covers you for incidents that happen after coverage becomes effective. The claim, however, must be reported while your policy is in force. Claims filed after your coverage ends may be covered by purchasing an extended reporting period often referred to as a "tail."

The two example policies included as Appendix B and Appendix C are claims-made policies.

> **Note:** The verbiage contained in an insurance policy is critical in determining coverage. The problem is that most professionals who purchase policies do not take the time to read them carefully. The legal maxim in insurance policies is that "the big print giveth and the small print taketh away." Therefore, read the policy and understand exactly what it covers. Only covered and nonexcluded items are within the purview of the policy. If there are obscure or oblique terms, ask your lawyer or insurance agent for an interpretation. Determine with certainty what items are covered and what items are not covered. This determination is critical when a claim is made.

The verbiage contained in an insurance policy is critical in determining coverage.

Malpractice Exclusions: Practicing without a License

A license is generally a prerequisite to coverage. Scott, the psychologist, would not be covered by his APA-sponsored professional liability insurance policy because the malpractice action was brought against

A license is generally a prerequisite to coverage.

him for professional services he rendered while his license was suspended. It is irrelevant that his license was fully reinstated and that he was cleared of the misconduct charges and any ethical violations. When the services were rendered that constituted the basis of the action, his psychologist's license was suspended and he was prohibited from practicing psychology. Consider the exclusions contained in the sample professional liability policies that follow.

Allied Healthcare Providers Professional and Supplemental Liability Insurance Policy

2. EXCLUSIONS

This insurance does not apply to Claims or Suits for Damage: . . .

v. any Claim arising from professional services that you provide when:

(1) you are not properly licensed or certified by the laws of the state(s) in which you provide such services;

(2) such services are not authorized or permitted by the laws of the state(s) in which your professional services are provided.
(Offered by Philadelphia Insurance Companies through CPH & Associates, Chicago, Illinois: www.cphins.com; see Appendix B).

American Home Assurance Company, Social Workers Professional Liability Insurance Policy

VI. EXCLUSIONS FOR ALL INSURING AGREEMENTS

shall not defend or pay any against under Insuring Agreements A, B, and C . . .

Q. Arising from any lawful act committed while you did not have a license required by law or while your license was suspended.
(Offered by American Home Assurance Company through the NASW Insurance Trust, Washington, DC: www.naswinsurancetrust.org and administered by American Professional Agency, Inc., Amityville, New York: www.americanprofessional.com; see Appendix C).

Malpractice Exclusions: Sexual Misconduct

Most professional liability insurance policies contain exclusions for therapists' sexual

Most professional liability insurance policies contain exclusions for therapists' sexual misconduct with clients and family members or persons in close relationship to clients. Sexual misconduct is a clear ethical violation and can lead to substantial damages being awarded against the mental health professional (see Chapter 12, "Sexual

Misconduct"). Plaintiffs' lawyers often refer to sexual exploitation cases as "slam-dunk" lawsuits. Once the plaintiff establishes the sexual relationship, the only question remaining for the jury to decide is how much money to award. Juries are very generous when the violation is clearly a client breach or exploitation and the therapist should have known better.

Some policies provide a limited liability benefit when sexual misconduct is alleged whereby the insurance company will pay damages awarded up to a maximum monetary limit, that is, $25,000, or pay defense costs up to a maximum monetary limit, that is, $25,000, without any obligation to pay for damages assessed (see Appendix C). Allen, the licensed marriage and family therapist, would be entitled to a defense under this type of professional liability insurance policy, but once $25,000 in legal fees and expenses were incurred, coverage would cease. If a judgment were entered against Allen or if he decided to settle the case, regardless of the amount agreed on, Allen must pay the money from his personal assets or out of his future earnings. It might be noted that in many states, once a judgment is received and properly recorded, it remains a lien for 10 years and is renewable. Therefore, if litigation is ever commenced against a therapist, legal representation is essential. Lawsuits cannot be ignored.

Typical professional liability insurance policies also contain provisions that exclude claims arising out of "any criminal, dishonest, fraudulent or malicious act or omission" (see Appendix B).

Because many state statutes criminalize sexual exploitation by mental health professionals, ethical violations of this type involving direct sex or sex once removed (i.e., family, friends, or business associates) are doubly excluded from the policy coverage. The message has always been clear—avoid sexual relationships with clients and those in close relationships with clients. A mental health professional engaging in this kind of misconduct will stand alone, unprotected by the insurance carrier and its policy. Sex of this nature is unprotected sex from any perspective.

Consider the clauses related to sexual misconduct in the following sample policies:

misconduct with clients and family members or persons in close relationship to clients.

Because many state statutes criminalize sexual exploitation by mental health professionals, ethical violations of this type involving direct sex or sex once removed are doubly excluded from the policy coverage.

Allied Healthcare Providers Policy: Appendix B

2. EXCLUSIONS

This insurance does not apply to Claims or Suits for Damage: . . .

u. physical abuse, sexual abuse or licentious, immoral or sexual behavior whether or not intended to lead to, or culminating in any sexual act, whether caused by, or at the instigation of, or at the direction of, or omission by any Insured. However, the Company will defend any civil Suit against an Insured seeking amounts that would be covered if this exclusion did not apply. In such case, the Company will only pay Fees, Costs and Expenses of such defense. (Note: The declaration sheet issued with this policy will include a monetary limit.) Our duty to defend will cease upon admission of guilt by the Insured, or if the Insured is adjudicated guilty. We will have no obligation to appeal any such judgment or adjudication.

Social Worker's Policy: Appendix C

Section IV. Sexual Misconduct Provision

A. Our limit of Liability shall not exceed $25,000.00 in the aggregate for all damages with respect to the total of all claims and against you involving any actual or alleged erotic physical contact, or attempt thereat or proposal thereof:

1. By you or by any other person for whom you may be legally liable; and
2. With or to any former or current client of yours or with or to any relative or member of the same household as any said client, or with or to any person with whom said client or relative has an affectionate personal relationship.

B. In the event that any of the foregoing are alleged at any time, either in a complaint, during discovery, at trial or otherwise, any and all causes of action alleged and arising out of the same or related courses of professional treatment and/or relationships shall be subject to the aforesaid $25,000 aggregate Limit of Liability and shall be part of, and not in addition to, the Limits of Liability otherwise afforded by this Policy.

C. . . . We shall not be obligated to undertake nor continue to defend any claim or proceeding subject to the $25,000 aggregate Limit of Liability after the $25,000 aggregate Limit of Liability has been exhausted by payment of judgments, settlements and/or other items included within the Limits of Liability. . . .

Making Sense of the Policies

The Allied Healthcare Providers policy provides no payment for assessed damages for sexual misconduct but does provide for a defense up to a stated maximum benefit. What this means is that the insurance carrier will retain an attorney and pay court costs and legal expenses incurred in defending the suit against the insured but will not be obligated to fund any resulting settlement or judgment. The NASW-sponsored policy provides for payment of damages up to a maximum of $25,000.

Malpractice Exclusions: Billing

The NASW Code of Ethics Section 3.05 "Billing" states, "Social workers should establish and maintain billing practices that accurately reflect the nature and extent of services provided and that identify who provided the service in the practice setting." Susan, while trying to assist her clients and maximize her income, violated her canon of ethics, which enabled her insurance carrier to deny coverage under her professional liability insurance policy. Under these facts, her insurance carrier would not even provide a defense, and she must hire and pay her own attorneys and costs. And the fees? Most lawyers charge a minimum of $200 per hour. Thus, an 8-hour day in court can cost at least $1600 in addition to preparation time, which may consist of hours waiting for the trial to begin or waiting for the jury to reach a decision. Hiring an attorney is not for the faint of heart.

Consider what the following professional liability insurance policies say about billing issues and coding insurance claim forms:

Allied Healthcare Providers Policy: Appendix B

2. EXCLUSIONS

This insurance does not apply to Claims or Suits for Damage: . . .

o. arising out of an Insured gaining any personal profit or advantage to which they are not legally entitled; . . .

Social Worker's Policy: Appendix C

VI. EXCLUSIONS FOR ALL INSURING AGREEMENTS

We shall not defend or pay any claims against you under Insuring Agreements A, B, and C . . .

D. For matters involving over billing, miscoding, reimbursement requests, and other fee related matters or inquiries, unless the action involves an actual disciplinary proceeding where your license or your ability to practice is threatened; . . .

Clearly succumbing to temptation to get paid for services that are not provided or through miscoding a billing invoice or misdiagnosing a client's condition or problem is unethical and illegal. It will also render the malpractice policy of no benefit or protection to the mental health professional.

Malpractice Insurance: Other Exclusions

Professional liability insurance policies exclude coverage for claims arising from wrongful acts committed while under the influence of an illegal substance or drug or while intoxicated.

Other ethical violations are excluded in malpractice policies. For example, professional liability insurance policies exclude coverage for claims arising from wrongful acts committed while under the influence of an illegal substance or drug or while intoxicated. Professional liability insurance policies exclude coverage for claims arising out of any business relationship or venture with any prior or current client. They will exclude coverage for claims arising from discrimination.

Regardless of the alleged complaint, offense, or negligent act, some other interesting exclusions come into play. This is true even if the alleged wrongful acts of commission or omission are covered under the policy. Some examples of additional exclusions included in malpractice policies follow.

A common and extremely broad exclusion eliminates coverage for intentional wrongful acts—the result being that only negligent or unintentional acts will be covered by the policy. Consider the following policy provisions:

Allied Healthcare Providers Policy: Appendix B

2. EXCLUSIONS

This insurance does not apply to Claims or Suits for Damage: . . .

f. arising out of intentional wrongful acts of the Insured;

Social Worker's Policy: Appendix C

VI. EXCLUSIONS FOR ALL INSURING AGREEMENTS

We shall not defend or pay any claims against you under Insuring Agreements A, B, and C . . .

M. For any wrongful act committed with knowledge by you that it was a wrongful act . . .

This same policy defines wrongful act as "any actual or alleged negligent act, error, or omission, or any actual or alleged defamation." Mental health professionals are presumed to know the ethical canons promulgated by their national and local organizations and their licensing boards. You could argue then that any violation of an ethical canon constitutes a wrongful act committed with knowledge thereby eliminating the insurance carrier's obligation to defend and pay claims.

Every policy will include a list of 20 or more exclusions. Many, however, are for risks that would be covered under other types of insurance coverage. Every professional in private practice should consider whether to carry premises liability, general liability, and automotive liability coverage. A good insurance agent should be engaged and is a necessary resource for the practicing professional.

Malpractice Insurance: Punitive Damages Provision

Intentional, malicious, or particularly offensive misconduct can lead to the imposition of damages against the defendant that are intended not to compensate the plaintiff for loss or harm but to punish the defendant. These are called *punitive* or *exemplary* damages. Sexual misconduct or financial exploitation of a client could easily lead to the award of punitive damages. These types of damages are often excluded from the coverage of a professional liability insurance policy or the coverage is severely limited. Consider the following policy provisions:

Allied Healthcare Providers Policy: Appendix B

2. EXCLUSIONS

F. **Damages** means a monetary:

1. judgment,
2. award, or
3. settlement,

but does not include fines, sanctions, penalties, punitive, or exemplary damages or the multiple portion of any damages.

Punitive or exemplary damages are often limited or excluded from the coverage of a professional liability insurance policy.

Social Worker's Policy: Appendix C

IX. PUNITIVE DAMAGES PROVISION

We shall not pay for fines or penalties or punitive, exemplary or multiplied damages; wherever permitted by law we shall pay up to $25,000 in the aggregate for all damages with respect to the total of all claims and suits against you involving punitive, exemplary or multiplied damages as part of and not in addition to the applicable Limits of Liability of this Policy.

It is not hard to imagine a jury awarding millions of dollars in punitive damages against a mental health professional for conspicuous exploitative conduct even if the plaintiff's actual damages are nowhere near as great. A jury, riled up or angry after a lawyer's stirring emotional appeal, can easily award significant punitive damages, especially if the sensitivity of the moment makes them generous with the therapist's money. Awarding another's cash seems easier than awarding one's own. Under the aforementioned NASW-sponsored policy language, the carrier is limiting its exposure to $25,000.

Licensing Board or Other Regulatory Authority Cases

The increasing number of complaints filed against mental health professionals with state and federal regulatory authorities makes it crucial for mental health professionals to secure professional liability insurance coverage for expenses incurred in connection with these cases and investigations. These regulatory authorities may require travel to their location for appearances and hearings. Travel costs alone for the mental health professional, legal representative(s), and witnesses can be prohibitive. There is a far greater likelihood that therapists will have complaints filed against them with a licensing board or the Office of Civil Rights than a malpractice suit. When considering malpractice insurance coverage, carefully review and consider the benefits offered for expenses in responding to and defending against a complaint to a regulatory authority.

Consider the following provisions from the specimen policies, the first providing expense reimbursement but not the actual defense (have to hire your own attorney) and the second providing the actual defense for administrative hearings:

Allied Healthcare Providers Policy: Appendix B

C. Additional Policy Benefits . . .

2. State Licensing Board Investigation Expenses

We shall pay reasonable expenses that you incur resulting from an investigation or proceeding by a state licensing board or other regulatory body provided that the investigation or proceeding arises out of events which could result in Claims covered by this Policy. We will not be responsible for conducting such investigation or providing such defense. The maximum amount we will pay for this benefit is $25,000.

Social Worker's Policy: Appendix C

I. Insuring Agreements

C. Administrative Hearing

We shall pay reasonable administrative expenses arising out of an administrative hearing, arising solely out of your performance of professional services as a social worker, even if the basis for that administrative hearing is groundless or fraudulent. The request or notification for the administrative hearing must take place on or after the retroactive date, but before the end of the policy period. . . .

IV. Defense Costs, Charges and Expenses

The following shall apply to Insuring Agreement C:

A. We shall defend you and pay administrative expenses at an administrative hearing arising solely out of your profession as a social worker up to our Limit of Liability stated in the Declarations.

Ethical Flash Points

- Practical considerations make acquiring professional liability insurance a necessity for the mental health professional.

- The cost of defense of even a fabricated claim could bankrupt an uninsured therapist. The angst caused by protracted and expensive litigation could easily result in the therapist withdrawing from the profession. Litigation, when the professional provider is a defendant, is an emotional and often debilitating experience.

- The professional liability insurance coverage purchased should include defense of licensing board complaints and administrative hearings. Read each insurance policy
(*continued*)

(Continued)

carefully and determine individually if coverage is provided for attorneys while representing the mental health professional before the licensing board, an ancillary administrative agency or before a national organization.

- Although professional liability insurance policies provide needed coverage, the typical policy contains over 20 policy exclusions. Exclusions are part of the policy and indicate what is *not* covered.

- Sexual offenses result in severely limited policy coverage. The maximum coverage is stated in the policy.

- Coverage for punitive damages is often greatly restricted.

- Many ethical violations are not covered by professional liability insurance policies.

- Knowledge of and compliance with ethics codes are critical to a successful mental health practice.

- If operating in an agency, school, managed care setting, or other venue where malpractice insurance is provided as part of employment, the same rules apply. The policy must be read, understood, and digested. Only then can the line provider truly understand the nature and extent of the coverage. Coverage for representation before a disciplinary board of any type is not universal or required.

- In the authors' perspective, an appearance before a disciplinary committee without representation is not a wise move. As soon as a complaint of any type from any source is determined, consult with an attorney familiar with mental health rules and regulations.

- Read the policy carefully. Coverage for an agency does not automatically indicate coverage for the individual.

- Policies must be maintained in force. Employees have been held liable when the agency "forgot" to pay the premium and the policy was cancelled. Likewise individual policies must be scrupulously paid according to their terms.

- When making a referral, check to determine that the individual or agency you are referring to has a current policy in force.

- Make sure your policy covers you if you inadvertently make a negligent referral.

- If assembling an association, determine that all members of the group have individual policies in force. (If coverage has been denied, investigate the reason for the denial.)

Summary

Each mental health discipline presumes therapists are thoroughly familiar with their profession's ethics codes, and ignorance has never been an excuse for violations. An ethical violation not only will lead to licensing board complaints, malpractice lawsuits, and criminal prosecutions, but also can result in the assertion of a policy exclusion to deny professional liability insurance benefits. Knowledge of and compliance with Ethics Code provisions are as critical to a mental health practice as obtaining a professional liability insurance policy.

Ethical violations can limit or in many cases eliminate an insurance carrier's obligation to defend and pay claims under a professional liability insurance policy. Sexual misconduct is not the only violation excluded from coverage. A knowing violation of any ethical canon that gives rise to a claim can leave the unfortunate mental health professional in the undesirable position of having to pay for the defense and damages from personal assets or future earnings. As with all insurance policies, beware of the fine print and be sure to read and understand all of the policy's stated exclusions and definitions.

As with all insurance policies, beware the fine print and be sure to read and understand all of the policy's stated exclusions and definitions.

> **Note:** In this chapter, we reviewed some of the more common policy clauses contained in malpractice insurance policies utilized by mental health practitioners. We understand that a malpractice insurance carrier might, under numerous circumstances, interpret the policy differently. When a question arises concerning coverage under a policy of insurance of any type, it is helpful to contact the insurance carrier itself, communicate in writing with a knowledgeable officer of the company or employee, and obtain the position of the company. Insurance companies are ready, willing, and able to clarify possible or potential ambiguities in their policies. All the insured has to do is ask. We have no authority to speak on behalf of any insurance carrier.

Suggested Research Assignments

1. Contact mental health professionals in your area and find out whether they carry professional liability insurance and if so, through what company or sponsoring agent. Ask the following questions:

   What type of policy was purchased (claims made or occurrence)?

   What is the benefit for licensing board representation?

   What are the policy limits?

   What are the policy exclusions?

   What is the cost of the policy?

   Does the policy cover all agents, servants, and employees as well as independent contractors?

2. Research the various professional liability insurance options available to you in your state and discuss the pros and cons of the coverages or programs offered by each company. For example, what services are available other than just insurance coverage (i.e., insured hotlines, educational resources available, bundled coverages)?

3. Research case law in your state for cases that involved professional liability insurance policy coverage or exclusion issues.

4. Contact marketing agents for professional liability companies to determine what factors would preclude the company from issuing or renewing a policy to a mental health professional.

Discussion Questions

1. What features would you look for in a professional liability insurance policy?

2. A client is complaining about the quality of your services. Should you contact your professional liability insurance carrier and advise the claims office? If not, at what point should you contact the insurance company?

3. How might a mental health professional's employability be impacted by his or her inability to secure professional liability insurance coverage?
4. What do you tell a client who wants to know about your malpractice insurance coverage? Is the client entitled to this information?
5. Are you more likely to be sued if you have professional liability insurance coverage? And if so, should you carry this insurance?

25

Record Keeping

After many years in private practice, Bob, a licensed psychologist, developed an adversarial attitude when it came to the legal profession and attorneys' seemingly endless demands to access client records for litigation purposes. Bob began to believe that his profession's exceptions to confidentiality were compromising his clients' rights to privacy and impeding the therapeutic process. He devised a method to combat the legal system's intrusions into his files and to protect his clients' privacy and the confidentiality of their work together by keeping minimal notes of his sessions. He limited his note taking to documenting the date a session occurred, the payment, and a phrase such as ''worked toward client's stated goals utilizing agreed-upon therapeutic techniques.'' When one particular attorney secured a court order for one of Bob's client's files, he was appalled at what he considered inadequate record keeping. The attorney filed a complaint against Bob with the state board. Are Bob's stated intentions sufficient to prevent a licensing board sanction?

Carol, a social worker, made an extraordinary effort to record in her session notes virtually everything her clients told her. At the end of each day, she had a habit of reviewing her notes and fleshing them out when she remembered the content of discussions she did not have time to record earlier. In the context of one therapy session, a client mentioned that she and her husband had seen a married neighbor, a local judge whom she mentioned by name, coming out of a gay bar with a very young-looking man on his arm. Carol dutifully recorded the remark and the judge's name in her notes. Two years later, the client and her husband became ensnared in a messy, media-centered divorce and custody case. The husband successfully subpoenaed Carol's file and introduced her notes into evidence at their final custody hearing. Before long the courthouse was buzzing with delicious gossip about the recorded remarks concerning the judge and the gay bar. The judge in question was furious. Carol's records were admitted into evidence and became part of the public record. Does he have grounds to complain against Carol for recording the remarks in a clinical file in which he had no involvement?

When Bill, a licensed professional counselor, decided to retire, he moved all his client files home and stored them in the garage. But Bill had forgotten about two boxes of files on the top shelf of his basement storage room. When the building manager sent in a cleaning crew to prepare the office space for lease to a new tenant, they discovered the boxes and, overwhelmed with curiosity, began reviewing their contents. One unsavory cleaning person recognized the name on one of the files as belonging to a local television news anchorperson. He took the file home that night and attempted to blackmail the anchorperson, who contacted the police. The cleaning person was ultimately arrested and charged with criminal offenses. Bill faced a licensing board complaint as well as a malpractice lawsuit.

Sheila was Dr. Blanque's client for three years. One day she reported to Dr. Blanque's office for her usual therapy session and was informed that Dr. Blanque had committed suicide. In a panic, Sheila called Dr. White, another competent therapist in Dr. Blanque's office. When Dr. White reviewed Dr. Blanque's clinical record of Sheila's treatment, he should have been able to determine with reasonable accuracy the status of Sheila's treatment (i.e., the diagnosis, prognosis, and treatment plan).

Dr. Stanford, a professional counselor, kept meticulous records of all clients. The statute in his state mandated that records be maintained for 10 years before they could be destroyed. Every year, Dr. Stanford shredded his

11-year-old files. Out of the blue, a client filed a complaint that Dr. Stanford had sex with her during treatment 12 years ago. Dr. Stanford had no file and could not even remember whether she had ever been a client. He denied having sex with any client, but he was vulnerable when forced to defend a credible-sounding story without any documentation to prove the client wrong.

Mary Lou, a social worker, worked with several managed care panels. With the approval of her managed care gatekeeper, she treated clients and was reimbursed for the services provided. One day the managed care auditor called wanting to inspect Mary Lou's files to determine if the treatment offered was consistent with what the company had authorized and if the diagnosis was consistent with the treatment plan (i.e., when a covered diagnosis was indicated, were the clients receiving the authorized treatment and was this reflected in the progress notes?). Mary Lou would be responsible for reimbursing the managed care company for any treatment that the company paid for but did not authorize.

Tom and Mary brought their 5-year-old, acting-out son to Rosemary, a licensed professional counselor, for therapy. Rosemary treated the son for about a year, and then the therapy was terminated by mutual agreement. All parties signed a termination letter that contained the clause: "Should further treatment be needed, Tom and Mary will call Rosemary." How long should this file be preserved by Rosemary? According to the law in her state, the file must be maintained until the child turns 25 (i.e., until the child turns 18, age of majority, plus 7 years). In most jurisdictions, files must be maintained at least until children reach their majority.

Why Keep Records?

Mental health professionals have always maintained clinical records for their practice. Before licensing boards and professional associations published their canons of ethics and codes of conduct, clinicians maintained records of appointments, pricing and billing procedures, and financial records concerning income and disbursements for tax purposes and to determine the profitability of their practice. Therapists can make sound business decisions only if they maintain accurate records according to normally accepted accounting procedures.

Clinical records are another matter. For years, mental health providers resisted generating copious clinical notes, and most were unfamiliar with medical professionals' standard practice of charting. Although therapists jotted down occasional notes to record significant facts or events, generally, clinicians were not taught or inclined to record information that might be harmful or embarrassing to them or their clients in the future. They were especially paranoid about becoming involved in the judicial system, where their record keeping might be subject to examination, cross examination, and peer review in a public forum, such as a courtroom.

We attended a cocktail party during which we talked about record keeping procedures with a psychiatrist. We argued for maintaining accurate files in case another therapist assumed responsibility for a client's treatment. The psychiatrist said she had been practicing for 30 years and had never been sued nor had her clinical records ever been audited. She was unwilling to change her method of documenting treatment and preserving files. She did not contemplate dying or becoming incapacitated soon and was not worried if she did. Later, we discussed privately the psychiatrist's incredible vulnerability should any of her patients have committed suicide or homicide, or had any patient made an unjustifiable claim against her. It is unlikely a judge or jury would have taken the psychiatrist at her word. Without written evidence to corroborate her testimony, they would assume whatever she said to defend herself was self-serving dialogue to "win" the case. Most judges and juries rely on the maxim, "Absence of evidence is evidence of absence." Without evidence that the psychiatrist did anything appropriate or helpful to the client, they can assume the psychiatrist did nothing.

A client record may be the only tangible evidence available to a licensing board or a jury in assessing an alleged ethics code violation or malpractice allegation. The file is the therapist's first line of defense. Licensing boards and ethics committees usually review the clinical record under professional scrutiny to determine if the complaint is valid. The authors have defended numerous providers whose records were examined and who were disciplined, not because the complaint was valid, but because the record, as considered and examined by a professional board of peers, was found not to be adequate or in accordance with professional ethical standards. Thus, if for no other reason than self-interest or self-preservation, good record keeping makes common sense. Even if a therapist believes that meticulous, thorough, and complete record keeping is unnecessary and doesn't make good sense, the ethics codes of the mental health disciplines at both the state and national level require it. When clinicians try to justify incomplete, sketchy, or limited record keeping as being justifiable, licensing boards tend to discount the testimony as being self-serving. The true professional maintains a file, which would serve, if needed, to bring a subsequent treatment provider up to date concerning the client/patient. Any incomplete records are considered slothful and negligent. Memories are fallible, while good records are a permanent record or memorial of events as they took place.

A client record may be the only tangible evidence available to a licensing board or a jury in assessing an alleged ethics code violation or malpractice allegation.

Licensing boards and ethics committees usually review the clinical record under scrutiny to determine if the complaint is valid.

Maintaining Clinical Files

The clinical file serves many purposes, and many parties have a stake in its contents. Thus, maintaining accurate records is important for more than just the provider's sake.

For clients, the clinical file serves as a permanent record of their entire mental health history. Although the file may be destroyed after a certain number of mandated years, when preserved, it is an accurate information source and an invaluable record of the client's diagnosis, treatment plan, and therapeutic outcome. A well-organized and faithfully maintained file indicates the client's baseline condition and treatment goals. It is also a memorandum concerning whether these goals were accomplished. Clients may review their files and may request that they be shared with subsequent mental health providers.

For clients, the clinical file serves as a permanent record of their mental health history.

Therapists use progress notes from the client file to refresh their memories between therapy sessions. Often clients visit therapists with intense frequency, then drop out of treatment only to return months or years later. Only a complete and up-to-date record will provide the needed background for continuing treatment. This is especially true

Therapists use progress notes from the client file to refresh their memories between therapy sessions.

when therapists retire, become ill, disabled, or die. The new clinician will be more comprehensively informed if treatment was thoroughly documented and the file is still available. In fact, if the new clinician does not review an available file, it might be grounds for a malpractice action or an ethical complaint. Perusing the file can indicate to the therapist what helped a particular client and what methods did not work. Knowing either or both would be helpful.

To insurance companies and managed care organizations who audit provider records, the clinical files or case notes indicate whether the provider is offering the authorized therapy in the prescribed manner. The authorized treatment is usually stated in a diagnosis and projected treatment plan. The recorded treatment must conform to that diagnosis and plan. If not, insurance companies may refuse payment, or if they have already paid for treatment, the insurance company may bill the provider for reimbursement.

To disciplinary boards, ethics committees, courts, and juries, the clinical records or case notes reflect what transpired between the patient/client/consumer and the provider/clinician/therapist. In their minds, as peers review the file, what is recorded is what happened, and what is not recorded did not happen. When providers are called to account for professional actions, the first records examined are the clinical case notes, the intake history, and the informed consent and intake forms. If the case notes reveal unethical or negligent conduct on their face, disciplinary action will follow and the vulnerable provider will be even more vulnerable. Thus, therapists should maintain clinical records beyond the state-mandated retention limits. It is worthwhile to spend a few dollars a month for a secure storage facility. Defending a claim without proper documentation is difficult. The careful provider never knows when a client will become unhappy and demand a record review by another expert.

What Constitutes a Well-Documented Client Record?

Conscientious record keeping requires more than jotting down a few descriptive notes about a session. A well-documented client file should include the following:

- *Diagnosis:* What the problem is
- *Treatment plan:* What the therapist is going to do about it
- *Prognosis:* As a result of what is done, what is expected to happen and, perhaps, when it is expected to happen

As these elements change, the case notes must evolve accordingly. A diagnosis can shift slightly as time progresses or can turn dramatically. A treatment plan, once thought effective, may have to be altered, changed completely, or disregarded if it is not efficacious. A prognosis, which depends on the correct diagnosis and treatment plan, may have to be updated to reflect the client's changing situation and condition. The clinical file should include the facts, as stated by the client, the reactions, as determined by the professional, and all the necessary times, dates, and information to obtain a complete mental picture of a particular client.

National Guidelines for Record Keeping

American Association for Marriage and Family Therapy (AAMFT) Code of Ethics (2001)

Principle III: Professional Competence and Integrity . . .

3.6 Marriage and family therapists maintain accurate and adequate clinical and financial records.

American Counseling Association (ACA) Code of Ethics (2005)

A.1. Welfare of Those Served by Counselors

A.1.b. Records

Counselors maintain records necessary for rendering professional services to their clients and as required by laws, regulations, or agency or institution procedures. Counselors include

(*continued*)

(Continued)

sufficient and timely documentation in their client records to facilitate the delivery and continuity of needed services. Counselors take reasonable steps to ensure that documentation in records accurately reflects client progress and services provided. If errors are made in client records, counselors take steps to properly note the correction of such errors according to agency or institutional policies.

A.12.g. Technology and Informed Consent

As part of the process of establishing informed consent, counselors do the following:

7. Inform clients if and for how long archival storage of transaction records are maintained.

B.6. Records

B.6.a. Confidentiality of Records

Counselors ensure that records are kept in a secure location and that only authorized persons have access to records.

B.6.d. Client Access

Counselors provide reasonable access to records and copies of records when requested by competent clients. Counselors limit the access of clients to their records, or portions of their records, only when there is compelling evidence that such access would cause harm to the client. Counselors document the request of clients and the rationale for withholding some or all of the record in the files of clients. In situations involving multiple clients, counselors provide individual clients with only those parts of records that related directly to them and do not include confidential information related to any other client.

B.6.f. Disclosure or Transfer

Unless exceptions to confidentiality exist, counselors obtain written permission from clients to disclose or transfer records to legitimate third parties. Steps are taken to ensure that receivers of counseling records are sensitive to their confidential nature.

B.6.g. Storage and Disposal after Termination

Counselors store records following termination of services to ensure reasonable future access, maintain records in accordance with state and federal statutes governing records, and dispose of client records and other sensitive materials in a manner that protects client confidentiality. When records are of an artistic nature, counselors obtain client (or guardian) consent with regards to handling of such records or documents.

American Psychological Association (APA) Ethical Principles of Psychologists and Code of Conduct (2002)

6. Record Keeping and Fees

6.01 Documentation of Professional and Scientific Work and Maintenance of Records

Psychologists create, and to the extent the records are under their control, maintain, disseminate, store, retain, and dispose of records and data relating to their professional and scientific work in order to (1) facilitate provision of services later by them or by other professionals, (2) allow for replication of research design and analyses, (3) meet institutional requirements, (4) ensure accuracy of billing and payments, and (5) ensure compliance with law. (See also Standard 4.01, Maintaining Confidentiality.)

6.02 Maintenance, Dissemination, and Disposal of Confidential Records of Professional and Scientific Work

(a) Psychologists maintain confidentiality in creating, storing, accessing, transferring, and disposing of records under their control, whether these are written, automated, or in any other medium.

(b) If confidential information concerning recipients of psychological services is entered into databases or systems of records available to persons whose access has not been

(continued)

(Continued)

consented to by the recipient, psychologists use coding or other techniques to avoid the inclusion of personal identifiers.

(c) Psychologists make plans in advance to facilitate the appropriate transfer and to protect the confidentiality of records and data in the event of psychologists' withdrawal from positions or practice.

4. Privacy and Confidentiality

4.01 Maintaining Confidentiality

Psychologists have a primary obligation and take reasonable precautions to protect confidential information obtained through or stored in any medium, recognizing that the extent and limits of confidentiality may be regulated by law or established by institutional rules or professional or scientific relationship.

4.04 Minimizing Intrusions on Privacy

(a) Psychologists include in written and oral reports and consultations, only information germane to the purpose for which the communication is made.

American School Counselor Association (ASCA) Ethical Standards for School Counselors (2004)

A8. Student Records

The professional school counselor:

a. Maintains and secures records necessary for rendering professional services to the counselee as required by laws, regulations, institutional procedures, and confidentiality guidelines.

National Association of Social Workers (NASW) Code of Ethics (1999)

3.04 Client Records

(a) Social workers should take reasonable steps to ensure that documentation in records is accurate and reflects the services provided.

(b) Social workers should include sufficient and timely documentation in records to facilitate the delivery of services and to ensure continuity of services provided to clients in the future.

(c) Social workers' documentation should protect clients' privacy to the extent that is possible and appropriate and should include only information that is directly relevant to the delivery of services.

(d) Social workers should store records following the termination of services to ensure reasonable future access. Records should be maintained for the number of years required by state statute or relevant contracts.

Texas State Board of Professional Counselors Subchapter C Code of Ethics*

Rule §681.41 General Ethical Requirements

(o) For each client, a licensee shall keep accurate records of the dates of counseling treatment intervention, types of counseling treatment intervention, progress or case notes, intake assessment, treatment plan, and billing information.

(p) Records held by a licensee shall be kept for seven years for adult clients and seven years beyond the age of 18 for minor clients.

(q) Records created by licensees during the scope of their employment by educational institutions; by federal, state, or local governmental agencies; or their political subdivisions or programs are not required to comply with subsections (o) and (p) of this section.

Note: Extract (p) is a concise statement of the minimum records that should be maintained and the minimum length of time for preservation in Texas. Check your state regulations.

Source: The provisions of this §681.41 adopted to be effective September 1, 2003, 28 TexReg 4143; amended to be effective November 21, 2004, 29 TexReg 10512; amended to be effective September 1, 2005, 30 TexReg 4978.

HIPAA Record Keeping Requirements

The major emphasis of the HIPAA Privacy Rule is the protection of individually identifiable health information that is also referred to as protected health information (PHI). Protected health information is defined as: any information that has been created or received by a health-care provider, health plan, public health authority, employer, life insurer, school or university, or health-care clearinghouse and that relates to:

- The past, present or future health information of an individual;
- The provision of health care to an individual; or
- The past, present, future payment for the provision of health care. (45 C.F.R. §160.103)

The Privacy Rule further defines psychotherapy notes as the "notes recorded (in any medium) by a health care provider who is a mental health professional documenting or analyzing the contents of conversation during a private counseling session or a group, joint, or family counseling session that are separated from the rest of the individual's medical record." By definition, psychotherapy notes do not include "medication prescription and monitoring, counseling session start and stop times, the modalities and frequencies of treatment furnished, results of clinical tests, and any summary of the following items: diagnosis, functional status, the treatment plan, symptoms, prognosis, and progress to date" (45 C.F.R. §164.501).

Although protected health information and psychotherapy notes are defined, the Privacy Rule does not provide much specific direction as to what health information should be recorded in a client's record by the health-care professional. There are a few requirements, though. Two involve a client's right to insert information into his or her health-care record. First, if clients wish to restrict the use and disclosure of their protected health information, they may make the request and if agreed to by the health-care provider it must be documented in the client record (45 C.F.R. §164.522).

Clients can also request changes to their health-care record and if the health-care provider disagrees with the requested change the client has two options: (1) Submit a written statement disagreeing with the denial that must be appended to or linked to the actual record, and (2) require the health care provider to include the client's request for amendment and the denial with each disclosure of the client's record (45 C.F.R. §164.526).

Another record keeping requirement of the Privacy Rule deals with requests for disclosures of the client's protected health information. Clients are entitled to an accounting of disclosures of their protected health information made in the 6 years prior to the date on which the request is made. The health-care provider is required to document and retain information regarding the disclosure. This documentation must include the date of disclosure, identity, and address if known of the recipient, a brief description of the information that was disclosed, and a brief statement of the purpose of the disclosure or a copy of the request itself (45 C.F.R. §164.528). This accounting for disclosures is often referred to as a disclosure log.

All HIPAA-required documentation must be retained for a period of 6 years (45 C.F.R. §164.530(j) (2)). Therapists practicing in a jurisdiction in which state law only requires client records be maintained for a period of 5 years should consider maintaining client files for a minimum of 6 years. The Privacy Rule does not provide for an extended reporting period for a minor's records, however. It just sets forth a 6-year rule for all required documentation.

All HIPAA-required documentation must be retained for a period of 6 years.

Commonalities among Ethics Requirements for Record Keeping

- Every mental health discipline requires a clinical record for both business and therapeutic purposes, but the exact information to be recorded remains within the clinician's discretion.
- The length of time a record must be maintained differs from discipline to discipline and from jurisdiction to jurisdiction.
- State guidelines have to be checked meticulously. They are altered and amended from time to time.
- Although records may be destroyed after a certain number of years, a better practice would be to preserve them for a greater length of

time, perhaps forever. (Some ethics complaints have no statute of limitations. Some malpractice actions have a discovery rule: The statute of limitations does not begin to run until the client "discovers" that the actions of the therapist were negligent. That could occur 20 years after the negligence or bad conduct arose.)

- Clinical records may be written, computerized, or automated, but all must be preserved according to statute. The clinician should note that the computer used today, and the tape, hard drive, or disc that preserves the information may not be able to "save" the information for the requisite number of years required by the preservation statute. In this case, as computers are updated and substituted, information must be transferred to an instrument that ensures that it will be available for the length of time mandated by the law.
- A disposition cycle may be established.
- Confidentiality of clinical records survives the death of the therapist and the client.
- Client records should only contain information pertinent to the client's treatment.

Avoiding Ethics Violations

A therapist can commit an ethical violation related to record keeping in several ways. First, therapists are professionally obligated to generate, preserve, and maintain complete, accurate, thorough, and professionally competent client records. Records must be meaningful and essentially establish a road map of the therapeutic process from initial intake to the present time. The notes should make obvious what has transpired in therapy and where the process is headed. A subsequent therapist should be able to review a file and determine the goals, progress to date, and current needs of the client (diagnosis, treatment plan, and prognosis) at any given time. If this information is not in a client record, the record is inadequate and the therapist has violated the records provisions of the applicable ethics code.

Records must be meaningful and essentially establish a road map of the therapeutic process from initial intake to the present time.

Thus, in the first vignette, Bob, although well intentioned, violated the APA Ethics Code by failing to thoroughly document his client sessions. He failed to document therapy so that he or another therapist could easily continue the client's treatment later. His concern that the legal system might compromise his client's rights of privacy and confidentiality caused him to take action exactly the opposite of what was ethically required. Bob's record keeping did not rise to the level required of psychologists, and he would be subject to licensing board sanctions.

Another way therapists may violate ethics codes is by failing to secure client files and maintain, preserve, and protect confidentiality of client records. Even accidentally leaving behind a box of files during a move violates ethical requirements. Bill, the counselor mentioned earlier, violated the ACA ethics code because he was "responsible for securing the safety and confidentiality of any counseling records" (ACA Code of Ethics, 2005, B.6.a. Confidentiality of Records) he created. It doesn't matter what medium is used to create the record. The therapist has full and complete responsibility to ensure that prying eyes do not obtain access to the files. Locked file cabinets and password-protected computers are a minimum practice to protect records. Allowing anyone access to client files without client consent is a breach of confidentiality and an ethical violation. Files must be protected from the cleaning staff, temporary help, and others who are not involved in clients' treatment, including other curious clients who have a tendency to peer over a counter or around a door, or other therapists or friends who visit the office. Only those individuals who need to know about a file should perceive that a particular client file even exists. Bob's failure to protect and secure his patient records also constituted violations of the HIPAA Privacy and Security Rules.

Another way therapists may violate ethics codes is by failing to secure client files and maintain, preserve, and protect confidentiality of client records.

Therapists must preserve not only a file's confidentiality but also the physical integrity of the file itself. Ethics codes and the HIPAA Security Rule mandate this obligation. Each state requires records to be maintained for various lengths of time, typically 5 to 7 years for adults and for 5 to 7 years past the age of 18 for a minor client. HIPAA requires 6 years for its required documentation. Files must be safeguarded from fire, theft, flood damage, rodents, mildew, and disintegration or decay. Special care should be taken with files kept on audio- or videotape and computer tape or discs. These mediums may be more sensitive to temperature, humidity, and air pressure variations than paper records.

Therapists must preserve not only a file's confidentiality but also the physical integrity of the file itself.

Computer-generated records must be maintained for the same length of time as paper records. With technology evolving at a fast pace, therapists may be unable to access some files that were preserved using outmoded processes and hardware. The therapist bears total responsibility for maintaining the client file and its physical integrity for the requisite period, even if it means converting files from one type to another to keep pace with technology. Failure to do so is an ethical violation and a violation of the HIPAA Security Rule.

Maintaining Accuracy

Inaccurate entries should be crossed out, corrected, dated, and initialed, so that the record clearly reveals what was recorded, the new entry, the date the new entry was made, and the person making it.

Client records must be accurate and reflect the services provided. Incorrectly recording information, even inadvertently, can be an ethical violation. Each entry should be reviewed and any errors should be corrected. A simple change from "he" to "she" can alter the entire meaning of an entry, and pronouns are easy to miss in the editing process. Too often, errors are discovered only after a file has been copied and provided to a third party for review. Once that happens, an ethical complaint is sure to follow. Inaccurate entries should be crossed out, corrected, dated, and initialed, so that the record clearly reveals what was recorded, the new entry, the date the new entry was made, and the person making it. The same is true for computer files. Never delete information. Client records must reveal the new corrected entry and the former inaccurate documentation.

Overdocumentation

Can a therapist violate an ethics code for recording too much information? Carol, the social worker who recorded her client's remarks about the local judge, seemingly violated the NASW Ethics Code provision that states the social workers should record only information that is "directly relevant to the delivery of services" (NASW Code of Ethics, Sec. 3.04(c)). The information about the judge had no direct relevance to the therapeutic services Carol was providing to her client. When case notes include information irrelevant to treatment, therapists may face licensing board sanctions for recording too much information.

Ethical Flash Points

- Documenting therapy in client records and files is a basic tenet of therapy. Being cavalier about the clinical file, and what it contains, is unwise, unprofessional, and unethical.

- Entries in a clinical file should be timely—made at or near the time of the service. Notes are always suspect when they are added as an afterthought, days, weeks, or months later.

- Laziness or concern for client confidentiality is not an acceptable excuse for a sloppy or incomplete record.

- Recording irrelevant information in a client file can lead to an ethics code complaint.

- The therapist bears complete responsibility to maintain the confidentiality of the client file. Locked file cabinets and password-protected computers are a minimum protection for client files.

- It is important to preserve the physical integrity of the client file at least for the length of time prescribed by law. Make a record of all files destroyed. Better still, cull files rather than destroying them. Preserve informed consent and intake forms along with other significant documents including the termination interview, memo, or letter. Create a summary of the file's contents. This can reduce the preserved file to a few pages. Keep culled files permanently.

- The therapist is responsible for the accuracy and completeness of all information in the client file. While all disciplines require providers to maintain clinical files, they are vague in stating exactly what to include in each file.

- Files should be reviewed periodically for accuracy and ethical compliance. Any corrections to client records should be documented and initialed and the inaccurate information crossed out but not deleted. Electronic records must be periodically tested for corruption.

- When files are requested, review them first. If entries require clarification or explanation, add the additional description or information as a dated addendum to the file. Do not delete information before surrendering files.

- When an ethical complaint is filed or registered, the clinical record is often the first item requested by the disciplinary board.

(continued)

(*Continued*)

- Insurance companies can audit clinical records for completeness and accuracy, and to verify that the authorized treatment took place. Auditors may report inconsistencies to disciplinary boards.

- If the therapist makes a referral to a psychiatrist or vice versa, and medication is needed, the file should reflect the coordination between therapy and the medication. Case notes should reflect consultations between the two mental health disciplines.

- Always keep the original file if the client requests a copy or if the client transfers to another therapist. Send out copies only with a signed release of information form.

- Covered entities have additional record keeping requirements mandated by the HIPAA Privacy Rule.

- All HIPAA-required documentation must be maintained for 6 years.

Summary

Record keeping is critical from an ethical and legal perspective as well as for the therapist's personal protection. Conceptualizing the file as the first line of defense against an accusation of an ethical violation, a HIPAA complaint or a suit for malpractice should motivate mental health professionals to keep thorough records. Therapists should consider the client file a road map of the therapy that can fully inform subsequent therapists of the client's problems, progress, and therapeutic needs and ensure a successful therapy transition.

Suggested Research Assignments

1. Locate and discuss the provisions of the ethical codes promulgated by the mental health profession licensing boards and the law in your state with regard to record keeping.
2. Locate and discuss any state and national professional association rules with regard to record keeping. What are their similarities and differences?
3. Compare and contrast the obligations imposed by the state licensing boards in your state with the rules promulgated by the state professional associations.

4. Compare and contrast state licensing board and professional association obligations with the guidelines of national professional associations.

5. Research the decisions of your state licensing boards and state and national professional association ethics committees for sanctions imposed for violations relating to record keeping.

6. Research legal civil case decisions for your state involving improper record keeping or record keeping related–negligence by mental health professionals.

7. Talk to practicing mental health professionals in your area and ask them about their record keeping practices.

8. Research HIPAA Privacy and Security Rule requirements with respect to record keeping and protecting the privacy and ensuring the integrity of client files.

9. Create a protocol for your practice with respect to record generation, maintenance, and security.

Discussion Questions

1. A licensed mental health professional informs you over lunch that she is leaving private practice for a teaching position and is going to destroy all files that exceed the minimum legal retention period. What do you advise her to do with respect to her files?

2. A client specifically instructs you during your second therapy session with him not to include in his patient file any notes about information that he will share with you during therapy sessions. What do you say and do?

3. What do you do when you discover that you have somehow lost two pages of notes from a client file?

4. What would you tell a colleague who shares with you his practice of not recording any information in his client files that could be harmful or embarrassing to the client if he was compelled to turn over the file to a third party?

5. What are the reasons that accurate and thorough record keeping is in the therapist's best interest?

PART IV

PROFESSIONAL ISSUES

26

Drug and Alcohol Use, Impairment

Suzanne, a therapist in private practice, had a reputation for being a fine clinician. Her colleagues also knew her to be a liberal drinker although her criminal and professional records were clean. A gossipy cloud seemed to follow Suzanne in this small town, but no one could find hard evidence of a drinking problem. One day, on the way to her office, she stopped in a bar to have a soft drink with friends. Suzanne did not take so much as a sip of alcohol, but when she left for the office, her clothing had picked up the smoky smell that permeated the bar along with the odor of stale beer. Ten minutes into her first session, her client accused her of coming to the office drunk and stormed out of the office in a fit of rage. How does Suzanne defend herself if a complaint is filed? What does she do now?

Jack, a therapist for 20 years, has just had major dental surgery. His dentist has prescribed pain medication, which he warned could make Jack a little woozy. Jack has a client scheduled for a weekly appointment and knows the client becomes very upset if appointments are canceled. Just as he is about to go into the session, the pain becomes severe. His options: take a pill before his client arrives, cancel the session, or conduct the session without medication while trying to hide the pain that is affecting his concentration. Which option is most acceptable? Does Jack have other options?

Karen, a licensed professional counselor, had been in private practice for over 15 years. She enjoyed professional success and a satisfying personal life. As she started her 16th year in practice, her mother died from a massive stroke and 6 weeks later her father died from a heart attack. In between, her husband left her for a younger woman. Karen was emotionally devastated and severely depressed but continued to go into her office each day. One day during a therapy session with a new client who was depressed and had been expressing suicidal ideation, Karen lost it. She broke down and began crying uncontrollably, upsetting the client who ran out of the office. Did Karen wait too long to address her own problems?

Substance Abuse and Ethics

Using drugs and alcohol, individually or in any combination that impairs the clinician's judgment, constitutes an ethical violation, and disciplinary action will follow a substantiated claim.

Using drugs and alcohol, individually or in any combination that impairs the clinician's objective, clinical, and professional judgment, constitutes an ethical violation, and disciplinary action will follow a substantiated claim. In addition to the case vignettes, what other circumstances might generate complaints of ethical infractions to licensing boards and state and national organizations?

The inappropriate use of drugs or alcohol is a recurring problem to which mental health providers, like any other professionals, are not immune. Professional publications, especially state licensing board and bar association reports, list the names and circumstances of professionals who injure clients or patients while under the influence of drugs or alcohol or while their clinical or legal judgment is impaired. Intemperate drug or alcohol use compromises their competent treatment of clients. Clients suffer when drugs, alcohol, or a controlled substance of any type have become an inappropriate part of the provider's life and adversely affect his or her therapeutic skills.

Mental health professionals, like other substance abusers, will often deny a problem exists. Inappropriate use of alcohol or drugs can take many forms, including:

- Taking a controlled substance without a prescription
- Taking a higher dosage of prescription medication than is recommended or combining it with other medications
- Consuming an amount of alcohol that impairs judgment
- Using alcohol in a manner that might lead clients to *think* that the provider is under the influence and therefore the therapy offered *appears* to be unsound
- Having alcohol (even if disguised by enormous amounts of breath spray or mouthwash) on your breath during a session
- Using a combination of medication and alcohol (both legal) in a manner that causes an overall harmful effect on the clinician's judgment
- Practicing while under the influence of a legally prescribed medication that impairs judgment in any way

When to Say No

Some drugs are totally acceptable in reasonable dosages, including all prescription drugs taken according to a physician's order. Drinking alcohol is also legal under most circumstances, including having a drink in your own home. Drinking alcohol or taking prescribed medication becomes a problem for therapists only when it impairs their clinical and professional judgment. Pilots, for example, have strict rules concerning the length of time they should abstain from alcohol before flying. Likewise, therapists should not have so much as one drink before a session if it will even slightly impair their judgment. This is a self-policing policy. Only the individual can know his or her limits as far as drinking and driving or carrying on a conversation are concerned.

Therapists must raise the bar when thinking about taking alcohol or medication while seeing clients, who are often vulnerable, dependent, and hypersensitive. Even a hint of a lack of concentration when coupled with a whiff of alcohol could create a situation that would compromise the entire therapeutic relationship. If the client perceives an impairment, real or imagined, and files a complaint with either the licensing board or a national organization, the therapist could face serious repercussions. Thus, mental health providers should never use

This is a self-policing policy.

Mental health providers should never use any alcohol, drug, or controlled substance that might in any way, no matter how slight, affect their judgment while dealing with clients.

any alcohol, drug, or controlled substance that might in any way, no matter how slight, affect their judgment while dealing with clients.

National Guidelines for Recognizing Impairment

American Association for Marriage and Family Therapy (AAMFT) Code of Ethics (2001)

3.3 Marriage and family therapists seek appropriate professional assistance for their personal problems or conflicts that may impair work performance or clinical judgment.

American Counseling Association (ACA) Code of Ethics (2005)

C.2.g. Impairment

Counselors are alert to the signs of impairment from their own physical, mental, or emotional problems and refrain from offering or providing professional services when such impairment is likely to harm a client or others. They seek assistance for problems that reach the level of professional impairment, and, if necessary, they limit, suspend, or terminate their professional responsibilities until such time it is determined that they may safely resume their work. Counselors assist colleagues or supervisors in recognizing their own professional impairment and provide consultation and assistance when warranted with colleagues or supervisors showing signs of impairment and intervene as appropriate to prevent imminent harm to clients.

American Psychological Association (APA) Ethical Principles of Psychologists and Code of Conduct (2002)

2.06 Personal Problems and Conflicts

(a) Psychologists refrain from initiating an activity when they know or should know that there is a substantial likelihood that their personal problems will prevent them from performing their work-related activities in a competent manner.

(b) When psychologists become aware of personal problems that may interfere with their performing work-related duties adequately, they take appropriate measures, such as obtaining professional consultation or assistance, and determine whether they should limit, suspend, or terminate their work-related duties.

National Association of Social Workers (NASW) Code of Ethics (1999)

4.05 Impairment

(a) Social workers should not allow their own personal problems, psychosocial distress, legal problems, substance abuse, or mental health difficulties to interfere with their professional judgment and performance or to jeopardize the best interests of people for whom they have a professional responsibility.

(b) Social workers whose personal problems, psychosocial distress, legal problems, substance abuse, or mental health difficulties interfere with their professional judgment and performance should immediately seek consultation and take appropriate remedial action by seeking professional help, making adjustments in workload, terminating practice, or taking any other steps necessary to protect clients and others.

Ethical Responsibilities

If the therapist feels unable to provide effective therapy, or the ability to provide therapy is limited or impaired in any way, treatment must be terminated or suspended.

Clients are entitled to effective treatment from educated and well-functioning therapists. Thus, therapists should be aware at all times of their physical and mental condition. If at any point, regardless of the cause, the therapist feels unable to provide effective therapy, or the ability to provide therapy is limited or impaired in any way, treatment must be terminated or suspended. Any act that interferes with the goal of effective treatment could easily be considered unethical and inappropriate, and subject the provider to disciplinary action.

In the third vignette, Karen waited too long to seek treatment for her own problems, and this delay could have resulted in serious consequences for her. Fortunately the unnerved client only decided to seek help from another therapist and did not file a complaint against Karen. Even more fortunate for Karen, the suicidal client did not take any action to harm herself after the upsetting incident in Karen's office. Karen should not have been attempting to treat clients in her condition.

After decades of work with mental health professionals who have committed serious ethical violations, we have observed that the majority of these individuals have been impaired in some manner, which affected their competence to practice and rendered them vulnerable to commit an ethics violation. This has been particularly true for mental health professionals who have become sexually or romantically involved with clients or former clients. When we examined what was going on in the violating mental health professionals' lives we found that often they were a mess, physically, mentally, or emotionally. Their problems made them more susceptible to advances from clients or former clients who maneuvered them into having incredibly poor judgment. It is imperative for therapists to regularly and objectively analyze their level of competence and to seek professional assistance quickly when they have serious problems that impair their judgment.

Mental health professionals also have a duty to address and report the impairment of colleagues and their delivery of incompetent services. For example, see the ACA Ethics Rule, C.2.g. Impairment, set forth previously and the following provision from the NASW Code of Ethics (1999):

2.09 Impairment of Colleagues

(a) Social workers who have direct knowledge of a social work colleague's impairment that is due to personal problems, psychosocial distress, substance abuse, or mental health difficulties and that interferes with practice effectiveness should consult with that colleague when feasible and assist the colleague in taking remedial action.

(b) Social workers who believe that a social work colleague's impairment interferes with practice effectiveness and that the colleague has not taken adequate steps to address the impairment should take action through appropriate channels established by employers, agencies, NASW, licensing and regulatory bodies, and other professional organizations.

The protection of the public and the integrity of all mental health disciplines demand competency of both the provider and the services provided. Nothing less will be tolerated.

The following are practice guidelines regarding misuse of alcohol or other substances and impairment:

- All mental health professionals should regularly take stock of their ability to provide competent therapy in their own judgment and in accordance with the client's expectations.
- The impaired professional must seek professional help as soon as the impairment is discovered.
- Until professional help is obtained and the problem of impairment overcome, professional responsibilities must be limited, suspended, or terminated.
- Each mental health professional is individually responsible for determining whether drugs, alcohol, or some other substance, controlled or not, or their physical, emotional, or mental condition affects professional competence.
- The abuse of any controlled substance as well as the intemperate use of alcohol can lead to an ethical disaster.
- The earlier the professional discovers the impairment and seeks help the better.
- Treating a client while impaired is both unethical and grounds for a malpractice suit if the client is injured. The treatment of clients while impaired is unethical whether or not drugs or alcohol led to personal problems or personal problems led to the substance abuse. The client's perception of the therapist's condition will be given great weight. The provider is the vulnerable person. (*Note:* Recently, a state licensing board member indicated that complaints took about a year to process. The threat of disciplinary action

hanging over a therapist's head is unpleasant and produces anxiety. Even a dismissal of a complaint may not be a finding of innocence. It may simply indicate that the case could not be proved to the satisfaction of the ruling body. The black cloud of suspicion could follow the provider for the rest of his or her career.)

- Malpractice and unethical conduct are determined by two different systems. Injury must be proved in a malpractice suit. In a complaint for unethical conduct, the board need only find that the practitioner practiced while impaired thus endangering clients while not necessarily injuring them.

- Therapists have an ethical obligation to help impaired colleagues and to report evidence of unethical conduct resulting from their impairment. This may include reporting the colleague to the licensing board.

- A clinician should never take a client out for a drink and should never accept an invitation to go for a drink from a client.

Ethical Flash Points

- Impairment can come from many sources. Use of a substance, even a legal substance such as prescription drugs or alcohol, may represent an ethical infraction if it impairs the clinician's ability to function effectively.

- "Functioning effectively" is in the eyes of the consumer of mental health services. Perception is everything. If the client perceives the therapist is "under the influence" as that phrase is commonly understood, the therapist could be disciplined if a complaint is filed.

- As soon as impairment is detected, arrangements must be made to protect clients and client records. Other competent therapists must be consulted to carry the client load so that all clients are served and protected on a continuing basis.

- If impairment is permanent, proper termination procedures must be followed (see Chapter 13, "Terminating Therapy"). The impaired therapist may have to close the practice (see Chapter 22, "Closing or Interrupting a Practice").

- If impairment is temporary, the therapist must make arrangements for clients while the therapist is receiving treatment.

- If therapy is terminated or suspended, the therapist should consider and address clients' abandonment issues, especially if the client requires continuous care and treatment.

- An act can be unethical and still be legal.

- An illegal act is generally unethical, although this depends on the circumstances. (A clinician might drive while under the influence—an illegal act—but if all clients are seen while the clinician is sober and functioning perfectly, the clinician has not committed an ethical violation.)

- Ethical conduct requires that the client receive competent, effective treatment. Any drug or alcohol use that dilutes therapeutic effectiveness is unethical.

- If the clinician feels "woozy," impaired, or unable to function in any way, cancel the session, regroup, consider the options, and consult any applicable ethical standards. A clinical session should not take place if the therapist is functioning at 90 percent. The client is entitled to 100 percent of the therapist's concentration and attention.

- An impaired therapist is much more likely to commit a serious ethical violation than a therapist who is operating with all his or her faculties.

- Taking chances courts ethical disaster.

Summary

Not all drugs are forbidden. Over-the-counter drugs are legal as are prescription drugs and all the "natural" supplements found in health food stores. What is unethical is taking medication or any drug or substance that prevents the mental health professional from performing with 100 percent clarity and efficiency and thereby *potentially* injuring a client in the process. Legitimate medications can become inappropriate when taken in higher than physician recommended dosages or when taken in combination with other substances that cause impairment.

Some substances are illegal and defined as such by state and federal penal codes. The clinician who takes a controlled substance that alters his or her ability to function is acting unethically in addition to acting criminally.

Alcohol is generally legal, and the mental health professional who has wine or champagne with dinner or imbibes within tolerable limits is free to exercise his or her right to drink with impunity. Unethical conduct only takes place when any illegal substance is used or when the active provider is adversely affected by alcohol intake while practicing as a professional. Clients take a dim view of the provider/clinician who comes to the office with the odor of alcohol surrounding him or her. Our advice: Don't see clients after a champagne dinner or a one-martini lunch.

Providers are skating on thin ethical ice if they use alcohol, drugs, or controlled substances of any type, especially if they use them in a manner that adversely affects the provider's ability to provide effective therapeutic services or treatment. Also, it is unethical, as well as illegal, to use illegal drugs of any kind or to promote, encourage, or concur in the illegal use or possession of illegal drugs.

Strange as it may seem, there is a small but impressive roster of therapists who have lost their licenses because of their inability or unwillingness to seek and receive the help offered by well-meaning friends and colleagues. "I don't have a problem," they said. But they did, and the board disciplined them for their problem because it adversely affected their clients.

As lawyers, we are constantly reminded of how bad things can happen to good people. Even the most experienced and careful mental health professionals can be overwhelmed with physical or emotional problems that will render them vulnerable and cause them to commit acts of poor judgment. Treating a client when you are not competent to do so is just one possibility—often, other serious ethical violations result. Mental health treatment providers must be objective and realistic and frequently assess their abilities when determining their level of competence and ability to competently treat clients.

Denial, in the therapeutic sense, is not limited to clients. The mental health professional should know better.

Suggested Research Assignments

1. Locate and discuss the provisions of the ethical codes promulgated by the mental health profession licensing boards and the law in your state with regard to impairment due to the abuse of alcohol or drugs or for other reasons. What rules and duties do they impose?

2. Locate and discuss any state and national professional association rules with regard to impairment. What are their similarities and differences?

3. Compare and contrast the obligations imposed by the state licensing boards in your state with the rules promulgated by the state professional associations.

4. Investigate whether there are programs offered by the licensing boards in your state for impaired licensees.

5. Compare and contrast state licensing board and professional association obligations with the guidelines of national professional associations.

6. Research the decisions of your state licensing boards and state and national professional association ethics committees for sanctions imposed for violations relating to alcohol or substance abuse and impairment.

7. Research legal civil case decisions for your state that involve abuse of alcohol or substance abuse and impairment.

8. Talk to practicing mental health professionals in your area and ask them about how they would handle an incompetent colleague.

9. Create a protocol that you will implement if you determined a colleague was incompetent to treat clients or was providing incompetent services.

Discussion Questions

1. A colleague tells you over lunch that she is having a difficult time focusing during afternoon therapy sessions and often does not hear or remember what clients are telling her. What do you advise? What do you do when you find out the colleague has ignored your advice regarding a perceived impairment?

2. After a painful period of self-analysis, you have determined you
   have a problem with alcohol and that it is affecting your professional and personal life. You have decided to enter into treatment
   that initially will require 30 days of inpatient care. What do you do
   about your practice clients? What do you tell them? What do you
   document in their files?

3. You are a licensed professional counselor who receives a large number of referrals from a local psychiatrist. Several of the referred clients have told you that the psychiatrist often appears intoxicated
   when they see him for their medication-related follow-ups. What
   do you do? What do you advise the clients? What, if anything, do
   you document in the clients' files? Would your answer be different
   if the psychiatrist involved was not someone who regularly referred
   clients to you?

27

Duty to Warn

An agitated client began a fourth therapy session with Karen, a licensed psychologist, with the statement, "If my boss doesn't get off my back soon, I don't know what I'm going to do!" When Karen asked him what he meant, he responded, "You know. Like those post office cases." Control went downhill from there. Karen learned the client had a state-issued concealed handgun permit and several firearms and knew how to use them. Karen tried to get the client to agree to contact her or present himself to a hospital emergency room if he felt sudden homicidal urges coming over him. She tried to obtain the written or oral commitment that he would immediately see a psychiatrist on leaving her office. Karen also asked him to allow another family member to take possession of his guns and his permit for the weapons. She even sought consent from the client to notify his boss that the boss might be in danger. The client refused all her requests, and after 30 frustrating, frightening, and unproductive minutes, he abruptly ran out of the office. After 45 more uncomfortable and difficult minutes of contemplation, Karen elected to breach confidentiality. She phoned the client's boss and warned him of the threats. The boss was so frightened by the warning that he terminated the client's employment immediately and sent a telegram to the client's home to advise him of the fact. Is Karen free from any liability *for breaching confidentiality? Has she created a hornet's nest of legal-ethical concerns?*

Sylvia is a patient in marital and individual therapy with Kevin, a licensed marriage and family therapist. She told Kevin in an individual counseling session that she was on the verge of killing herself. She said that her marital problems, her kids, and her job were all more than she could handle at one time. After an extended therapy session, Sylvia said she felt much better and did not feel suicidal. She contracted with Kevin to call him should she become overwhelmed again and said she would see her family doctor the next day and ask for a prescription for an antidepressant. After Sylvia left the office, Kevin phoned her husband and advised him to watch Sylvia very closely because she had indicated she felt like killing herself. The husband called his lawyer and told him to proceed with a divorce and custody lawsuit and to subpoena Kevin and his wife's records. When Sylvia learned that Kevin called her husband, she was incensed and promised to pursue all legal remedies against the therapist. Does Kevin have anything to worry about?

Case Law Regarding Duty to Warn

In 1976, the California Supreme Court established what many perceived to be the national standard for mental health professionals when a client poses a threat to an identified person. In *Tarasoff v. Regents of the University of California* (17 Cal. 3d 425, 551 P2d 334, 131 Cal. Rep. 14, 1976), the highest California state court ruled that the psychotherapist of a potentially violent patient had a duty to protect the identifiable intended victim from the patient's threatened violence. The California Supreme Court opined that *society's need for protection outweighed a client's right to confidentiality.* Over the past several decades, the trend around the country has been to follow the ruling of *Tarasoff* although it has by no means been universally applied. Courts in states such as Texas and Florida have specifically rejected the holding in *Tarasoff.* Therefore, whether Kevin and Karen, the mental health professionals in the previous vignettes, acted appropriately depends on the state in which the practice is located.

In 1976, the California Supreme Court opined that society's need for protection outweighed a client's right to confidentiality.

National ethics codes lean in the direction of the *Tarasoff* holding, requiring a breach of confidentiality to prevent harm by the client to third persons or to the client, but fall short of imposing the *obligation* to contact the identified potential victim. The HIPAA Privacy Rule provides an option consistent with the *Tarasoff* case, but it too contains permissive rather than mandatory options. It reads as follows:

(j) Standard: uses and disclosures to avert a serious threat to health or safety.

(1) Permitted disclosures. A covered entity may, consistent with applicable law and standards of ethical conduct, use or disclose protected health information, if the covered entity, in good faith, believes the use or disclosure:

(A) Is necessary to prevent or lessen a serious and imminent threat to the health or safety of a person or the public; and

(B) Is to a person or persons reasonably able to prevent or lessen the threat, including the target of the threat. . . .

National Guidelines Regarding Duty to Warn

American Association for Marriage and Family Therapy (AAMFT) Code of Ethics (2001)

Principle II: Confidentiality . . .

2.2 Marriage and family therapists do not disclose client confidences except by written authorization or waiver, or where mandated or permitted by law. . . .

American Counseling Association (ACA) Code of Ethics (2005)

Section b: Confidentiality, Privileged Communication and Privacy . . .

B.2. Exceptions

B.2.a. Danger and Legal Requirements

The general requirement that counselors keep information confidential does not apply when disclosure is required to

(*continued*)

(Continued)

protect clients or identified others from serious and foresee-able harm or when legal requirements demand that confidential information must be revealed. Counselors consult with other professionals when in doubt as to the validity of an exception. Additional considerations apply when addressing end-of-life issues.

B.2.b. Contagious, Life-Threatening Diseases

When clients disclose that they have a disease commonly known to be both communicable and life threatening, counselors may be justified in disclosing information to identifiable third parties, if they are known to be at demonstrable and high risk of contracting the disease. Prior to making a disclosure, counselors confirm that there is such a diagnosis and assess the intent of clients to inform the third parties about their disease or to engage in any behaviors that may be harmful to an identifiable third party.

American Psychological Association (APA) Ethical Principles of Psychologists and Code of Conduct (2002)

4. Privacy And Confidentiality

4.05 Disclosures . . .

(b) Psychologists disclose confidential information without the consent of the individual only as mandated by law, or where permitted by law for a valid purpose such as to (1) provide needed professional services; (2) obtain appropriate professional consultations; (3) protect the client/patient, psychologist, or others from harm; or (4) obtain payment for services from a client/patient, in which instance disclosure is limited to the minimum that is necessary to achieve the purpose.

American School Counselor Association (ASCA) Ethical Standards for School Counselors (2004)

A.2. Confidentiality

The professional school counselor . . .

b. Keeps information confidential unless disclosure is required to prevent clear and imminent danger to the student or others or when legal requirements demand that confidential information be revealed. Counselors will consult with appropriate professionals when in doubt as to the validity of an exception.

c. In absence of state legislation expressly forbidding disclosure, considers the ethical responsibility to provide information to an identified third party who, by his or her relationship with the student, is at a high risk of contracting a disease that is commonly known to be communicable and fatal. Disclosure requires satisfaction of all of the following conditions:

> Student identifies partner or the partner is highly identifiable.
>
> Counselor recommends the student notify partner and refrain from further high-risk behavior.
>
> Student refuses.
>
> Counselor informs the student of the intent to notify the partner.
>
> Counselor seeks legal consultation as to the legalities of informing the partner.

National Association of Social Workers (NASW) Code of Ethics (1999)

1.07 Privacy and Confidentiality . . .

(c) Social workers should protect the confidentiality of all information obtained in the course of professional service, except

(continued)

(*Continued*)

for compelling professional reasons. The general expectation that social workers will keep information confidential does not apply when disclosure is necessary to prevent serious, foreseeable, and imminent harm to a client or other identifiable person. In all instances, social workers should disclose the least amount of confidential information necessary to achieve the desired purpose; only information that is directly relevant to the purpose for which the disclosure is made should be revealed. . . .

Mandated Disclosure versus Duty to Warn

The professional association ethics code provisions allow for disclosure of confidential information when the client or a third party is in imminent danger but do not specifically provide authority for contacting the identified potential victim. The cited ACA and ASCA rules contain exceptions in certain circumstances for persons who may be exposed to a communicable life-threatening disease by a client. The AAMFT provisions were the most general of all. Each code states that confidentiality must be breached when "mandated by law" or "when laws require disclosure." These codes create a situation whereby the mental health professional must be cognizant of the specific state statutes and the case law of the state in which the mental health services are being provided.

The HIPAA Privacy Rule permits contact with the potential victim but its rules do not supersede state law that is more protective of privacy. *State law is controlling on the issue of duty to warn.* It is apparent that in situations involving danger to self and others, confidentiality may be breached. What is not clear and is not universal is the *duty to warn* and which person or persons should or can be warned or contacted. Does the therapist have a duty to contact the identified victim? Can the therapist contact the identified victim? Can the therapist contact medical or law enforcement personnel? The answers to these questions vary from state to state, although the consensus is that imminent danger to a client or another person generally gives rise to an exception to confidentiality. The following is a sampling of states that have imposed a duty by statute on mental health professionals to warn identifiable potential victims:

Alaska (Alaska Stat. Sec. 08.86.200, 1986),

California (Cal. Civ. Code Sec. 43.92, West Supp. 1988),

Colorado (Colo. Rev. Stat. Sec. 13-21-117, 1987),

Indiana (Indiana Code Ann. Sec. 3.4-4-12.4-1, Burns Supp., 1988),

Kansas (Kan. Stat. Ann. Sec. 65-5603. Supp, 1987),

Kentucky (Ky. Rev. Stat. Ann. Sec. 202A400, Baldwin, 1987),

Louisiana (La. Rev. Stat. Ann. Sec. 9:2900.2, Supp. 1989),

Minnesota (Minn. Stat. Ann. Sec. 148.975, West Supp., 1989),

Montana (Mont. Code Ann. Secs. 27-1-1101, 2, 3, 1987),

New Hampshire (N.H. Rev. Stat. Ann. Sec. 329:31),

Utah (Utah Code Ann. Sec. 78-14a-102, Supp., 1986), and

Washington (Wash. Rev. Code Ann. Ch. 212 and 301, Cum. Supp. 1987).

Many of these statutes require notification of the identified potential victim as well as local law enforcement personnel. Many require that the client, whose right of confidentiality has been superseded by state law, be advised of the information disclosed and the identities of the person(s) to whom disclosure was made. More states impose a *Tarasoff* duty than do not. Many experts in the area believe that, regardless of specific state statutes, the *Tarasoff* holding is a national standard. Robert I. Simon (1992), in his treatise, *Clinical Psychiatry and the Law*, writes, "practitioners should practice as if the *Tarasoff* duty to protect is the law . . . the duty to protect is, in effect, a national standard of practice" (pp. 312–313). We would pose two questions to a therapist practicing in a state that does not follow *Tarasoff* or that does not have a duty-to-warn statute:

It is apparent that in situations involving danger to self and others confidentiality may be breached.

1. Would you prefer to be sued for breaching confidentiality, by warning the identifiable potential victim or a family member if the client is suicidal, and perhaps saving a life or preventing harm?

2. Would you prefer to be sued for not breaching confidentiality and allowing harm to be suffered by a third party or the client?

Any clear-thinking person would pick the first question as the lesser of two evils, but courts and legislatures are still debating these issues. Whenever a case of duty to warn presents itself in practice, put the client on hold. Call a lawyer, your insurance liability carrier, or a knowledgeable colleague at once. Duty to warn is a serious and evolving area of law, and an immediate technical understanding is essential to making an informed judgment.

Exceptions to the Tarasoff Rule

The threats of imminent danger by a client to himself, herself, or a third party create an immense ethical conflict for therapists. When state law clearly defines the therapist's duty, the correct course of action is obvious. The therapist follows the statute and warns each person to whom warnings are required to be given. Ethics codes impose a duty on therapists to breach confidentiality when mandated by law. Failing to do so to preserve confidentiality under those circumstances is an ethical violation that could lead to sanctioning by a licensing board or professional organization. This would be true even if the client or a third party suffers no harm and no civil or criminal action is brought against the therapist. Failure to follow the law is an ethical violation. When state law is not specific or in fact precludes contacting identified potential victims, the therapist's resolution of the ethical conflict is not clear.

As stated earlier, *Tarasoff* is not universally applied. Texas has clearly departed from the holding of the California Supreme Court in the *Tarasoff* case. Texas statutory law gives a mental health professional the option of notifying medical or law enforcement personnel if the mental heath professional reasonably believes that the client or a third person is in imminent physical danger or the client is in imminent emotional danger. The statute doesn't authorize disclosure or warning to the identified victim. It uses the word "may" in connection with notifying medical or law enforcement personnel so it does not even create a duty to notify those persons (Texas Health and Safety Code Sec. 611.004(a)(2)).

On June 24, 1999, the Texas Supreme Court, in *Thapar v. Zezulka* (994 S.W.2 635) (Texas 1999), reversed a lower court's decision imposing a duty on mental health professionals to warn identifiable victims when a client reveals an intention to harm a third party. In this case, a psychiatrist was sued when one of his patients, after threatening to kill his stepfather, did so. The Texas Supreme Court held, "Because the Legislature has established a policy against such a common law cause of action, we refrain from imposing on mental health professionals a duty to warn third parties of a patient's threats." The court carefully reviewed Texas statutory law on confidentiality and although many exceptions and duties were legislated, a duty to warn identifiable potential victims was conspicuously absent. Because the applicable statute did not impose a duty to contact medical or law enforcement personnel, the court refused to hold the psychiatrist liable for his failure to do so. The court held that the legislature had given the mental health professional the option, but not the duty, to contact medical or law enforcement personnel.

Differentiating between Homicide and Suicide Threats

Even states following *Tarasoff* distinguish between cases of threats of homicide and suicide. A therapist's duty to warn is less straightforward when a client threatens to commit suicide. Can a family member be contacted? Is there a duty to warn family members? The therapist may simply have to consider all available information; consult with colleagues, an attorney, the professional liability insurance provider, and the licensing board; and then balance the potential risk of each option in deciding which will best serve the client, the therapist, and society. The current national consensus regarding duty to warn seems to favor notifying potential victims when harm is threatened to a third party (potential homicide), or family members in the event of suicidal ideation. The therapist must be knowledgeable of all applicable laws, case precedents, and ethics code provisions regarding duty to warn before a client ever walks into the therapist's office.

The current national consensus regarding duty to warn seems to favor notifying potential victims when harm is threatened to a third party (potential homicide), or family members in the event of suicidal ideation.

Waiting until a duty-to-warn crisis situation is presented in therapy may be too late to correctly, ethically, and effectively handle the situation.

Ethical Flash Points

- Threats by a client to harm a third party or the client should be taken very seriously, carefully documented, and a serious rationale outlined that substantiates the route taken to ameliorate the condition.

- National ethics codes do not establish a clear, mandated "duty to warn potential identified victims" but do require confidentiality to be breached when mandated by law. A few codes provide for warning to be made to persons who may be exposed to a life-threatening communicable disease by a client. New state statutes and ethics codes are being promulgated to control this situation.

- The HIPAA Privacy Rule provides a permissive option to notify an identified intended victim, but more protective state laws would supersede its provisions.

- Since not all states impose a duty to warn, the *Tarasoff* case cannot be considered the universal standard of care.

- It is critical to acquire and keep updating thorough knowledge of the statutory law and case law regarding the duty to warn applicable in the state in which the therapist provides mental health services. An understanding of the statute and case law must be evaluated in the risk-reward context each time a problem arises.

- Even when potential victims cannot be specifically notified, a therapist is usually authorized to contact law enforcement personnel.

- Since this area of law is not well settled in many states, therapists should annually seek an advisory opinion from their licensing board before a situation raises the question about the duty to warn.

- Depending on the state where services are provided, the failure to warn or warning and breaching confidentiality could each be an ethical violation.

- When state law is not specific or does not authorize warning potential victims, therapists must balance each risk when making a decision concerning what action to take, if any.

- Breaking new ground and becoming a test case is not always professionally helpful.

- Therapists need to keep abreast of current case law concerning duty to warn because such situations constitute an emergency, allowing the therapist little time to reflect and ponder the options. When a client threatens homicide or suicide, the threat is usually immediate, serious, and emotional and requires the therapist to decide quickly what action to take, if any.

- Consent to warn an identifiable or identified potential victim or the family, friends, or physician of a potential suicidal client might be considered by utilizing a carefully drafted intake and consent form. In this form, reviewed by an attorney in each jurisdiction, the client might consent in writing, in advance, waiving confidentiality in the event of possible homicide or suicide dangers. (See p. 45 of *The Portable Lawyer for Mental Health Professionals*, Bernstein and Hartsell 2004, for a discussion of such language in an intake and consent form.)

- In situations where the practitioner is arranging continuing education seminars, consulting with a lawyer or insurance expert on the therapist's duty-to-warn problem on an annual basis is advisable. Practitioners are often not apprised of this issue when the ethical and legal standards are discussed and up-to-date information must be presented.

Summary

Most therapists practice in a state that either follows *Tarasoff* or has enacted specific legislation that imposes a duty to warn and identifies those persons who are to be contacted. The ethical considerations are less complicated for these particular therapists. For those who do not practice in such states, the therapist is left with choices to ponder and a multitude of options. The Texas *Thapar* case indicates that in some jurisdictions there is *no* duty to warn the identifiable potential victim.

The national consensus seems to favor notifying potential victims when harm is threatened to a third party (potential homicide), or family members in the event of suicidal ideation. Knowledge of all applicable laws and ethics code provisions is essential before a client ever walks into a therapist's office. Waiting until a duty-to-warn crisis situation is presented in therapy may be too late to correctly, ethically, and effectively handle the situation. Whichever option is exercised, the clinical record must reflect the reasons for the choice. Indeed, the client record is the best evidence to substantiate whichever action is taken.

Suggested Research Assignments

1. Locate and discuss the ethical provisions of the mental health profession licensing boards and the law in your state with respect to issue of duty to warn. What are the rules and duties they impose?
2. Locate and discuss any state and national professional association rules with regard to the duty to warn. What are their similarities and differences?
3. Compare and contrast the obligations imposed by the state statutes and licensing boards in your state with the rules promulgated by the state professional associations.
4. Compare and contrast state statute and licensing board and professional association obligations with the guidelines of national professional associations.
5. Research the decisions of your state licensing boards and state and national professional association ethics committees for sanctions imposed for violations relating to the duty to warn.
6. Research legal civil case decisions for your state that involve the duty-to-warn issue. What damages if any were assessed? How have these cases evolved over the years?
7. Talk to practicing mental health professionals in your area and ask them about how they would handle the duty-to-warn issue and ask them to describe the kinds of cases in which it has been presented in their practices.
8. Create a protocol that you will implement if a client is expressing serious homicidal or suicidal ideation.

Discussion Questions

1. The husband of a longtime client calls you at the office and tells you that his wife is threatening to kill herself. He is so worried that

he has stayed home from work to keep an eye on her. What do you advise? What do you do? What do you document in the client's file? How much can you reveal about the wife, your client?

2. A seriously depressed client continues to express suicidal ideation and refuses to see a psychiatrist for medication. What do you advise? What do you do? What do you document in the client's file?

3. A client sent you an e-mail telling you that he has just gotten to work and can't take the "abuse" his boss keeps giving him. The client thanks you for all your help, but there is no other choice now but to "take out" the boss. What do you do? What do you document in the client's file?

4. You are having coffee with another therapist with whom you went to graduate school. She is telling you about a difficult client who may be suicidal and is not cooperative in therapy. What do you advise?

28

Interprofessional Issues

A few years ago in a major midwestern city, an argument concerning the relative effectiveness of psychiatry versus psychology became part of the local media scene. Psychiatrists and psychologists were publicly criticizing each other while each profession defended its perceived turf. Eventually the conflict fizzled out, but not until after the debate had sullied the dignity and reputation of both professions in the eyes of the public. What should have been a quiet negotiation ended in a noisy, media-inspired discourse that confused rather than clarified. Leading questions by reporters seemed to force each discipline to take positions that were extreme and that did not clearly state the reasonable position of the profession. However, the conflict made good copy and sold newspapers.

Jane consulted an open forum of mental health providers representing members of each of the major mental health professions. She indicated that her marriage was in trouble, she had difficulty keeping a job, her son "might" be using a controlled substance, and her attractive 14-year-old daughter was sexually active and only chuckled when Jane wanted to talk to her about sex. Jane felt terribly depressed as a result. Jane's insurance covered therapy, but she was confused by her treatment options. Should she consult a social *worker, a job counselor, a marriage and family therapist, or a psychologist? She received a different answer from the practitioner of each discipline represented.*

Alike Yet Different

No one really knows what Sigmund Freud was thinking when he began his quest to understand the human mind. We'll never know whether he foresaw the diverse group of mental health providers or the incredible variety of treatment options available to consumers. Today, there are several major categories of mental health practitioners, and subgroups too numerous to mention within those categories. Therapists practice hypnosis, play therapy, music therapy, and animal therapy. Others offer marriage counseling, addictions counseling, substance abuse counseling, or career counseling. To the consuming public in need of mental health help, the options can be mind-boggling. If testing is needed, a psychologist should be engaged. If the presenting problem concerns a family, does one call a pastoral counselor, a relationship counselor, or a marriage and family therapist? If an addiction surfaces in the middle of couple therapy, should the individual be referred to an addiction counselor or can the marriage and family therapist call in a consultant for the addiction problem and continue to offer counseling to the couple? In the hospital setting, where cost-conscious administrators make every effort to cut expenses, does it make a difference whether a psychiatrist, psychologist, counselor, hospital chaplain, or social worker is consulted, considering that the hourly rate can vary considerably between and among disciplines? If someone were to examine a well-documented diagnosis and treatment plan, could that person determine to which discipline the mental health provider belonged?

Common Threads: Ethics

The ethics codes of the various disciplines indicate that the common ground far outweighs the differences among them. Common to all the mental health professions is a responsibility to the public, confidentiality, professional competence and integrity, a responsibility to research participants, and responsibilities to the different professions. Financial arrangements with clients, limits on advertising, the requirements for advanced degrees and constant continuing education, and, in most cases, obtaining and maintaining a license also represent common ground among the professions. There are some differences. For example, psychological testing in some jurisdictions is restricted to being done by psychologists, and addictions counseling in some jurisdictions can be limited to individuals with special background and training, but in general the concepts are the same.

Other commonalities among the professions include:

- A vulnerability to malpractice suits and ethical complaints. In addition, the elements of a malpractice suit (i.e., duty, breach of duty by an act of commission or omission, negligence, proximate cause, and damages) among the disciplines are almost identical.
- Using ethical codes as evidence of the appropriate standard of conduct in a malpractice suit. Licensing board rules and regulations are also admissible evidence to indicate negligence in a malpractice suit.
- Malpractice policy exclusions. For example, most policies will not cover, except up to a certain set limit, sexual activities with a client, criminal accusations such as fraudulent billing or insurance claims, and intentional wrongful acts.
- Limitations on bragging rights in literature, advertising, introductions, and publicity.
- Insisting on truth in articles, introductions, and promotional material.
- Specific and general elements of informed consent.
- Limitations on the treatment that can be offered and the need to back up the treatment modality by research, the literature, or sufficient education or experience.
- Prohibitions against kickbacks.
- Prohibitions against boundary violations, dual relationships, or any hint of client exploitation.
- Duty-to-warn provisions for potentially homicidal or suicidal clients.
- Record keeping and documentation procedures.

Common to all the mental health professions is a responsibility to the public, confidentiality, professional competence and integrity, a responsibility to research participants, and responsibilities to the different professions.

- Billing records including correct procedures for missed appointments, court appearances, and other services rendered.
- The need to interview clients in person.
- Rules against sexual misconduct.
- Policies for reporting an impaired provider and practicing while impaired.
- Rules for maintaining confidentiality.
- Guidelines for supporting suppressed and recovered memory.
- Policies for addressing special problems within group settings.
- Guidelines for avoiding potential discrimination accusations.
- Procedures for managing turf disputes.
- Policies for reporting colleagues' unethical conduct.

Protecting One's Professional "Turf"

Most mental health practitioners see clear boundaries between the mental health disciplines, but the differences among them may be less clear to the consuming public. Picking and choosing intelligently from among the many types of providers is difficult. The boundaries of the mental health disciplines are not clearly defined for the layperson, nor can they be identified with enough specificity to be totally separated.

What might be considered a turf problem actually represents healthy competition for the mental health dollar.

What might be considered a turf problem actually represents healthy competition for the mental health dollar. The number of licensed mental health professionals continues to grow, and many large metropolitan areas are saturated with qualified providers who are seeking their fortune in a managed care, controlled mental health environment in which only the strongest survive. The mental health professions will continue to protect what they perceive to be their turf if they can, but in many cases control of the mental health environment has slipped out of providers' hands and into the hands of insurance companies, conglomerates, and other gatekeepers.

Avoiding Turf Battles

Some differences between mental health disciplines are well recognized. Psychiatrists are able to prescribe medication, whereas most psychologists are not. Other specialties also have protected turf, but most mental health providers practice under a wide umbrella whose services compete with other mental health professionals. Every provider has a proprietary interest in protecting his or her turf. But is it worth it? The last thing the larger mental health profession and its practitioners need is interdisciplinary discord, especially public discord. Mental health professionals should avoid public turf battles. A large segment of society already views the mental health profession and its practitioners with skepticism, cynicism, or uncertainty. Public expressions of mutual respect and support among the disciplines will increase public confidence in the profession and induce more people to seek services.

The current reality is that mental health professionals often find themselves working as one member of an interdisciplinary team. In these circumstances, it is crucial for all team members to understand each other's roles and to work to provide the highest quality of services possible for the client. Achieving the best result for the client requires interdisciplinary respect and a knowledge about other disciplines and cooperation among all treating practitioners. The ACA Code of Ethics (2002) includes an entire section on relationships with other professionals that reads in part as follows:

Section D: Relationships with Other Professionals

Introduction
Professional counselors recognize that the quality of their interactions with colleagues can influence the quality of services provided to clients. They work to become knowledgeable about colleagues within and without the field of counseling. Counselors develop positive working relationships and systems of communication with colleagues to enhance services to clients.

D.1. Relationships with Colleagues, Employers, and Employees

D.1.a. Different Approaches
Counselors are respectful of approaches to counseling services that differ from their own. Counselors are respectful of traditions and practices of other professional groups with which they work.

D.1.b. Forming Relationships
Counselors work to develop and strengthen interdisciplinary relations with colleagues from other disciplines to best serve clients.

D.1.c. Interdisciplinary Teamwork

Counselors, who are members of interdisciplinary teams delivering multifaceted services to clients, keep the focus on how to best serve the clients. They participate in and contribute to decisions that affect the well-being of clients by drawing on the perspectives, values, and experiences of the counseling profession and those of colleagues from other disciplines.

Counselor members of ACA are prohibited from engaging in turf war kinds of behaviors. They are required to be knowledgeable and respectful of other disciplines and they endeavor to develop the kinds of relationships that will enhance the services clients receive. This is clearly an enlightened and sensible approach, one that should be emulated by all disciplines.

There is also a potential for media involvement if a conflict does arise. Ever vigilant for a juicy story, the media often goad disputing parties to cross the lines of professionalism to heat up their broadcasts. In such cases, practitioners should consider the adage "Stop! Look! Listen!" before jumping into the fray.

Ethical Flash Points

- Engaging in public turf conflicts with other mental health professionals can be mutually disastrous and should be avoided. Counselors must be aware that the purpose of newspapers is to sell newspapers. Reporters have a way of gathering information from professionals and then presenting it in a manner different from that intended by the interviewee. Be careful when a reporter asks you if you will just answer a "few simple questions." These "simple" questions seldom have simple answers.

- To mental health consumers, differences among mental health disciplines are ill defined, unnecessary, and confusing.

- "Bad mouthing" a competitive discipline is unethical and demonstrates a clinician's bad judgment. It could also be libelous, slanderous, or both.

- Personal success makes turf battles unnecessary.

- Understanding, cooperation, and respect for practitioners of other mental health disciplines on an interdisciplinary team are essential if the client is to receive the best possible treatment.

Summary

In the field of psychiatry, only medical doctors can prescribe medications. Psychologists are seeking to obtain the same privileges in their field of expertise, but to date the ability of nonmedical people to write prescriptions is not widely supported and is severely limited.

Some specialties have protected turf that is well recognized, acceptable, and accepted. Many mental health providers are under a wide umbrella and provide overlapping services. The provisions of licensing laws that define the various disciplines are not always clear.

Every professional has a proprietary interest in protecting his or her turf. The last thing the mental health profession and mental health professionals need, however, is interdisciplinary discord, especially public discord. A large segment of our society already views the mental health profession and its practitioners with limited and controlled skepticism, not to mention cynicism and uncertainty. Public expressions of mutual respect and support will increase confidence in the profession and induce more people to seek professional services. All disciplines will benefit.

Note: We continue to view movies and television programs, ever optimistic that somewhere, somehow, movies will be made and shows will be produced that portray a mental health professional as the hero, endowed with mental health healing qualities of profound benefit to the public. There have been very few.

Suggested Research Assignments

1. Locate and discuss the provisions of any ethical codes promulgated by the mental health profession licensing boards in your state with respect to relationships with other professionals. What rules and duties do they impose?

2. Locate and discuss any state and national professional association rules with regard to relationships with other professionals. What are the similarities and differences?

3. Compare and contrast the obligations imposed by the licensing boards in your state with the rules promulgated by the state professional associations.

4. Compare and contrast state licensing board and professional association obligations with the guidelines of national professional associations.

5. Research the licensing acts for the various mental health disciplines in your state and compile a list of unique and different services each discipline is legally authorized to provide to consumers.

6. Talk to practicing mental health professionals in your area and ask them about their relationships with professionals of different mental health disciplines.

7. Create a protocol that you will implement in your practice for interacting with other kinds of mental health professionals.

Discussion Questions

1. A potential client seeking services for depression asks you what kinds of help are available from you and how does that compare with what she could expect from other kinds of mental health professionals. What do you tell her? What do you document in the client file regarding this conversation if you are hired?

2. You are a licensed professional counselor working in a state hospital. A psychologist working in this same hospital continuously demeans and belittles your services and your discipline to patients and other staff members. What do you say? What action do you take?

3. What other professionals would you anticipate working with in your practice? What steps could you take to ensure the best possible outcome for clients when working with these other professionals?

29

Professional Vulnerability

Dick was a therapist in private practice. One of his clients suffered from borderline personality disorder and was dependent, needy, and vulnerable. Several times during treatment, she directly and indirectly implied that their common interest in art and art history transcended therapy and suggested they attend openings and other cultural events together. Dick always indicated that any relationship other than their professional one was a clear boundary violation, a prohibited dual relationship, and inappropriate as well as unethical. He also reminded her that there were published ethical codes that prohibited such relationships. One evening, after a particularly stressful session for Jane, she again suggested a liaison. Without thinking about it too much, Dick replied, "It might be nice, but I can't." Jane only heard the "it might be nice" part and conveniently forgot the rest. Building on her selective memory, Jane convinced herself that she and Dick had actually attended an art exhibit together, and although she was fuzzy about the details, she convinced herself that some sort of a sexual encounter had taken place. She was furious when, after a few more sessions, Dick indicated that he had helped her as much as he could and that she was ready to terminate their professional relationship and, if she felt she needed more help, she should seek another therapist. He offered her several competent referral sources

*should she wish to continue the therapeutic process, all of which she could
afford and all of whom were competent and available recognized professionals. Jane's fury turned to anger, and the anger became that of a woman
scorned. Jane would show Dick. No one could reject her without consequences. So she lashed out in every direction she could find or create: civil, criminal, and ethical. Even though Dick had done nothing inappropriate,
unethical, immoral, illegal, questionable, evil, unprofessional, or indecent,
he was still vulnerable.*

Criminal Vulnerability

*The legal process
begins when a client
makes an allega-
tion. If a district at-
torney or grand
jury finds the cli-
ent's testimony be-
lievable, the
defendant is
indicted.*

In Dick's state, as in many others, sex with a client is a felony. The
legal process begins when a client makes an allegation. If a district
attorney or grand jury finds the client's testimony believable, the defendant (in this case, Dick) is indicted. An indictment only means
there is probable cause of guilt. A jury trial would follow. Assuming
justice triumphed, Dick would be found not guilty after several years
of pending litigation, thousands of dollars in legal fees, countless
hours away from his practice, and colleagues who snickered quietly
thinking, "Where there's smoke, there's fire." Even if Dick is found
not guilty, the damage to his professional reputation and credibility
can never be repaired. Many people believe that "not guilty" does not
mean innocent, and "not liable" does not mean the transaction was
totally above suspicion. There would always be a cloud over Dick's
head.

Civil Vulnerability

*Civil litigation for
money damages in
a malpractice suit is
common practice.*

In our litigious society, civil litigation for money damages in a malpractice suit is common practice. Plaintiff's attorneys usually accept
these cases on a contingent fee (i.e., for a percentage of the recovery) and often advance their client's court costs and other litigation
expenses. Jane's attorney would have to prove that Jane was one
of Dick's clients, thereby acquiring a duty, both legal and ethical,
toward her. Further, they must prove that Dick breached his duty to
Jane by an inappropriate or negligent proposition and that the

proposition caused physical or psychological damage or both to her. If malpractice is determined, the jury then decides what money damages will compensate Jane for the provable damage she suffered.

As in the criminal trial, Dick's professional reputation could be ruined even if the jury finds in his favor. He is forced to spend additional time in court, becomes a minor celebrity on the evening news during the trial, and receives only limited exposure or publicity when found innocent. Moreover, he must pay the deductible on his malpractice insurance (assuming he had it—otherwise he would have had to pay all the trial expenses) in addition to suffering lost income from spending time out of the office. Finally, he will experience terrible anxiety while waiting for a jury to deliberate and report the verdict. On the other hand, Jane has nothing to lose by filing suit. Although she may not receive a settlement, she also does not have to pay attorney fees. Nor does she owe Dick anything for the inconvenience and expense to him. She just smirks as she leaves the courtroom and waves her gloved hand to Dick. "Adios," she says, with smug satisfaction, well aware of the inconvenience and embarrassment she has caused him.

Ethical Vulnerability

Jane located Dick's local professional organization, which indicated it did not have jurisdiction to discipline members. The local organization referred her to the state organization, which referred her to the national organization, which requested that she submit a written complaint to the national disciplinary committee responsible for overseeing complaints and taking action when an ethics violation is determined. By now, conversant with the jargon of the trade and knowledgeable concerning the terminology relative to dual relationships, boundary violations, and sex with clients, she embellished what had never happened to create a scenario of sordid events to further her goal: having Dick expelled from the national organization. She also recognized that she was not jeopardized in any way if her complaint were dismissed. Her only reaction could be, "Oops."

The national committee, after reviewing all the "he said" and "she said" evidence, concluded that no infraction had taken place and dismissed the complaint. Finally, after almost a year of interviews, letters, affidavits, and legal expenses, Dick was exonerated. He retained his membership in the national organization and continued to hold office in his supportive local chapter.

When a complaint in writing is filed, it is referred to the association's ethics committee and then forwarded to a local committee where the member resides.

Dick belongs to several other national organizations, each with a Code of Ethical Conduct and each with a mechanism in place to discipline members who violate the published ethical standards of the profession. When a complaint in writing is filed, it is referred to the association's ethics committee and then forwarded to a local committee where the member resides. Committee members review the facts and the member's written response and then, if the complaint is sustainable, expel the member from the organization and publish notice of the expulsion in the organization's annual publication and in their quarterly newsletter. Or, they can come to some compromise, mediate the dispute, or both. Jane located all of Dick's memberships and wrote to all the parent organizations explaining her situation. The national organizations also investigated, found nothing inappropriate, and dismissed her complaints. Dick spent agonizing hours defending himself and won the battle, but did he win the war?

Licensing Board Vulnerability

Jane also filed a complaint with Dick's state licensing board, consisting of eight individuals: six professional and two lay members. The board's ethics committee oversees any violations of the canons of ethics issued by the state board of examiners of Dick's discipline. After Jane filed a written complaint, they compared the complaint with the licensing law, board rules, and, in some cases, published ethical opinions of the state's attorney general. If the complaint states a violation, they send it to the licensee who must respond within 10 to 20 days. The board quotes the sections of the licensing law canons on ethics that include the alleged violation and ask the licensee to respond to the alleged violation. Based on their review of the licensee's response, they can dismiss the complaint or continue their investigation if the complaint merits further examination.

Dick answered fully, openly, and completely, and sent his response to the board after sending a rough draft to his attorney for approval (paying more than $200+ per hour in legal fees). After reviewing the circumstances, the rules, the evidence, and the allegations, the board dismissed Jane's complaint. Dismissing the complaint does not return Dick to his previous status of unfettered professional. Should the question ever be asked in an application of any type if he ever had a complaint filed against him, he would have to answer in the affirmative, and then explain. Complaints filed and then dismissed do not enhance a reputation. Rather, they may imply an unproved accusation.

Media Vulnerability

Each time Jane left the courtroom, reporters besieged her with questions. She was even asked to address various civic organizations concerning therapeutic ethics and the vulnerability of clients when they are in the hands of predatory professionals. With a publicist in tow, she glibly and intelligently answered all questions, offering to the media the picture of a wronged person. Some of her interviews appeared as sound bites on the evening news for a few seconds, and her words often found their way into the print media. As each accusation vaporized and Dick was found not guilty, not culpable, or not liable, media and public interest in her vanished, the speaking invitations were withdrawn, and the visibility of the situation dissolved. But although the media hounded Dick during his ordeal, his vindication received little press. Vindication did not seem to be newsworthy. Vindication by a jury, the press, or a judge does not seem to find itself easily into the public consciousness.

Overcoming Professional Vulnerability

Every forum hearing the evidence realized nothing had taken place that was in any way culpable. No evidence of an inappropriate dual relationship, a boundary violation, or a sexual proposition could be proven. Yet there was significant professional damage to Dick. Despite being cleared of any wrongdoing, his problems are not over. He now has trouble applying for hospital privileges and renewing his malpractice insurance because they always ask if there have been any complaints filed against him alleging ethical violations. He also has to grapple with slyly placed personal questions when considering a new job opportunity or a different association with professional colleagues. There is often skepticism when reading the required explanation that vigorously denies inappropriate conduct. Making an accusation is easy. Explaining it away is much more difficult, and writing a believable exculpatory letter is a Herculean challenge.

In addition, Dick still owes significant fees to his attorney and will be saddled with a public record, a media history, and the apparently unshakable questionable reputation of "*did he or did he not*" following him the remainder of his professional life. It is unlikely that he will ever completely recover emotionally, financially, and psychologically from the ordeal.

Now consider Jane. She is perfectly happy. She achieved her 15 minutes of fame, and now retires with a full scrapbook and memories of how the world is full of voracious therapists, none of whom are ever punished. No one can ever prevent her from telling her tale to anyone who will listen and, because her version of the relationship will go on unchallenged by any listener, the rumor mill will have a grand time embellishing the story and passing it on to interested gossipers. In fact, it could be reported in the press as an unconfirmed and unsubstantiated rumor and placed firmly in the literature.

> **Note:** In this fictitious case, Dick is the alleged perpetrator and Jane is the alleged victim. This is not to imply that in such situations men are always the wrongdoers and women are always the victims.

Ethical Flash Points

- As soon as the hint of an interpersonal connection arises, the professional must set the record straight, explain the strict boundaries, and document the event and the method by which it was handled.

- Attach a copy of the ethical standards to the initial intake form signed by the client so the client knows the distances and boundaries that must be observed between client and therapist.

- Be careful with casual offhand remarks. They may return to haunt you. Between a therapist and a client there is no such thing as an innocent, offhand remark. The therapist never knows which remarks a client may take seriously, out of context, be insulted by, offended, and angered. Any of these emotions can result in a complaint, litigation, and resentment.

- The client who has lunch with his lawyer, plays golf with his banker, and goes sailing with his broker is trying to blur the boundaries with his therapist. Don't do it! You are a very special category of helping professional.

- For a premium, good malpractice insurance exists. Unethical conduct insurance does not.

- There is no insurance to cover the loss of a license and, hence, a career.

- Income disability insurance does not cover the loss of a professional license or reputation.

Summary

There is no professional practice without risk, and many of the risks to mental health professionals are discussed in this chapter. These risks include civil liability, criminal vulnerability, and administrative controls such as licensing boards and state enforcement organizations. In addition, professional people join numerous national, state, and local organizations too numerous to mention without thinking of whether these organizations have published ethical standards and without realizing that when a person joins an organization with published standards they are bound by those standards and might be negligent if those principles are not honored. Published ethical standards are admissible evidence in court concerning minimum standards of conduct.

Then there are the ever-intrusive eyes of the free press. This makes every person's life, when that person becomes a "public" figure, the object of an open, publicly viewed, hunting season. A newspaper or television station can fill the pages or the screen with "unsubstantiated allegations," which is a true statement, but when the emotional and hotly contested allegations prove to be totally untrue and absolutely without legitimate foundation, the media is under no obligation to offer equal time to the vindication. All the innocent professional can do is show his scrapbook to colleagues, family, and friends who are interested.

So in summary: Know the rules, regulations, and ethical codes, practice within those rules, and, when an *ethical flash point* becomes a reality or a potential reality, honor and respect your gut reaction. Take immediate notice and respond seriously. Review the entire file, check the codes, and consult a colleague and a lawyer.

The potential consequences far exceed the obvious. Remember the case of poor Dick who did nothing wrong.

Suggested Research Assignments

1. Locate and discuss a case in which a mental health professional has been accused of misconduct that resulted in two or more of the following kinds of investigations: criminal, civil, administrative, and professional association. What were the outcomes of each?
2. Locate and discuss any story involving misconduct by a mental health professional that received extensive media coverage. Was the media coverage consistent in terms of its scope and prominence throughout the media life of the story?
3. Talk to practicing mental health professionals in your area and ask them about how vulnerable they feel as practicing professionals and what makes them feel the most vulnerable?

4. Create a protocol that you will implement if a client comes at you from all angles and a list of other professionals you can call on to assist you.

5. Examine your malpractice insurance policy to see how much protection it affords you with respect to each area of vulnerability discussed in this chapter.

Discussion Questions

1. A former client is interviewed by a reporter for a local newspaper about mental health issues and makes disparaging remarks about you and your services that appear in the article when it is published. Prior to publication of the article, you refused based on confidentiality concerns to discuss the former client's comments with the reporter. What are your options now?

2. What are the risks and benefits of joining professional associations?

3. You are accused by a client in an ethical complaint of having sex with her, and this same client has filed a criminal complaint and a civil malpractice case against you as well. You are required to respond to the licensing board within 20 days. The attorney you consult directs you to assert your Fifth Amendment privilege against self-incrimination in connection with your response to the licensing board. What do you do? What are the consequences of this action?

30

Supervision

Dr. Livingston heads a college campus counseling clinic utilized by both students and faculty who have problems they wish to discuss. On staff are psychology and marriage and family counseling graduate students who see clients under Dr. Livingston's clinical supervision. Unknown to Dr. Livingston, his niece, a student at the school, sought counseling and was assigned to one of the graduate student intern counselors for consultation. Dr. Livingston only learned about his niece's therapy after the niece had seen the counselor for three sessions and indicated the counseling in an informal family discussion. A fourth session is scheduled. To appropriately supervise the intern, Dr. Livingston must review his niece's clinical file. What should Dr. Livingston do?

Jane attends a college that requires psychology students to complete a certain number of supervised hours of clinical training. The supervisor who would normally be assigned to her is a former employer with whom she has had a rocky relationship. She feels reluctant to enter a supervision relationship with him because she is aware of the control a supervisor has over her future career. What are her options?

The graduate school caters to mature adults returning for postgraduate degrees. Dr. Smythe, an available bachelor, is in charge of the school's counseling program. He supervises a divorced graduate student who, over the period of supervision, appears to show personal interest in him, although they have never discussed this. Ethically, can Dr. Smythe date her, or even request a date, while she is under his supervision? Would it be ethical to ask her for a date after she completes her supervisory hours? What if he waited to ask her out until she graduates in two years? Would it be better to wait until after she graduates, is employed, and independent? Should Dr. Smythe assume that the risk of seeking a social relationship with a supervisee, current or former, is too risky and unethical and seek a social life elsewhere? Does it matter if she is the one pursuing the relationship?

Dr. Goldberg is a professor who operates a small private practice on Monday evenings. Joy, a practicum student-intern whom he supervises, calls one day and asks if he will see her as a client because she has some severe personal problems that she believes only he is competent to handle. Joy is an outstanding student, and Dr. Goldberg thinks she will eventually become a distinguished professional colleague. He has consulted with her in his capacity as a caring professor, but is reluctant to take her on as a client. What should he do?

Dr. O'Hara supervised Sue while she was in graduate school. They engaged in no inappropriate behavior during supervision, although each could sense the other's attraction. Following graduation, Dr. O'Hara wrote Sue a recommendation letter for a job she ultimately accepted. Soon after, they met coincidentally at a national conference and began to date. The social arrangement ended badly, however, and they went their separate ways. Sue decided to look for a new job two years later, but Dr. O'Hara refused to write another recommendation letter. Sue complained to the university and the licensing board. Dr. O'Hara would probably be called on the carpet for unprofessional conduct. Supervisors are always vulnerable to disciplinary action when they become involved with supervisees or former supervisees.

When Is Supervision Advisable?

In mental health practice, supervision is often part of a future clinical practitioners' initial education. During their training, students treat clients under the watchful eyes of credentialed, savvy, and experienced clinician-supervisors. Later, as individuals apply for state licenses and seek other advanced professional credentials, supervision is often a prerequisite and is or becomes a part of providers' continuing education as they develop and utilize new skills. The disciplinary committees of many national organizations and licensing boards use supervision to reeducate practitioners who have committed ethical infractions. Their misconduct may not be sufficient to revoke or suspend their licenses, but the committees find that therapists who violate a rule or regulation benefit from additional supervision and ethical training either to increase knowledge, correct a bad habit, or augment their awareness and sensitivity. Thus, boards often discipline providers by requiring additional supervision hours to bring them up to ethical standards.

Committees find that therapists who violate a rule or regulation benefit from additional supervision and ethical training either to increase knowledge, correct a bad habit, or augment their awareness and sensitivity.

Experienced clinical supervisors are in an excellent position to explain and illustrate current ethical principles, review published standards, and relate these rules to the situation at hand or to future problems as they arise. In addition, the cultivated informality provides a nonthreatening forum for the supervisor and supervisee to discuss concerns that would be difficult if these personal concerns were public knowledge or if the parties began a course of conduct that could be headed off without incident, but that develops after a time and is harder to correct than it would have been to avoid in the first place. Supervision is more like tutoring. Bad habits or concepts can be corrected at once. They can be corrected, augmented, or restructured before any client is hurt or injured. And this can all be done in the privacy of a clinical office.

Supervisor-Supervisee Relationships

The supervisor-supervisee relationship is one-sided in terms of authority, power, and position. The supervisor oversees the supervisee's work, and the supervisee is expected to learn, emulate, and accept feedback from the supervisor. The supervisor must be fair and competent, but the supervisee must follow the supervisor's directives and respect his or her limits, boundaries, and guidelines. In a broad sense, the supervisor is a guru. Although the relationship may eventually be characterized by friendship, the essential ingredient initially is professionalism. No friendship, no matter how well established or fostered, can interfere with the professional objectivity so essential to the supervision relationship.

The supervisor-supervisee association is a close professional relationship with serious ethical overtones that affect all of the individuals involved.

As a general rule, the supervisor-supervisee association is a close professional relationship with serious ethical overtones that affect all of the individuals involved. These individuals include the supervisor, the supervisee, and the client or, in the event of family therapy, the clients. The state licensing boards and the national organizations for the mental health disciplines have clearly stated principles for supervision. These guidelines are constantly being amended, revised, and republished. Should a problem arise requiring immediate attention, therapists should consult the appropriate organization and obtain the most current published rules and regulations.

National Guidelines for Supervision

American Association for Marriage and Family Therapy (AAMFT) Code of Ethics (2001)

Principle IV: Responsibility to Students, Employees, and Supervisees

Marriage and family therapists do not exploit the trust and dependency of students, employees, and supervisees.

4.1 Marriage and family therapists are aware of their influential position with respect to students, and supervisees, and they avoid exploiting the trust and dependency of such persons. Therapists, therefore, make every effort to avoid conditions and multiple relationships that could impair professional judgment objectivity or increase the risk of exploitation. When the risk of impairment or exploitation exists due to conditions or multiple roles, therapists take appropriate action.

4.2 Marriage and family therapists do not provide therapy to current students or supervisees.

4.3 Marriage and family therapists do not engage in sexual intimacy with students or supervisees during the evaluative or training relationship between the therapist and student or supervisee. Should a supervisor engage in sexual activity with a former supervisee, the burden of proof shifts to the supervisor to demonstrate that there has been no exploitation or injury to the supervisee.

4.4 Marriage and family therapists do not permit students or supervisees to perform or to hold themselves out as competent to perform professional services beyond their training, level of experience, and competence.

4.5 Marriage and family therapists take reasonable measures to ensure that services provided by supervisees are professional.

4.6 Marriage and family therapists avoid accepting as supervisees or students those individuals with whom a prior or existing relationship could compromise the therapist's objectivity. When such situations cannot be avoided, therapists take appropriate precautions to maintain objectivity. Examples of such relationships include, but are not limited to, those individuals with whom the therapist has a current or prior sexual, close personal, immediate familial, or therapeutic relationship.

4.7 Marriage and family therapists do not disclose supervisee confidences except by written authorization or waiver, or when mandated or permitted by law. In educational or training settings where there are multiple supervisors, disclosures
(continued)

(Continued)
are permitted only to other professional colleagues, administrators, or employers who share responsibility for training of
the supervisee. Verbal authorization will not be sufficient except in emergency situations, unless prohibited by law.

American Counseling Association (ACA) Code of Ethics (2005)

Section F: Supervision, Training, and Teaching

Counselors aspire to foster meaningful and respectful professional relationships and to maintain appropriate boundaries
with supervisees and students. Counselors have theoretical
and pedagogical foundations for their work and aim to be fair,
accurate, and honest in their assessments of counselors-in-
training.

F.1. Counselor Supervision and Client Welfare

F.1.a. Client Welfare

A primary obligation of counseling supervisors is to monitor
the services provided by other counselors or counselors-in-
training. Counseling supervisors monitor client welfare and
supervisee clinical performance and professional development. To fulfill these obligations, supervisors meet regularly
with supervisees to review case notes, samples of clinical
work, or live observations. Supervisees have a responsibility
to understand and follow the *ACA Code of Ethics*. . . .

F.2. Counselor Supervision Competence

F.2.a. Supervisor Preparation

Prior to offering clinical supervision services, counselors are
trained in supervision methods and techniques. Counselors
who offer clinical supervision services regularly pursue continuing education activities including both counseling and
supervision topics and skills. . . .

F.3. Supervisory Relationships

F.3.a. Relationship Boundaries with Supervisees

Counseling supervisors clearly define and maintain ethical professional, personal, and social relationships with their supervisees. Counseling supervisors avoid nonprofessional relationships with current supervisees. If supervisors must assume other professional roles (e.g., clinical and administrative supervisor, instructor) with supervisees, they work to minimize potential conflicts and explain to supervisees the expectations and responsibilities associated with each role. They do not engage in any form of nonprofessional interaction that may compromise the supervisory relationship.

F.3.b. Sexual Relationships

Sexual or romantic interactions or relationships with current supervisees are prohibited.

F.3.c. Sexual Harassment

Counseling supervisors do not condone or subject supervisees to sexual harassment.

F.3.d. Close Relatives and Friends

Counseling supervisors avoid accepting close relatives, romantic partners, or friends as supervisees.

F.3.e. Potentially Beneficial Relationships

Counseling supervisors are aware of the power differential in their relationships with supervisees. If they believe nonprofessional relationships with a supervisee may be potentially beneficial to the supervisee, they take precautions similar to those taken by counselors when working with clients. Examples of potentially beneficial interactions or relationships include attending a formal ceremony; hospital visits; providing support

(continued)

(Continued)

during a stressful event; or mutual membership in a professional association, organization, or community. Counseling supervisors engage in open discussions with supervisees when they consider entering into relationships with them outside of their roles as clinical and/or administrative supervisors. Before engaging in nonprofessional relationships, supervisors discuss with supervisees and document the rationale for such interactions, potential benefits or drawbacks, and anticipated consequences for the supervisee. Supervisors clarify the specific nature and limitations of the additional role(s) they will have with the supervisee.

F.4. Supervisor Responsibilities

F.4.a. Informed Consent for Supervision

Supervisors are responsible for incorporating into their supervision the principles of informed consent and participation. Supervisors inform supervisees of the policies and procedures to which they are to adhere and the mechanisms for due process appeal of individual supervisory actions.

F.4.b. Emergencies and Absences

Supervisors establish and communicate to supervisees procedures for contacting them or, in their absence, alternative on-call supervisors to assist in handling crises.

F.4.c. Standards for Supervisees

Supervisors make their supervisees aware of professional and ethical standards and legal responsibilities. Supervisors of postdegree counselors encourage these counselors to adhere to professional standards of practice.

F.4.d. Termination of the Supervisory Relationship

Supervisors or supervisees have the right to terminate the supervisory relationship with adequate notice. Reasons for withdrawal are provided to the other party. When cultural, clinical, or professional issues are crucial to the viability of the supervisory relationship, both parties make efforts to resolve differences. When termination is warranted, supervisors make appropriate referrals to possible alternative supervisors.

F.5. Counseling Supervision Evaluation, Remediation, and Endorsement

F.5.a. Evaluation

Supervisors document and provide supervisees with ongoing performance appraisal and evaluation feedback and schedule periodic formal evaluative sessions throughout the supervisory relationship.

F.5.b. Limitations

Through ongoing evaluation and appraisal, supervisors are aware of the limitations of supervisees that might impede performance. Supervisors assist supervisees in securing remedial assistance when needed. They recommend dismissal from training programs, applied counseling settings, or state or voluntary professional credentialing processes when those supervisees are unable to provide competent professional services.

Supervisors seek consultation and document their decisions to dismiss or refer supervisees for assistance. They ensure that supervisees are aware of options available to them to address such decisions.

F.5.c. Counseling for Supervisees

If supervisees request counseling, supervisors provide them with acceptable referrals. Counselors do not provide counseling services to supervisees. Supervisors address interpersonal competencies in terms of the impact of these issues on clients, the supervisory relationship, and professional functioning.

F.5.d. Endorsement

Supervisors endorse supervisees for certification, licensure, employment, or completion of an academic or training

(continued)

(Continued)

program only when they believe supervisees are qualified for the endorsement. Regardless of qualifications, supervisors do not endorse supervisees whom they believe to be impaired in any way that would interfere with the performance of the duties associated with the endorsement.

F.6. Responsibilities of Counselor Educators

F.6.a. Counselor Educators

Counselor educators who are responsible for developing, implementing, and supervising educational programs are skilled as teachers and practitioners. They are knowledgeable regarding the ethical, legal, and regulatory aspects of the profession, are skilled in applying that knowledge, and make students and supervisees aware of their responsibilities. Counselor educators conduct counselor education and training programs in an ethical manner and serve as role models for professional behavior. . . .

F.9. Evaluation and Remediation of Students

F.9.a. Evaluation

Counselors clearly state to students, prior to and throughout the training program, the levels of competency expected, appraisal methods, and timing of evaluations for both didactic and clinical competencies. Counselor educators provide students with ongoing performance appraisal and evaluation feedback throughout the training program.

F.9.b. Limitations

Counselor educators, throughout ongoing evaluation and appraisal, are aware of and address the inability of some students to achieve counseling competencies that might impede performance. Counselor educators

1. Assist students in securing remedial assistance when needed,

2. Seek professional consultation and document their decision to dismiss or refer students for assistance, and

3. Ensure that students have recourse in a timely manner to address decisions to require them to seek assistance or to dismiss them and provide students with due process according to institutional policies and procedures.

F.9.c. Counseling for Students

If students request counseling or if counseling services are required as part of a remediation process, counselor educators provide acceptable referrals.

F.10. Roles and Relationships between Counselor Educators and Students

F.10.a. Sexual or Romantic Relationships

Sexual or romantic interactions or relationships with current students are prohibited.

F.10.b. Sexual Harassment

Counselor educators do not condone or subject students to sexual harassment.

F.10.c. Relationships with Former Students

Counselor educators are aware of the power differential in the relationship between faculty and students. Faculty members foster open discussions with former students when considering engaging in a social, sexual, or other intimate relationship. Faculty members discuss with the former student how their former relationship may affect the change in relationship.

F.10.d. Nonprofessional Relationships

Counselor educators avoid nonprofessional or ongoing professional relationships with students in which there is a risk of potential harm to the student or that may compromise the training experience or grades assigned. In addition, counselor educators do not accept any form of professional services, fees, commissions, reimbursement, or remuneration from a site for student or supervisee placement.

(continued)

(Continued)

F.10.e. Counseling Services

Counselor educators do not serve as counselors to current students unless this is a brief role associated with a training experience.

American Psychological Association (APA) Ethical Principles of Psychologists and Code of Conduct (2002)

7. Education and Training

7.01 Design of Education and Training Programs

Psychologists responsible for education and training programs take reasonable steps to ensure that the programs are designed to provide the appropriate knowledge and proper experiences, and to meet the requirements for licensure, certification, or other goals for which claims are made by the program . . .

7.04 Student Disclosure of Personal Information

Psychologists do not require students or supervisees to disclose personal information in course- or program-related activities, either orally or in writing, regarding sexual history, history of abuse and neglect, psychological treatment, and relationships with parents, peers, and spouses or significant others except if (1) the program or training facility has clearly identified this requirement in its admissions and program materials or (2) the information is necessary to evaluate or obtain assistance for students whose personal problems could reasonably be judged to be preventing them from performing their training- or professionally related activities in a competent manner or posing a threat to the students or others.

7.05 Mandatory Individual or Group Therapy

(a) When individual or group therapy is a program or course requirement, psychologists responsible for that program allow students in undergraduate and graduate programs the option of selecting such therapy from practitioners unaffiliated with the program.

(b) Faculty who are or are likely to be responsible for evaluating students' academic performance do not themselves provide that therapy. (See also Standard 3.05, Multiple Relationships.)

7.06 Assessing Student and Supervisee Performance

(a) In academic and supervisory relationships, psychologists establish a timely and specific process for providing feedback to students and supervisees. Information regarding the process is provided to the student at the beginning of supervision.

(b) Psychologists evaluate students and supervisees on the basis of their actual performance on relevant and established program requirements.

7.07 Sexual Relationships with Students and Supervisees

Psychologists do not engage in sexual relationships with students or supervisees who are in their department, agency, or training center or over whom psychologists have or are likely to have evaluative authority.

National Association of Social Workers (NASW) Code of Ethics (1999)

3.01 Supervision and Consultation

(a) Social workers who provide supervision or consultation should have the necessary knowledge and skill to supervise or consult appropriately and should do so only within their areas of knowledge and competence.

(b) Social workers who provide supervision or consultation are responsible for setting clear, appropriate, and culturally sensitive boundaries.

(c) Social workers should not engage in any dual or multiple relationships with supervisees in whom there is risk of exploitation of or potential harm to the supervisee.

(d) Social workers who provide supervision should evaluate supervisees' performance in a manner that is fair and respectful.

General Rules for Supervision

Although the published guidelines differ in nature and scope of detail, certain principles may be extrapolated to form the following 16 general rules. Some are ethical referring only to published guidelines, whereas others refer to legal principles that bind the supervisor-supervisee relationship and create controlling standards:

1. The supervisee's actions are the supervisor's actions when the supervisee is acting in the course and scope of the supervision.

2. Supervisees' negligent, malpractice, or perhaps criminal activities will be shifted to the supervisor if the supervisor knew, or, with reasonable diligence should have known of the negligent, malpractice, or criminal acts. "Don't ask, don't tell" does not apply to the supervisory relationship. For example, a supervisor could be held responsible if a supervisee has sex with a client or breaches confidentiality.

3. Supervision requires a periodic review of the file, a consultation concerning each case subject to supervision, and notations made in the supervisor's and supervisee's files indicating the effect supervision had on the diagnosis, prognosis, or treatment plan of each case.

4. All supervision must be documented. The documentation must be complete regardless of the method used (i.e., printed hard copies, computer-generated records, or oral and taped documentation) and must all indicate the therapeutic realities. Corrected documentation should likewise indicate the original record, the corrections, dates, the initials of the individual creating the record, and all changes made.

5. Where supervision is conducted, a review of the supervisor's malpractice policy is essential to ensure that both the individual supervisor's policy and the agency's or university's covers the supervisee's actions if that is the structure being utilized.

6. Just as a therapist cannot treat a good friend, relation, or business associate, neither can the therapist supervise such persons. Another supervisor must be located to serve when a therapist's relative, friend, or associate requires supervision.

7. When a potential supervisee feels a supervisor might have compromised or might have a tendency to compromise clinical or supervision objectivity, another supervisor must be obtained before supervision is commenced and a record created.

8. Clinical judgment and objectivity might be compromised in any worst-case scenario if a supervisor asks a supervisee for a date. This can place all future supervision in jeopardy and has the appearance of a dual relationship, which is prohibited. The supervisor cannot ask a supervisee for a date, go on a date with a supervisee, or have any social or sexual relationship with a supervisee. The codes are unclear as to whether supervisors may ethically date their supervisees following the supervisee's completion of the supervision.

9. Dual relationships are clearly prohibited. A current student or a supervisee cannot become a client.

Dual relationships are clearly prohibited.

10. Supervisors must use self-discipline when conducting supervision in specialty areas. Each supervisor must be cognizant of his or her own professional limitations. For example, if a client presents with an alcohol problem and the supervisor is inexperienced in this area, he or she should consult a more learned professional. You never want to be accused of exceeding your level of competence or expertise.

11. Supervisors must establish boundaries with their supervisees. Going out for a business lunch might be appropriate, whereas a postclinical drink at a local bar or the supervisor's apartment or home might blur the boundaries. Although supervisors should use common sense when establishing boundaries, common sense is hardly a national standard and can vary with each individual. The appearance of a boundary violation or dual relationship is often as harmful as the violation itself.

12. Any business relationship (e.g., buying a car from a supervisee or selling one) has a potential for exploitation. Anything that might affect objectivity must be avoided.

13. Supervisors should avoid informality with their supervisees. The power differential between supervisors and supervisees must have clearly defined boundaries. Sharing a cup of coffee occasionally

Supervisors should avoid informality with their supervisees.

after a session to discuss a case might be acceptable, whereas meeting for coffee after or before each consultation has a tendency to shift the relationship from clinical to social, at least in the mind of the supervisee, and is to be avoided.

14. Supervision may be, but is not always, reactive. The supervisor must prepare for the supervisory session by reviewing clinical notes, appraising each specific situation, and noting that the diagnosis, treatment plan utilized, and possible prognosis is appropriate. Misdiagnosis is a common ground for malpractice suits as well as an ethical complaint. The supervisor is responsible for the efficacy of the treatment.

15. Supervisors should respect supervisees' confidentiality. The concept of danger to self or others presents a constant problem, and the duty-to-warn scenario is always in flux. Supervisors should take every available precaution when forced to breach a confidence. For self-protection, therapists should consult the licensing rules, the state boards, the malpractice carrier, and an attorney in their jurisdiction. A carefully drafted and lawyer-approved contract is essential and necessary before supervision begins. Most historically vulnerable areas can be anticipated by a contract between the parties. When there is a difficulty between a supervisor, a supervisee, and the client, most of the time the problem was anticipated and then ignored.

Note: We receive more inquiries concerning duty to warn than any other subject. Each fact situation is slightly different. We advise practitioners to keep current with their state's laws as well as national and state standards regarding duty to warn. When a question arises, there is usually little time for thorough inquiry and research.

---

16. Supervisees are entitled to fair and respectful feedback on a regular basis. Supervisors should systematically review all case files subject to supervision.

Ethical Flash Points

- Supervisees are not friends or professional colleagues; they are interns learning their profession.

- The supervisor is the teacher.

- The supervisee is the student.

- Clinical objectivity should never be compromised by dual relationships, blurring of boundaries, strong emotions, or kinship.

- The supervisor has the duty and obligation to establish clear and enforceable boundaries. The supervisee must respect those boundaries.

- Many of the prohibited relationships between therapist and client are likewise prohibited between supervisor and supervisee.

- The supervisor has the ultimate responsibility to the client. If the supervisee acts inappropriately, the supervisor is likely to be held responsible.

- Even if not set out specifically in the national or state standards, the compromising situations described at the beginning of this chapter would likely be considered unprofessional conduct subject to sanctions.

- Exploitation in any disguise is still exploitation. Beware of free tickets, dinner invitations, gifts, and offers of preferential treatment by influential spouses.

- A malpractice policy might cover therapists in their capacity as clinician or provider. If they act as supervisors, however, they should review their policies to ensure that they are covered if a supervisee is negligent and the supervisor is ultimately held responsible.

Summary

Most graduate programs provide for an internship, practicum, or supervised clinical contact with clients. Although the supervisee has the major client contact, supervisors accept responsibility for the supervisee's actions through their primary role by making suggestions, offering examples, and approving or tinkering with the supervisee's treatment plan, diagnosis, and methodology. Therefore, the supervisor must take the job seriously, relate to the client and the supervisee within professional guidelines, and ensure that the supervisee's treatment is in the client's long- and short-term best interest.

There has been a national movement toward a more formal and structured approach to supervision. Supervisor credentials are offered by both state licensing boards and national certification programs. Greater emphasis is being placed on training and continuing education for supervisors. Many states now require supervision to be provided by a person with the license the supervisee is attempting to attain. All of this is in recognition of the importance supervision plays in developing good practitioners who can safely and effectively deliver mental health services to the public.

Suggested Research Assignments

1. Locate and discuss the provisions of any ethical codes promulgated by the mental health profession licensing boards in your state with respect to supervision. What rules and duties do they impose? What are the qualifications for a supervisor?
2. Locate and discuss any state and national professional association rules with regard to supervision. What are the similarities and differences?
3. Compare and contrast the obligations imposed by the licensing boards in your state with the rules promulgated by the state professional associations.
4. Compare and contrast state licensing board and professional association obligations with the guidelines of national professional associations.
5. Research licensing board cases in your state involving supervision. What were the specific rules involved, and what sanctions if any were issued?
6. Research civil malpractice cases in your state involving supervision. What were the outcomes, and what damages if any were assessed?
7. Create a list of characteristics and qualifications a potential supervisee should look for in a supervisor.

8. Talk to local mental health professionals who do supervision and find out what problems they experience in supervision. Also learn what they perceive to be the benefits and risks associated with doing supervision.

Discussion Questions

1. What advice would you give a colleague who is considering accepting a dinner invitation from a former supervisee whom the colleague admits to being extremely attracted to? Would your advice differ if the supervision was provided during a graduate school practicum or if it occurred after graduate school when the supervisee was accumulating hours for licensure?
2. What advice would you give to a licensing applicant who is looking for supervision for licensing purposes?
3. Describe the documentation you would expect to be maintained by both the supervisor and supervisee with respect to the supervision relationship.
4. What are the risks and benefits of providing supervision services?
5. What are the risks for the supervisee of faulty supervision?
6. You are being supervised by a state-approved supervisor. You have only half of the supervised hours you need for licensure. You now realize your supervisor is addicted to methamphetamines and has been impaired the last two times you have met with her. What do you do? What do you document, if anything? How do you preserve and protect the documented supervision hours that might be forfeited if your supervisor loses her credentials and no longer has authority to record them properly?

PART V

SPECIAL THERAPY CONSIDERATIONS

31

Forensic Evaluation

Sharon, a licensed social worker, evaluated a 3-year-old girl for several weeks after her mother, a former client, suspected the child was being sexually abused. The child went into hysterics each time her mother attempted to bathe her and was having nightmares. A pediatric examination was inconclusive. After 10 play therapy sessions, the child indicated her father hurt her during his visitations. Her parents were in the middle of a contested divorce and bitter custody litigation. When asked to testify by the mother at a court hearing, Sharon testified that in her opinion the child's father had sexually abused his child. The father lost custody and was awarded only very limited and supervised visitation. Four months later, the parties learned that the girl's 13-year-old cousin on the mother's side of the family actually was committing the sexual abuse when his mother caught him in the act. The girl's father immediately filed a complaint with Sharon's licensing board and filed a malpractice suit. The facts showed that Sharon had very limited training and experience in sexual abuse cases. She was eventually sanctioned by the board and placed on probation and supervision. Her malpractice insurance carrier settled for an undisclosed sum.

After practicing 20 years as a psychologist and testifying in over 100 forensic cases for the state on the question of a criminal defendant's competency to stand trial, Mark learned that a complaint had been filed against him with the state licensing board. The attorney for a mentally retarded defendant charged with sexual assault learned that not once in over 100 cases had Mark ever rendered an opinion that a defendant was mentally incompetent. In each case, the district attorney prosecuting the case had hired and paid Mark. In the current case, the appellate court ultimately determined that the defendant was not competent to stand trial and reversed the conviction. Mark was accused of bias, unprofessionalism, and incompetence. After the licensing board began investigating the case, they moved to revoke Mark's license, which he surrendered voluntarily in lieu of a formal revocation hearing.

Jacob, a licensed professional counselor, was experienced working with sex offenders. He was court ordered to evaluate and treat a 19-year-old youth accused of having a sexual relationship with his 14-year-old sister. After 6 months of therapy, the boy admitted for the first time that he had entered his sister's room surreptitiously, gotten into bed with her, and fondled her. Jacob immediately notified the court, child protective services, and the police, who took the boy into custody. Jacob's later testimony helped send the client to the penitentiary for 5 years. While in prison, the client filed a complaint with the state licensing board, accusing Jacob of a breach of confidentiality, conflict of interest, and failure to warn him regarding the therapeutic limits to confidentiality. Although he was not severely sanctioned by the licensing board, Jacob was privately reprimanded for not securing informed consent from the client, documenting his relationship to the court, and disclosing to the client his duty to report sexual offenses prior to beginning therapy.

What Is Forensic Evaluation?

Forensic work involves an expert witness evaluating, reporting, and often testifying in legal proceedings.

Forensic work involves an expert witness evaluating, reporting, and often testifying in legal proceedings. An expert witness is a person who by education, learning, training, and experience is allowed to give testimony and render an opinion on facts or issues in a lawsuit. The court determines whether the individual is competent to testify as an expert in the case. If the court decides that the individual has sufficient learning, education, training, or experience to advise the court on the disputed issue or fact, then the court will find the witness competent and allow the testimony or report into evidence. The testimony will be admissible even over the objection of the other party. The judge, the jury, or both will hear it. Whether it will be believed is another question. Credibility is always a separate issue that depends on many factors, including presentation method, courtroom demeanor, individual preparation or lack thereof, or, sometimes, a judge or jury's general feeling that the witness is too glib to be believable. The weight to be assigned to admissible evidence is always personal to a judge or jury, and neither has to justify their personal reaction to anyone else. (See *The Portable Guide to Testifying in Court for Mental Health Professionals*, Bernstein and Hartsell 2005.)

Who Should Offer Forensic Services?

Many therapists actively seek forensic assignments from courts, litigants, and attorneys as part of their practice activities and in a few cases as the sum of their professional endeavors. Other mental health professionals get drawn into forensic work because of their prior work with a client who becomes involved in the legal system. Being asked to evaluate a client or render an opinion regarding a client or legal issues requires both caution and consideration.

Therapists offering expert testimony in court can usually assume that one of the parties is not going to like their opinion or testimony. The disagreeing party is usually the opposing counsel or the person against whom the expert testifies. Even in situations where therapists testify that they cannot reach an opinion, a client or party who expected a favorable opinion may become incensed. Because the mental health professional's recommendations or opinions can significantly impact the legal proceeding and a client's well-being, forensic work should be approached with heightened professionalism, sensitivity, increased theoretical and practical research, and the greatest possible competence.

As Sharon learned, exceeding your level of competence can be embarrassing and expensive. Rendering an expert opinion in a legal proceeding when you are not sufficiently experienced is unethical; moreover, it magnifies your incompetence. Numerous parties, including the judge, jury, and attorneys for both sides, will closely scrutinize

Because the mental health professional's recommendations or opinions can significantly impact the legal proceeding and a client's well-being, forensic work should be approached with heightened professionalism, sensitivity, and the greatest possible competence.

the mental health professional's competency to testify. Every word said under oath from the witness stand (even after swearing on a Bible) can be microscopically cross-examined by opposing counsel; and misstatements, exaggerations, allegations, or assumptions stated as truths can be revealed to the therapist's ultimate embarrassment and chagrin. Thus, therapists must be completely confident of their expertise in this area. Therapists must recognize their limits and resist being drawn beyond their professional competency levels by a pushy attorney or a needy client. It is unethical for a therapist to perform an evaluation or render an opinion if he or she does not have the requisite training, experience, or education.

Nationally, there has been a dramatic increase in the number of complaints being filed against mental health professionals by disgruntled family law litigants. Mental health professionals who volunteer for involvement in these cases or who are reluctantly subpoenaed and required to testify or produce records are extremely vulnerable to a licensing board complaint. Even greater care and consideration need to be given when the therapist or treating or retained forensic expert, becomes involved in family law litigation (see Chapter 10, "Risky Clients"). In the search for blame, losing litigants will rarely blame themselves for the loss. As they search about for a scapegoat, the therapist witness often becomes the target. The losing party thinks, "If only the testimony had been more resolute, more carefully presented, or more detailed, the litigant would have prevailed." Remember, in most litigation, someone loses.

National Guidelines for Competency to Testify as an Expert Witness

American Association for Marriage and Family Therapy (AAMFT) Code of Ethics (2001)

Marriage and family therapists do not diagnose, treat, or advise on problems outside the recognized boundaries of their competencies.

American Counseling Association (ACA) Code of Ethics (2005)

C.2.c. Qualified for Employment

Counselors accept employment only for positions for which they are qualified by education, training, supervised experience, state and national professional credentials, and appropriate professional experience. Counselors hire for professional counseling positions only individuals who are qualified and competent for those positions. . . .

American Psychological Association (APA) Ethical Principles of Psychologists and Code of Conduct (2002)

2. Competence

2.01 Boundaries of Competence

(a) Psychologists provide services, teach, and conduct research with populations and in areas only within the boundaries of their competence, based on their education, training, supervised experience, consultation, study, or professional experience. . . .

National Association of Social Workers (NASW) Code of Ethics (1999)

1.04 Competence

(a) Social workers should provide services and represent themselves as competent within the boundaries of their education, training, license, certification, consultation received, supervised experience, or other relevant professional experience.

(b) Social workers should provide services in substantive areas or use intervention techniques or approaches that are new to them only after engaging in appropriate study, training, consultation, and supervision from people who are competent in those interventions or techniques. . . .

Conducting a Forensic Assessment

Appropriate infor-
mation gathering
and proper testing
and therapy techni-
ques must be con-
ducted and utilized
to substantiate
opinions and
recommendations.

Assuming he or she has the competency to provide the forensic services requested, the mental health professional must then adequately
perform the services, whether it involves courtroom testimony or evaluation and written reporting. Appropriate information gathering and
proper testing and professional techniques must be conducted and utilized to substantiate opinions and recommendations. Examining and
interviewing the individuals involved in each case is almost always a
necessity.

We have been involved in several cases where a mental health professional has rendered an opinion concerning a custody or abuse issue
without ever having interviewed one of the parties in the case or the
accused perpetrator. It would be a very rare child custody case in which
a therapist could give an opinion concerning which parent should be
awarded custody without first clinically and thoroughly evaluating both
parents. If a therapist interviewed at least one of the parents, he or she
could offer an opinion on the mental health condition or the observed
parenting abilities of that parent but ethically could not offer expert testimony concerning the child's best interest without evaluating *both* parents. Likewise, in child abuse cases involving very young children in
which there is an absence of conclusive physical evidence or other corroboration, the failure to include the alleged perpetrator in the evaluation process could preclude a therapist from rendering an opinion of the
accused person's culpability. The accuracy of any testimony offered
would be so questionable as to be meaningless. If a court order or other
document or entity demands that a mental health professional render an
opinion for which adequate information, techniques, or testing have not
been obtained or utilized, then the therapist should fully disclose the
limitations of the opinion and lack of substantiation in testimony and
in every written report. Often opinions are requested where one of the
witnesses is either unavailable or totally uncooperative. In matters involving an unavailable witness, the forensic expert should state to the
court all the efforts made to complete the investigation and assessment,
then offer to testify on the information that was available and allow the
court to assess the weight to be given to the evidence.

National Guidelines for Conducting Forensic Assessments

American Association for Marriage and Family Therapy (AAMFT) Code of Ethics (2001)

3.13 Marriage and family therapists, because of their ability to influence and alter the lives of others, exercise special care when making public their professional recommendations and opinions through testimony or other public statements.

American Counseling Association (ACA) Code of Ethics (2005)

E.13. Forensic Evaluation: Evaluation for Legal Proceedings

E.13.a. Primary Obligations

When providing forensic evaluations, the primary obligation of counselors is to produce objective findings that can be substantiated based on information and techniques appropriate to the evaluation, which may include examination of the individual and/or review of records. Counselors are entitled to form professional opinions based on their professional knowledge and expertise that can be supported by the data gathered in evaluations. Counselors will define the limits of their reports or testimony, especially when an examination of the individual has not been conducted.

E.13.b. Consent for Evaluation

Individuals being evaluated are informed in writing that the relationship is for the purposes of an evaluation and is not counseling in nature, and entities or individuals who will receive the evaluation report are identified. Written consent to be evaluated is obtained from those being evaluated unless a

(continued)

(Continued)

court orders evaluations to be conducted without the written consent of individuals being evaluated. When children or vulnerable adults are being evaluated, informed written consent is obtained from a parent or guardian.

American Psychological Association (APA) Ethical Principles of Psychologists and Code of Conduct **(2002)**

2.04 Bases for Scientific and Professional Judgments

Psychologists' work is based upon established scientific and professional knowledge of the discipline. . . .

9. Assessment

9.01 Bases for Assessments

(a) Psychologists base the opinions contained in their recommendations, reports, and diagnostic or evaluative statements, including forensic testimony, on information and techniques sufficient to substantiate their findings

(b) Except as noted in 9.01c, psychologists provide opinions of the psychological characteristics of individuals only after they have conducted an examination of the individuals adequate to support their statements or conclusions. When, despite reasonable efforts, such an examination is not practical, psychologists document the efforts they made and the result of those efforts, clarify the probable impact of their limited information on the reliability and validity of their opinions, and appropriately limit the nature and extent of their conclusions or recommendations.

(c) When psychologists conduct a record review or provide consultation or supervision and an individual examination is not warranted or necessary for the opinion, psychologists explain this and the sources of information on which they based their conclusions and recommendations.

Documenting Forensic Evaluations

It is critical for mental health professionals to thoroughly document all information gathering, therapy techniques, and testing results obtained and relied on during the evaluation and on which they base their opinions. This documentation is necessary during the legal proceeding itself when presenting the case in chief and also when cross-examining lawyers scrutinize and challenge the therapist's competence, work, professionalism, and opinions. Documentation is critical when defending a therapist's actions or alleged inaction if a licensing board complaint or malpractice suit is later filed.

Documentation is critical when defending a therapist's actions or alleged inaction if a licensing board complaint or malpractice suit is later filed.

Avoiding Conflicts of Interest

Therapists should avoid conflicts of interest when providing any professional services to a client, including forensic services. When mental health professionals are hired for forensic evaluations and treatment, as is often the case with court appointments involving sex offenders, obvious potential conflicts of interest may arise. Therapists have an obligation to report honestly and objectively to the court and to assist the court in its duty to protect society. At the same time, therapists have an obligation to protect the client's rights and interests. Reporting recidivism to the court that results in clients being sent to the penitentiary dramatically highlights the conflict of interest.

At best, therapists in this situation should clearly document that they disclosed the potential conflict of interest to the client as well as the limits of confidentiality and possible consequences of those limits. Therapists should make such disclosures in writing and document their receipt with the client's signature and consent allowing the therapist to proceed with treatment in the dual role. In the opening example, Jacob's licensing board sanctioned him for failing to thoroughly document these disclosures and for failing to obtain his client's consent. Written documentation is important because trials can be delayed for years after an action or event occurs.

Oral discussions may be forgotten, distorted, and molded to fit the circumstance of the moment. A signed document speaks for itself.

The written documentation should be preserved in the permanent case folder and maintained and secured according to ethical standards. The wise therapist, upon entering practice, keeps and maintains up to date, a form file that covers all circumstances typically faced by therapists as they practice. The wise agency head always has at the fingertips of each agency practitioner, a form file that is up-to-date and available, which serves to confirm informed consent for each anticipated circumstance. Excellent form books are available with this information.

National Guidelines for Conflicts of Interest in Forensic Evaluations

American Association for Marriage and Family Therapy (AAMFT) Code of Ethics (2001)

Principle III: Professional Competence and Integrity

3.4 Marriage and family therapists do not provide services that create a conflict of interest that may impair performance or clinical judgment.

3.14 To avoid a conflict of interests, marriage and family therapists who treat minors or adults involved in custody or visitation actions may not also perform forensic evaluations for custody, residence, or visitation of the minor. The marriage and family therapist who treats the minor may provide the court or mental health professional performing the evaluation with information about the minor from the marriage and family therapist's perspective as a treating marriage and family therapist, so long as the marriage and family therapist does not violate confidentiality.

American Counseling Association (ACA) Code of Ethics (2005)

E.13.c. Client Evaluation Prohibited

Counselors do not evaluate individuals for forensic purposes they currently counsel or individuals they have counseled in the past. Counselors do not accept as counseling clients individuals they are evaluating or individuals they have evaluated in the past for forensic purposes.

E.13.d. Avoid Potentially Harmful Relationships

Counselors who provide forensic evaluations avoid potentially harmful professional or personal relationships with family members, romantic partners, and close friends of individuals they are evaluating or have evaluated in the past.

American Psychological Association (APA) Ethical Principles of Psychologists and Code of Conduct (2002)

3. HUMAN RELATIONS . . .

3.05 Multiple Relationships . . .

(c) When psychologists are required by law, institutional policy, or extraordinary circumstances to serve in more than one role in judicial or administrative proceedings, at the outset they clarify role expectations and the extent of confidentiality and thereafter as changes occur.

3.06 Conflict of Interest

Psychologists refrain from taking on a professional role when personal, scientific, professional, legal, financial, or other interests or relationships could reasonably be expected to (1) impair their objectivity, competence, or effectiveness in performing their functions as psychologists or (2) expose the person or organization with whom the professional relationship exists to harm or exploitation.

3.07 Third-Party Requests for Services

When psychologists agree to provide services to a person or entity at the request of a third party, psychologists attempt to clarify at the outset of the service the nature of the relationship with all individuals or organizations involved. This clarification includes the role of the psychologist (e.g., therapist,

(*continued*)

(Continued)

consultant, diagnostician, or expert witness), an identification of who is the client, the probable uses of the services provided or the information obtained, and the fact that there may be limits to confidentiality. . . .

National Association of Social Workers (NASW) Code of Ethics (1999)

1.6 Conflicts of Interest

1.06 Conflicts of Interest

(a) Social workers should be alert to and avoid conflicts of interest that interfere with the exercise of professional discretion and impartial judgment. Social workers should inform clients when a real or potential conflict of interest arises and take reasonable steps to resolve the issue in a manner that makes the clients' interests primary and protects clients' interests to the greatest extent possible. In some cases, protecting clients' interests may require termination of the professional relationship with proper referral of the client. . . .

Importance of Honest and Unbiased Opinions

Mental health professionals serving as expert witnesses should advise their clients in writing that ethical obligations require absolute honesty and

Clients hiring a mental health professional as an expert witness are hoping for, if not actually expecting, reporting and testimony favorable to their case. Clients are allowed to shop around for experts, particularly ones who are able to testify favorably in court. This smug "hired gun" theory permeates many facets of the lawyer/client/expert/therapist relationship. Can it be avoided? That is a question we cannot deal with in this book. Mental health professionals serving as expert witnesses should advise their clients in writing that ethical obligations require absolute honesty and accuracy and that clients may not be happy with their findings. Therapists should advise clients as early as possible regarding negative findings or opinions to allow them an opportunity to engage another expert.

If a therapist is hired and paid by one party to a lawsuit in any contested litigation and provides testimony favorable to that party, the opposing party will certainly challenge the report or testimony on bias and competency grounds. Paying an independent mental health professional a large fee for an evaluation and courtroom testimony does not guarantee favorable testimony. A therapist who gives the opinion a paying client requested, regardless of whether that opinion was warranted, is at risk of being sanctioned for ethical violations. In the second opening vignette, Mark testified over one hundred times in favor of the state. Mark's bias and lack of candor and accuracy seem at first glance to be blatant. On the other hand, any entity accusing Mark of bias or prejudice would still have to examine individual cases and prove that Mark was biased. Could it be that in each case Mark was clinically correct? Could it be that the district attorney only referred cases to Mark in which the defendant was competent?

We have represented several mental health professionals who were asked to sign affidavits by attorneys for therapy clients usually to support some extraordinary relief from a court involving access by a parent to a child. The attorneys explained that the affidavit would prevent the need for the therapist to testify in court. The problems arose when the affidavits contained conclusions and information that were not entirely accurate or for which a sound basis did not exist. If an affidavit is requested and the therapist is inclined to cooperate, never, ever let the attorney draft it. If anything, the attorney should only alter the document created into affidavit form. The information contained should be absolutely accurate and contain only information of which the therapist has personal knowledge, and any opinions should have a sound and adequate supporting basis.

accuracy and that clients may not be happy with their findings.

A therapist who gives the opinion a paying client requested, regardless of whether that opinion was warranted, is at risk of being sanctioned for ethical violations.

National Guidelines for Honest and Unbiased Opinions in Forensic Evaluations

American Association for Marriage and Family Therapy (AAMFT) Code of Ethics (2001)

Principle III: Professional Competence and Integrity

3.12 Marriage and family therapist make efforts to prevent the distortion or misuse of their clinical or research findings.

American Counseling Association (ACA) Code of Ethics (2005)

C.6.b. Reports to Third Parties

Counselors are accurate, honest, and objective in reporting their professional activities and judgments to appropriate third parties, including courts, health insurance companies, those who are the recipients of evaluation reports, and others. . . .

American Psychological Association (APA) Ethical Principles of Psychologists and Code of Conduct (2002)

6.06 Accuracy in Reports to Payors and Funding Sources

In their reports to payors for services or sources of research funding, psychologists take reasonable steps to ensure the accurate reporting of the nature of the service provided or research conducted, the fees, charges, or payments, and where applicable, the identity of the provider, the findings, and the diagnosis.

Ethical Flash Points

- Forensic work should be approached with extreme caution and care.

- Competency is critical both ethically and professionally in tackling any forensic assignment.

- Courts, attorneys, clients, and other interested parties will scrutinize the mental health professional's forensic work as well as the professional's overall competency.

- The mental health professional can expect to displease at least one party involved in a legal proceeding, and a licensing board complaint filed after the trial should come as no surprise.

- In forensic work, especially that which results in bitterly contested litigation, there is going to be a happy winner and an angry loser.

- Thorough documentation of all forensic activities is crucial in view of third-party reviews of the mental health professional's work and the defense against the inevitable licensing board complaint.

- Conflicts of interest should be avoided, but if unavoidable, the therapist should disclose them and obtain written consent. Providing therapy to a former forensic client or providing forensic testimony for a therapy client is almost always a bad decision.

- Mental health professionals must render unbiased, honest, and accurate reports and testimony.

- There is no substitute for complete and total preparation with an attorney prior to a court appearance.

- Being cross-examined concerning your competence, background, personal history, diagnosis, treatment plan, and changing prognosis is uncomfortable, to put it mildly.

- Role-playing the "withering crossfire of cross examination" is always a worthwhile exercise. This type of practice is very valuable. It is the lawyer's obligation to ensure that the witness is not surprised on the witness stand.

- Get paid prior to the trial for investigation, preparation, travel, and preparation time as well as the estimated time of the trial and any post-trial activities.

- Winners usually pay. Losers are reluctant to pay the forensic witness for his or her testimony.

Summary

Forensic work for many mental health professionals is both financially and professionally rewarding. However, it should not be pursued by anyone who is not unequivocally competent, thoroughly honest, and completely unbiased. Expert witnesses should also possess a controlled temper and a skin thick enough for them to accept being questioned about every facet of any given case. Cross-examination is far more intense than giving a lecture followed by a question-and-answer session. It is rapid, under oath, and usually unfriendly. Be prepared and beware. Most mental health services are provided in a relatively quiet office between a client and therapist. There is a total contrast when compared with forensic services where numerous third parties examine and challenge the services performed and the person performing them. Therefore, awareness and understanding of ethical codes are even more important for therapists interested in or drawn into providing forensic services. A therapist who thinks the courtroom is like a therapist's office is in for a rude awakening. The therapist controls what occurs in the clinical office setting, but has no control over what happens in the courtroom.

In a trial situation, the judge reigns supreme. Any therapist who regularly provides forensic services will experience an ethical complaint at some point in his or her career. It is an unfortunate cost of doing business. It is even more unfortunate if the complaint has merit. Competency, preparation, and detailed documentation of the process, data collected, and substantiation of the opinion rendered are critical in defending against the complaint.

A therapist who thinks the courtroom is like a therapist's office is in for a rude awakening.

Suggested Research Assignments

1. Locate and discuss the provisions of any ethical codes promulgated by the mental health profession licensing boards in your state with respect to forensic evaluation. What rules and duties do they impose? What are the qualifications for a supervisor?
2. Locate and discuss any state and national professional association rules with regard to forensic evaluation. What are the similarities and differences?

3. Compare and contrast the obligations imposed by the licensing boards in your state with the rules promulgated by the state professional associations.

4. Compare and contrast state licensing board and professional association obligations with the guidelines of national professional associations.

5. Research licensing board cases in your state involving forensic evaluations. What were the specific rules involved, and what sanctions if any were issued?

6. Research civil malpractice cases in your state involving forensic evaluations. What were the outcomes and what damages if any were assessed?

7. Create a set of guidelines for providing forensic services. Include all necessary documentation a practitioner should use and create.

8. Talk to local mental health professionals who volunteer to provide forensic services and find out what problems they experience in doing so. Also learn what they perceive to be the benefits and risks associated with doing supervision. What fees do they charge?

9. Talk to other mental health professionals who do *not* volunteer to provide forensic services and find out what they do to protect themselves when they are compelled to become involved in a client's lawsuit. What is their reaction when an unfriendly and unexpected subpoena *duces tecum* is served at their door?

10. Research options for increasing your competency and effectiveness as a provider of forensic services.

Discussion Questions

1. What advice would you give a colleague who is considering a request to testify for a therapy client in her child custody case?

2. If you do not want to testify on behalf of therapy clients, what steps can you take to limit this possibility?

3. Are you ethically obligated to testify for a therapy client if asked to do so?

4. What are the risks and benefits of providing forensic services?

5. What kinds of clauses might you want to include in a forensic client intake and consent form that you would not include in one for a therapy client?

6. A therapy client sends you an e-mail request asking if you would be willing to go to court and testify on her behalf at her custody trial. The client is coming in the next day for her regularly scheduled appointment. You know that if you testify honestly and objectively, you would end up giving very damaging and unfavorable testimony for the client and she could lose the case. What do you say to her when she comes in? What do you document in her file?

32

Group Therapy

Tracy, a group therapy participant, waited several months before opening up and discussing her problems and experiences in front of the group. She then consumed most of the session, sharing with her fellow members and therapist many intimate details about herself and the problems she was having with coworkers. The next week one of her coworkers confronted her concerning some remarks she made in the group therapy session. At first dumbfounded, Tracy collected herself long enough to find out that the coworker was dating one of the other group members. Tracy then called the therapist and reminded him of a conversation they had before she joined the group. He had assured her that she did not have to worry about confidentiality because he carefully screened each potential new member before asking the person to participate in the group. Tracy felt betrayed and complained to the agency that the group's therapist had failed to adequately disclose to her the potential for breaches of confidentiality. The participants in Tracy's group never signed any acknowledgments pertaining to the limits of confidentiality and the risks of disclosure in group therapy.

While working with a couple in marital therapy utilizing both joint and individual sessions, Robert, a licensed marriage and family therapist, learned from the husband that he was bisexual and occasionally had sex with men. His wife did not know about his extramarital sexual activity or his bisexuality. When Robert insisted that the husband either reveal this information to his wife or allow Robert to tell her, the husband refused on both accounts. Robert struggled with his options and finally decided to refer them to another therapist. The wife later called Robert to tell him how upset she was because she felt they had been making wonderful progress. She pressed him for a reason for the termination beyond his stated position that he was having trouble working with them and that he felt another therapist might be able to do a better job. Robert did not disclose his real reason for terminating therapy, and she hung up far less than satisfied with the conversation. She realized there was a hidden agenda but did not know what it was. The mystery was disconcerting.

Prior to a group therapy session, one of the participants, Joe, approached Dr. Kindheart, the therapist conducting the group, and complained about threatening remarks Jake, another group member, had made to him. Joe indicated that the altercations with Jake had occurred after several sessions when the participants were walking toward their cars in the parking lot. Dr. Kindheart promised to discuss the matter with Jake. After first confirming with several other participants that the altercations had indeed occurred, Dr. Kindheart decided to bring the matter up in group, hoping the peer pressure of the group would help Jake see the inappropriateness of his behavior. Rather than acknowledging his mistake, Jake became incensed and attacked Joe, breaking his jaw before the other group members could wrestle him down. Dr. Kindheart called the police, who arrested Jake and charged him with assault. Joe filed a civil suit against Jake for the damages he sustained as a result of the assault and against Dr. Kindheart for negligence. During the legal proceedings, Joe's attorney took depositions from each group member and Dr. Kindheart. Jake, out of jail on bond, filed a complaint against Dr. Kindheart with the licensing board alleging breaches of confidentiality for calling the police and providing them with information about him and for the information shared by each group participant as disclosed in their depositions, and as taken by a court reporter and transcribed.

Ethical Risks for Conjoint Therapy: Confidentiality

The national guidelines for conducting conjoint therapy indicate that confidentiality should be of the utmost concern for therapists and their clients. Therapists must thoroughly discuss confidentiality issues with each group participant and secure written commitments from them to preserve confidentiality with respect to all information disclosed during group sessions including the names of other participants in the group. Therapists could also ask group participants to sign a lawyer-drafted "hold harmless" agreement in which the participant agrees that if the facilitator is sued for breach of confidentiality, the participant who breached the confidentiality will hold the therapist harmless for any damages incurred, including attorney's fees and court costs. Moreover, each participant is personally responsible to the other group participants for breaches of confidentiality. This type of written instrument will have a sobering effect on the talkative or gossipy group member. For an example see *The Portable Lawyer for Mental Health Professionals* (Bernstein and Hartsell 2004, p. 84).

Therapists must thoroughly discuss confidentiality issues with each group participant.

Some agencies and individual practitioners have used the same standard consent forms for decades, without challenge or litigation. Nevertheless, these forms often do not reflect the developing needs of managed care, licensing board requirements, or the legal requirements that reflect emerging case law and statutory amendments, such as HIPAA. When a complaint is filed or a suit is put before the judicial system, obsolete forms do the therapist little good. The therapist and lawyer should jointly prepare all forms and review them regularly. Proper forms will ensure effective therapy as well as a consumer-oriented and, perhaps, a therapist-protective climate. Proper documentation and orientation will automatically protect the client. Every therapist and mental health agency should review all internal and external forms with an attorney at least annually.

In addition to asking clients to sign confidentiality agreements, therapists should clearly establish the consequences for a breach of confidentiality, which at a minimum should include expulsion from the group. Therapists should go one step further and advise each participant that although everyone involved in the group has made a

In addition to asking clients to sign confidentiality agreements, therapists should clearly establish the consequences for a breach of confidentiality, which at a minimum should include expulsion from the group.

confidentiality commitment, they (the therapist or facilitator) cannot guarantee that breaches of confidentiality will not occur. As a general rule, it is wise to remind the participants of the confidentiality rules and concept prior to each session. Such a reminder only takes a few minutes, but reinforces the facilitators' emphasis on the need and, indeed, the expectation of confidentiality.

In the first example, Tracy complained that her therapist did not adequately explain the limits to confidentiality before she participated in the group therapy. Without any written and signed documents, the therapist could not easily refute Tracy's allegations. Just as informed consent should be documented for individual therapy, so should it be for group or multiple client therapy. The informed consent should include the additional information that applies to multiple clients and disclosures ethically required by the ethics codes. Therapists should hold each participant personally and financially responsible for any inappropriate disclosure of information that comes out of the group (i.e., have them sign a "hold harmless" agreement). What is said in the group setting should remain there and cannot be disclosed to anyone, absent a legal exception to confidentiality.

A therapist is required to disclose whatever policy exists with respect to disclosure of confidential information. In the second case study, Robert struggled with the husband's confidential confession that he was bisexual and sexually active outside his marriage. The husband's right to confidentiality precluded Robert sharing that information with the wife or anyone else. This is not remotely a duty-to-warn situation. A good practice for a therapist offering family or marital therapy is to establish a policy that any and all information the therapist deems relevant and material to achieving the goals and purposes of the therapy will be disclosed to other participants. Couples and families then would acknowledge in writing their understanding of and consent to the disclosure policy and its consequences prior to the commencement of therapy, which will allow the therapist to avoid being limited by conflicting ethical interests. Robert was restricted by not receiving such written consent in advance.

National Guidelines for Confidentiality in Conjoint Therapy

American Association for Marriage and Family Therapy (AAMFT) Code of Ethics (2001)

Principle II: Confidentiality

Marriage and family therapists have unique confidentiality concerns because the client in a therapeutic relationship may be more than one person. Therapists respect and guard the confidences of each individual client.

American Counseling Association (ACA) Code of Ethics (2005)

B.4. Groups and Families

B.4.a. Group Work

In group work, counselors clearly explain the importance and parameters of confidentiality for the specific group being entered.

B.4.b. Couples and Family Counseling

In couples and family counseling, counselors clearly define who is considered "the client" and discuss expectations and limitations of confidentiality. Counselors seek agreement and document in writing such agreement among all involved parties having capacity to give consent concerning each individual's right to confidentiality and any obligation to preserve the confidentiality of information known.

National Association of Social Workers (NASW) Code of Ethics (1999)

1.07 Privacy and Confidentiality . . .

(f) When social workers provide counseling services to families, couples, or groups, social workers should seek agreement

(continued)

(Continued)

among the parties involved concerning each individual's right to confidentiality and obligation to preserve the confidentiality of all information shared by others. Social workers should inform participants in family, couples, or group counseling that social workers cannot guarantee that all participants will honor such agreements.

(g) Social workers should inform clients involved in family, couples, marital, or group counseling of the social worker's, employer's, and agency's policy concerning the social worker's disclosure of confidential information among the parties involved in the counseling.

Ethical Risks for Conjoint Therapy: Client Access to Therapy Records

Another problem facing a therapist with multiple clients is client access to records. We get numerous calls from therapists asking for legal advice after an individual involved in family or marital therapy requests a copy of his or her record when the therapists have not received written authorization from the spouse or other family members to disclose the information.

If therapists do not maintain separate files for each group member, they are faced with the problem of extracting confidential information pertaining to another family member or spouse.

If therapists do not maintain separate files for each group member, they are faced with the problem of extracting ("whiting out") confidential information pertaining to another family member or spouse. The simplest way for mental health professionals to deal with this problem is to secure written consent from each client that separate client files will be maintained for all individual sessions and one file will be maintained for joint sessions. Each participant then further consents that each participant has the right to access the joint file and the information in it. Another option might be to have all participants agree in advance that they will not seek the group's progress notes under any circumstances, nor will they subpoena them nor seek legal discovery of any type. A judge would have to be far reaching in order to permit the discovery of material that the litigant agreed in advance was inadmissible or undiscoverable.

National Guidelines for Client Access to Records in Conjoint Therapy

American Counseling Association (ACA) Code of Ethics (2005)

B.6. Records

B.6.d. Client Access

Counselors provide reasonable access to records and copies of records when requested by competent clients. . . . In situations involving multiple clients, counselors provide individual clients with only those parts of records that related directly to them and do not include confidential information related to any other client.

American Association for Marriage and Family Therapy (AAMFT) Code of Ethics (2001)

Principle II: Confidentiality . . .

2.2 Marriage and family therapists do not disclose client confidences except by written authorization or waiver, or where mandated or permitted by law. Verbal authorization will not be sufficient except in emergency situations, unless prohibited by law. When providing couple, family or group treatment, the therapist does not disclose information outside the treatment context without a written authorization from each individual competent to execute a waiver. In the context of couple, family or group treatment, the therapist may not reveal any individual's confidences to others in the client unit without the prior written permission of that individual.

(continued)

Ethical Risks in Conjoint Therapy: Conflicting Goals

It is not uncommon in multiple client therapy for participants to come into conflict with one another and have or develop different goals and objectives.

It is not uncommon in multiple client therapy for participants to come into conflict with one another and have different goals and objectives. Participants' therapeutic objectives may vary as the therapy progresses, sometimes without the therapist's or other participants' knowledge. This is often true in marital therapy where one or both spouses may decide that the marriage is irreconcilable and pursue a divorce.

The separate and confidential knowledge the therapist has about each participant makes continuing with one client problematic.

Under these circumstances, it is not uncommon for therapists to provide individual therapy to one or more participants; however, their susceptibility to accusations of breaches of confidentiality by the other member(s) is great. The separate and confidential knowledge the therapist has about each participant makes continuing with one client problematic under these circumstances. The better practice would be to discontinue therapy with each participant and refer each participant to a different provider. Make two separate referrals, in writing.

If it is apparent that the mental health professional will be asked to testify in any legal proceedings among group participants, immediate termination and referral is usually the best practice. The potential that the therapist's testimony may harm one client dictates this action.

National Guidelines for Conflict of Interest in Conjoint Therapy

American Counseling Association (ACA) Code of Ethics **(2005)**

A.5.e. Role Changes in the Professional Relationship

When a counselor changes a role from the original or most recent contracted relationship, he or she obtains informed consent from the client and explains the right of the client to refuse services related to the change. Examples of role changes include

1. changing from individual to relationship or family counseling, or vice versa; . . .

Clients must be fully informed of any anticipated consequences (e.g., financial, legal, personal, or therapeutic) of counselor role changes.

American Psychological Association (APA) Ethical Principles of Psychologists and Code of Conduct **(2002)**

10.02 Therapy Involving Couples or Families

(a) When psychologists agree to provide services to several persons who have a relationship (such as spouses, significant others, or parents and children), they take reasonable steps to clarify at the outset (1) which of the individuals are clients/ patients and (2) the relationship the psychologist will have with each person.

This clarification includes the psychologist's role and the probable uses of the services provided or the information obtained.

(b) If it becomes apparent that psychologists may be called on to perform potentially conflicting roles (such as family

(continued)

(Continued)

therapist and then witness for one party in divorce proceedings), psychologists take reasonable steps to clarify and modify or withdraw from, roles appropriately.

10.03 Group Therapy

When psychologists provide services to several persons in a group setting, they describe at the outset the roles and responsibilities of all parties and the limits of confidentiality.

National Association of Social Workers (NASW) Code of Ethics (1999)

1.06 Conflicts of Interest

(d) When social workers provide services to two or more people who have a relationship with each other (for example, couples, family members), social workers should clarify with all parties which individuals will be considered clients and the nature of social workers' professional obligations to the various individuals who are receiving services. Social workers who anticipate a conflict of interest among the individuals receiving services or who anticipate having to perform in potentially conflicting roles (for example, when a social worker is asked to testify in a child custody dispute or divorce proceedings involving clients) should clarify their role with the parties involved and take appropriate action to minimize any conflict of interest.

Note: Although this section does not specifically instruct a social worker to terminate a therapeutic relationship, it is probably a rare case where any other action would best minimize actual or potential conflict. Giving testimony in a lawsuit adverse to a client is not going to have a positive impact on therapy and often leads to a licensing board or ethics code complaint.

Ethical Risks of Conjoint Therapy: Group Member Safety

The therapist conducting the group is responsible for the safety and well-being of each participant. It is the therapist who admits participants; thus he or she is responsible for screening each person carefully before asking or allowing him or her to join the group. Failure to carefully study a person's background, characteristics, and suitability for the particular group can be a strong basis for liability if a participant is harmed by the inadequately screened member.

In the third case example, Joe argued that Dr. Kindheart did not properly screen Jake, failing to learn of his violent tendencies, before admitting him to the group. He also argued that Dr. Kindheart failed to protect Joe from Jake and in fact placed Joe in a potentially harmful situation by confronting Jake during a group session about his previous threats to Joe. Dr. Kindheart clearly failed to fulfill his ethical obligations to Joe and the other group participants.

National Guidelines for Group Member Safety in Conjoint Therapy

American Counseling Association (ACA) Code of Ethics (2005)

A.8. Group Work

A.8.a. Screening

Counselors screen prospective group counseling/therapy participants. To the extent possible, counselors select members whose needs and goals are compatible with goals of the group, who will not impede the group process, and whose well-being will not be jeopardized by the group experience.

(continued)

(Continued)

A.8.b. Protecting Clients

In a group setting, counselors take reasonable precautions to protect clients from physical, emotional, or psychological trauma.

American Psychological Association (APA) Ethical Principles of Psychologists and Code of Conduct **(2002)**

3.04 Avoiding Harm

Psychologists take reasonable steps to avoid harming their clients/patients, students, supervisees, research participants, organizational clients, and others with whom they work, and to minimize harm where it is foreseeable and unavoidable.

Ethical Flash Points

- Informed consent for group and other multiple client therapy should include all additional disclosures required by ethics codes and should be documented with a written and signed lawyer-approved consent form.

- Confidentiality must be thoroughly and completely discussed with each group participant.

- A weekly or session reminder is helpful.

- A written commitment to preserve the confidentiality of all information disclosed to the group should be secured from each participant.

- Consequences for breaches of confidentiality should be established and an understanding of them should be acknowledged in writing by each participant.

- The inability to guarantee absolute confidentiality should be disclosed to each participant.

- Separate records should be kept for all individual sessions held with each participant and a common file for all joint sessions.

- Secure written consent from each participant that all participants shall have access to the information in the group file and information pertaining to joint sessions.

- Policies regarding revealing information to other participants must be disclosed, as well as all the legal, statutory, and common-law exceptions to confidentiality. A lawyer-approved handout pamphlet would be advisable together with the acknowledgment that each participant has received a copy and understands the content of the copy.

- Securing written client consent in advance to share confidential information with other participants when deemed relevant and material to goals and purposes of the therapy can ward off a potential ethical quandary for the therapist.

- When conflicts between participants in marital and family therapy become apparent and cannot be reconciled, the therapist must consider terminating with each participant and offering appropriate referrals.

- If family or marital therapists learn that they may be asked to testify by one client in a lawsuit between two or more clients, they should consider terminating therapy with each family member or spouse.

- The therapist is responsible for adequately screening each group participant prior to admission.

- The therapist is responsible for the safety of each participant and must take reasonable precautions to prevent physical or psychological trauma.

- Beware of potential stalkers in any group. Participants may have hidden agendas.

- The reward of saving attorney's fees by failing to have a lawyer review the consent document is not worth the risk of utilizing a faulty, obsolete, and legally unenforceable form.

Summary

Individual therapy is risky enough, but multiple-client therapy compounds the risk to the therapist. The risks and responsibilities increase proportionately with each additional person who participates in the conjoint therapy. The desire of managed care companies to decrease

Careful screening and selective composition of the group are critical to a healthy and successful group therapy practice.

costs has led to an increase in group therapy. The stresses on the family are legion, and the need for marital and family therapy is also increasing. Multiple client therapy, therefore, is here to stay. Careful screening and selective composition of the group are critical to a healthy and successful group therapy practice. By understanding the ethical requirements and risks unique to multiple-client therapy, mental health professionals can safely treat these clients and enjoy more profitability in their practices. More forms will have to be drafted and reviewed by lawyers to protect confidentiality, but in the long run, such creative and defensive tactics are worth the effort.

Suggested Research Assignments

1. Locate and discuss the provisions of any ethical codes promulgated by the mental health profession licensing boards in your state with respect to multiple client therapy. What rules and duties do they impose?
2. Locate and discuss any state and national professional association rules with regard to multiple client therapy. What are the similarities and differences?
3. Compare and contrast the obligations imposed by the licensing boards in your state with the rules promulgated by the state professional associations.
4. Compare and contrast state licensing board and professional association obligations with the guidelines of national professional associations.
5. Research licensing board cases in your state involving multiple client therapy issues. What were the specific rules involved, and what sanctions, if any, were issued?
6. Research civil malpractice cases in your state involving multiple client therapy. What were the outcomes, and what damages, if any, were assessed?
7. Create a set of guidelines for providing multiple client therapy. Include all necessary documentation a practitioner should use and create.

8. Talk to local mental health professionals who offer multiple client therapy and find out what problems they experience in doing so. Also learn what they perceive to be the benefits and risks associated with doing multiple client therapy. What fees do they charge?

9. Research options for increasing your competency and effectiveness as a provider of multiple client therapy.

Discussion Questions

1. What advice would you give a colleague who is considering providing marital therapy to a couple? The colleague has been seeing the wife in individual therapy for several months.

2. Since you are the only marriage and family therapist in your church, the pastor asks you to lead a divorce recovery group for church members. What do you say and do?

3. You charge $100 for individual client sessions. Is there any reason you cannot charge each of five group therapy participants $50 per session thereby earning a total of $250 per session?

4. What are the risks and benefits of providing group therapy?

5. What kinds of clauses might you want to include in a group therapy intake and consent form that you would not include in one for an individual therapy client?

6. Can you maintain a single file for multiple client therapy sessions? What would be your record-keeping approach?

33

Don't Do Dumb Stuff

We were once invited to present a six-hour workshop to the local independent school district on the topic of "Ethics for the Mental Health Professional." We were introduced by a local superintendent who read our vitas with enthusiasm and then said, "You know, we will offer six hours of continuing education credit for this lecture and presentation, but, in truth, it can all be summed up in four words, Don't Do Dumb Stuff." This became the title for our presentation.

At first blush this sounded reasonable, and we were about to pass out our handouts, tell the group not to do dumb stuff, and go to an early lunch. Then we reviewed our outline and realized that much of what we had to say was more than just common sense laced with warnings of things to do and what not to do. To practice the mental health professions in peace, the clinician, therapist, provider of mental health services, psychologist, or counselor had to know much more than these four words. The counselors had to know the general rules of mental health practice, the board rules of the licensing board in their discipline and in their jurisdiction, malpractice case histories that defined what is or is not civil negligence conduct and the general criminal laws that may apply to mental health professionals of all disciplines. The problem, as we saw it, was that if dumb stuff were the only measure, or the only yardstick, then each professional would have the excuse to rely on his or her common sense alone and his or her own definition of what was dumb stuff, and all published information could be ignored.

Unfortunately, the practitioner has to be far more knowledgeable than that. By knowing what the cases, licensing boards, professional organizations, and publications guidelines set out in the literature, it is possible to avoid dumb stuff that is actionable civilly, criminally, and ethically.

The goal in this chapter is to summarize problematic acts and omissions the book has discussed in detail in the previous chapters. This information is not intended to be all-inclusive. However, this information is helpful as a checklist whenever a questionable problem occurs in real-life practice. By following the checklist, serious consequences can be avoided and difficult pitfalls can be eliminated. Dumb stuff *can* be avoided.

The categories of dumb stuff are somewhat arbitrary. You can review the listings and create priorities that relate more comfortably with your background, training, education, and experience. What is important is that when providing services in a litigious, complaining, and blaming society, you must be perpetually aware of legal, ethical, and criminal nuances.

Dumb Stuff

- Commencing therapy without a written contract, properly lawyer reviewed and signed by both the therapist and the client.
- Having an initial intake and consent form that does not comply with the requirements of the licensing law and HIPAA.
- Failing to obtain consent to contact the client at a specific phone number, address, or e-mail. *Note:* The fact that a client has given the provider his or her address does not indicate you can contact the client or leave a message at that location.
- Failing to properly document treatment or changes in treatment when indicated.

- Failing to keep and maintain separate files for each client, including children.
- Failing to obtain informed consent for the treatment from the parent, guardian, or conservator who has the legal authority to give such consent. (Review all legal documents that confer authority, that is, letters of guardianship, conservatorship, divorce decrees, recorded agreements, or papers issued from courts or social service agenciese—especially any documents that set out grandparent rights.)
- Failing to have a clear understanding of who owns a file when an employee leaves the agency, a corporation is dissolved, or a partnership or joint venture breaks up.
- Failing to define what happens to the client file on termination of the need for services when services to the client are no longer needed. Is it specified in the intake file or in the published rules or regulations?
- Failure to obtain specific client consent for video or audio recording a client session.
- Failing to properly supervise supervisees and documenting the supervision.
- Failing to obtain a new consent to treatment form when either the diagnosis, the treatment plan, or the prognosis changes.
- In play therapy, where a child is technically the client, dating either of the parents or soliciting a date from a parent of a child in therapy.
- Failing to adjust to a new consent form when the child client becomes an adult or is emancipated.
- Failing to obtain a new consent form when additional persons are introduced into the treatment program.
- Failing to discuss in detail the consequences of litigation and the effect of litigation on confidentiality.
- Failing to be very specific on the limits to confidentiality both within and without the judicial system.
- Failing to refer to a lawyer when it is clear that there is a legal problem that has an impact on the mental health relationship.
- Failing to discuss the incredible power of the court in the event litigation becomes inevitable.

- Using the same intake and consent form even though the modality of treatment has changed and a new consent form would be appropriate.
- Failing to require continuing education when indicated by either national or state licensing boards of professional associations.
- Allowing a front desk or intake system to be so open that incoming clients or visitors can see confidential information of clients (i.e., breaching the confidentiality of clients inadvertently).
- Using the original intake and informed consent form long after it has outlived its usefulness.
- Failing to get parental consent before treating a child and making sure the parent signing the consent has the legal authority to do so.
- Publishing an article about a case and revealing the identity of the client either directly or indirectly.
- Using identifiable examples in books, articles, videos, or case examples during presentations.
- Revealing more than is necessary for lectures, staffings, or examples.
- Receiving training in a modality of treatment and then fitting every diagnosis into that category.
- Thinking that if you incorporate, you have no liability for injuries to clients.
- Investing in a client's venture or having a client invest money in your venture, business, or other opportunity.
- Failing to comply with specific HIPAA rules.
- Failing to have a published protocol concerning the creation, maintenance, storage, protection, and destruction of client files and preserved documents.

Really Dumb Stuff

- Exceeding your level of competence with a particular client with a particular problem.
- Fudging or lying or gross exaggerations contained in applications for employment, provider panel applications, malpractice insurance applications, or hospital privilege applications.
- Failing to recognize and handle clients who are an actual or potential danger to themselves or others.

- Failing to seek and consult with previous therapists. Beware of the person who is therapist shopping. If they were dissatisfied with others, they are likely to be dissatisfied with you.
- Failing to explain the limitations of therapy: What it can and cannot do.
- Failing to mention that medication available through a psychiatrist is a treatment option.
- Offering serious advice at parties, seminars, social events, or any other venue where you don't have the time or do not have the atmosphere to take a proper history and make an effective evaluation.
- Failing to make a proper referral when a referral is indicated.
- Failing to consult with another therapist when a consultation would be helpful to the client.
- Failing to recommend a psychological or physical test when testing is indicated.
- Indicating to clients that a telephone answering service is available 24 hours per day when the provider only calls in every two or three days or so.
- Failing to respond to the answering service at all.
- Making a referral to a facility for treatment when the facility has not been checked out or investigated for appropriateness for this particular client or problem.
- Failing to properly monitor a client who requires constant or periodic supervision or follow-up.
- Failing to introduce an internal training program when indicated or required by HIPAA regulations.
- Delivering a computer to a computer repair facility without guaranteeing the confidentiality of the information on the hard drive.
- Allowing a repair technician access to confidential files on a hard drive without first obtaining a confidentiality agreement and a HIPPA required Bussiness Associate Agreement. (If a repair is to be accomplished in-house, be sure the technician does not compromise confidential files.)
- Attending a workshop that offers a more effective modality and then continuing to treat clients in the old-fashioned way.

- Failing to keep up with the latest literature in your specialty or assuming that the treatment plan recommended when you received your graduate degree is the best effective method to use today.
- Failing to explain in detail the risks of treatment.
- Failing to explain in detail the alternative treatments available.
- Failing to explain in detail the risks of forgoing treatment.
- Failing to recognize inappropriate dual relationships.
- Not recognizing and maintaining adequate boundaries between practitioners and clients. Engaging in any activity with a client that blurs or makes the boundary between a provider and a client somewhat fuzzy (such as attending a wedding, bar mitzvah, christening, engagement or bachelor party, house warming, or similar family celebration).
- Entering into a business with a client or utilizing the client's professional services, such as legal, accounting, medical, building or contracting, dental, house cleaning, or construction, real estate or insurance.
- Becoming pals with a client or establishing a personal friendship.
- Courting or marrying a client or former client, knowing that any social or sexual relationship is clearly prohibited.
- Giving or accepting gifts other than token gifts of more than a nominal amount.
- Trading out, bartering, or exchanging anything of value. *Note:* Professional services should be for cash using the customary community charges for like services. While there is some latitude here, trading is not a wise practice and should be avoided if at all possible.
- Any diagnosis must be justifiable and supportable by mental health theory and criteria. A misdiagnosis for the purpose of collecting third-party payments is fraud and the payor can recover the amounts advanced.
- Accepting kickbacks (i.e., payments made for the referral of clients where the recipient performs no useful service beyond the referral).
- Representing to a payor that the usual and customary rate is the published rate when in fact the rates charged are based on a sliding fee scale and rarely does the provider charge and receive the published "retail" amount.

- Terminating a client without a proper termination interview or a letter of termination or without proper notification and offering alternatives and continuing referral possibilities.
- Failing to have a plan in the event of either the death or disability of the client or the provider. This plan must provide for the continuing availability of the file to future therapists; the maintenance, confidentiality, preservation, and security of the file for a number of years; and ultimate destruction procedures when the file is no longer needed.

Unforgivable Dumb Stuff

- Failing to take a homicide or suicide threat seriously and making all arrangements possible and appropriate to protect the client or the potential victim.
- Failing to explain all the exceptions to confidentiality or leading the client to believe that everything said in a therapy session is absolutely confidential.
- Sex with a client, former client, or anyone associated with a client.
- Billing the insurance company or third-party payor for a "no show."
- Continuing to practice the profession after a license has been revoked, suspended, or placed under some restriction. (Many licenses have been lost because the licensee has paid for the registration with a hot check, failed to pursue continuing education credits, failed to respond to inquiries, or forgot to reregister.)

Potentially Dumb Stuff

- Protecting a client by failing to report, when required by law, child abuse, elderly abuse, or the abuse of a facility licensed by the state to provide services.
- Allowing an introducer to exaggerate your skills or credentials or allowing exaggerated publicity to be distributed.
- Failing to recognize a potentially dangerous client, such as a client whose early career goal was to be a therapist but who was unsuccessful

in completing graduate school or getting licensed and who second guesses all previous therapists, or who is jealous of your successful mental health career or who has an axe to grind with therapists, or who knows just enough about therapy to be dangerous, or who tells you his or her diagnosis and exactly what you should do about it, or who has taken a multitude of courses and is testing you constantly.

- Failing to obtain permission to contact former providers or family members when required.
- Failing to seek and comply with additional therapy sessions when indicated.
- Treating clients who complain about everyone and everybody and who blame every problem on an inadequate former therapist or an unjust world.
- Failing to consider clients diagnosed with borderline personality disorders with special care.
- Treating clients who demand a definite outcome as a result of therapy. No provider can make such a guarantee.
- Failing to involve both parents in a child's therapy.
- Treating clients who have been in treatment for years and who just don't get better.
- Treating clients who have filed numerous lawsuits or complaints against former providers.
- Treating other professionals with excellent licensed credentials without considering that these individuals have special concerns, needs, and interests. They will be analyzing you as you are analyzing them.
- Shading courtroom testimony so as to please a client.
- Accepting a position from a client in a business or mental health facility.
- Talking to investigators from the state who ask for information and then turn it around so that it becomes the basis of a complaint.
- Discussing any client information with anyone without written permission of the client (i.e., a waiver of confidentiality).
- Locking a client in the therapeutic office because the practitioner does not feel the session is over and has more to say or wants more conversation with the client.

- Failure to take seriously involvement in the judicial system, civil or criminal, or failure to respond to a letter from the licensing board which indicates that a complaint has been filed and a response is required, usually within a specific period of time. ("Seriously" means a lawyer should be contacted whenever there is even a hint of litigation, court involvement, or a client implies or states that judicial input is going to be part of his or her future problems.)

- Allowing the client to delay payment and then taking aggressive collection actions.

- Allowing substantial accounts receivable to build up when collection methods should be in place and satisfactory arrangements made for payment. Aggressive collection methods, turning accounts over to lawyers or collection agencies should be avoided. Collections are a business risk and some accounts just have to be written off. Not all valid bills are paid. Good judgment indicates that every business writes off a percentage of bad debts, and this is just part of the business of therapy.

- Not reading carefully the big and little print in your malpractice policy. Remember, the big print giveth and the small print taketh away. Language has the same value and legal effectiveness regardless whether it is in bold, italics, or underlined. If it is in the contract of insurance, it is part of the agreement and controls the agreement between the parties. Remember to review and renew the policy. Pay premiums promptly and see that the policy is in force until you choose to terminate coverage. Many policyholders have let a policy lapse by failing to pay a bill or sending in a check for payment on a closed or "insufficient funds" account. The prompt payment of bills can, but should not always be the full responsibility of staff. They make mistakes also, and the buck stops with the professional. Make sure the malpractice liability policy includes representation before licensing boards in the event a complaint is filed against you and you require representation.

- Failing to document when the diagnosis, treatment plan, or prognosis changes.

- Failing to handle minor complaints sympathetically, compassionately, patiently, respectfully, and with an eye to understanding the angst of the complaining client. Most misunderstandings can be solved using mediation principles. If all disputes can be reconciled before positions are polarized, the settlement is mutually beneficial. Since the professional provider is more vulnerable than the client, it is in everyone's best interest that differences be resolved quietly and quickly. It is better that the case be closed than it is important for the therapist to "win."

> **Note:** Litigation and licensing board hearings produce anxiety and can last for years without resolution. A common maxim is that a bad settlement is better than a good or winning lawsuit. When a conflict arises, work it out. When real parties assume antagonistic positions, everyone loses.

Summary

In the profession of counseling, therapy, or offering psychological services to clients, the general theory is that a client-serving attitude is paramount. In fact, serving clients is what the mental health disciplines are all about. That is true until the client who formerly thought the provider was wonderful and devoted suddenly shifts and becomes fault-finding, belligerent, hostile, blaming, and nonresponsive. At that time, the client becomes the provider's "enemy" and all the former goodwill is held in abeyance until there is a resolution to the dispute. Until a decision or ruling, the therapist must retreat to a defensive position. In this discourse, the therapist must understand that the former relationship between provider and client has changed. It is now the involvement in an adversarial system in which the complaining client wants self-defined satisfaction and the therapist wants, simply put, to practice in peace. We have indicated numerous vulnerable areas that, if complained about, might prove to indicate a criminal problem, a potential malpractice problem, or an ethical violation. When this occurs, it is the time to be a little less concerned about your client's well-being and a whole lot more concerned about your own.

Epilogue

Ethics in the Twenty-First Century

Karen is the unhappy consumer of mental health services. She wants to file an ethics complaint. She has not really been damaged, and several competent attorneys have already indicated to her that she does not have a viable case for a malpractice action. Most often lawyers accept malpractice cases on a contingent fee basis (i.e., for a percentage of the recovery should recovery occur). Therefore, after considering her complaint without charge, these attorneys refused to handle her case or represent her and offered her no encouragement for continuing with her suit. Her therapist may have committed an ethical wrong, but it is not a financially worthwhile lawsuit or an item for litigation. "File an ethics complaint," they said. "You will be vindicated."

To file an ethics complaint, Karen first had to locate the provider's state licensing board and the national organizations to which he belonged. That meant she had to determine just which license had been issued to her provider. Was it a PC, LPC, SW, LMSW, LMSW-ACP, LMFT, ACSW, MFT, LCDC, or some other license? Was the therapist a licensed psychologist? The therapist's business card and the letterhead on the bill contained more initials than Karen had ever thought about, and this even included some affiliations and registrations, such as RPT (Registered play therapist). Finally, Karen discovered four sympathetic disciplinary groups: (1) the complaints committee of one of the state licensing boards, (2) the complaints committee of another of the state licensing boards (this particular provider had two licenses: an LPC—Licensed Professional Counselor and an LMFT—Licensed Marriage and Family Therapist), and also (3) the disciplinary committee of AAMFT, and (4) ACA. The first two had in-state offices, and the second two maintained national offices out of state.

After researching these organizations on her computer and making several calls to their offices, she determined that each had a separate complaint procedure and a separate complaint form that needed to be completed, signed, and forwarded to the appropriate committee. That was just the beginning. After Karen filed her complaint, the therapist would have an opportunity to respond to each entity for each complaint, and Karen could be required to furnish additional details, perhaps answer questions and, in some cases, appear before these organizations and testify as if she were a prime witness in a litigated, hotly contested, lawsuit. Indeed, since a license is required to practice the profession, the complaint is serious. A revocation of a license often makes the provider unemployable in their chosen profession.

Karen already feels wounded by the provider. Nevertheless, to complete the complaint process and bring an alleged ethical wrong to conclusion, she must investigate the method used to discipline unethical providers, spend hours processing a claim or claims, and deal with multiple entities, each with its own turf to protect. Is there a better way?

Donald is a 35-year-old PhD, a psychologist, and licensed marriage and family therapist in his state. He has chosen to apply for and receive two licenses because it is good for business. He also belongs to two national organizations and has clarified with his malpractice insurance carrier that should a complaint arise, he would be covered for any injury to a client regardless of whether it is classified as the practice of marriage and family therapy or psychology. Now, after practicing 7 years, he faces a choice: either rent another office for storage or get rid of old files. He decides to begin culling or shredding his files but worries about his ethical responsibilities.

Each licensing board and perhaps each national organizations has different mandates regarding retention of files. Some are definite in terms of years: 5 to 10, while others are more difficult to determine with any degree of certainty. If a client is a minor, the rules change. The problem: Licenses conflict and national organizations are inconsistent. Both ignore the commonsense solution of keeping files forever in case some client "remembers" something 30 years later and wants to make Donald's life "interesting." Remember that discovery statutes may extend malpractice statutes of limitations.

Another preservation of records problem exists with rapidly changing technology. What happens if records are preserved on a disc and the disc self-destructs? Or if the problem occurs at a time when the new technology has made the current retrieval system obsolete? After all, Donald is only 35, and he might not retire for 30 years. By then, the whole computer-controlled system of record keeping and preservation will undoubtedly be entirely different. Certainly the technology used today won't be around in 30 years. It will be in the Smithsonian. State rules and the federal Security Rule require systemized backup systems and regularly scheduled testing of electronic data. Even backup systems can fail.

A National Ethics Code

There is a proposal to create a national *Ethics Code,* unanimously adapted, and suitable for all the nonmedical mental health professions. Certain footnotes or clarifications might have to be added to serve particular constituencies (e.g., addictions counselors or play therapists), but the general Ethics Code would be universal.

Establishing a common Ethics Code applicable to all "talking mental health professionals" would bring immediate clarity to the mental health professions and to consumers of mental health services. A careful review of Ethics Codes for the various mental health disciplines reveals that their concerns are essentially the same. All of the ethical problems outlined in Chapter 28, "Interprofessional Issues," and listed in the index of this book have been considered and processed by all the mental health professions as they consider what should be included in their codes of professional responsibility and what should be appropriate or permitted. The spirit of these codes is the same, only the wording and specifics differ.

No matter how it is said, mental health professionals must protect their clients' confidentiality; and dual relationships, boundary violations, and sex with clients are unethical for *all* clinicians. Discrimination is discrimination no matter how it is described, and the professional vulnerabilities remain essentially the same. So why are dozens of similar yet distinct national and state Ethics Codes necessary? The very thought creates a nightmare when you imagine

There is a proposal to create national ethical canons or codes, unanimously adapted and suitable for all the nonmedical mental health professions.

Establishing a common Ethics Code would bring immediate clarity to the mental health professions and to consumers of mental health services.

conscientious students and professionals seeking ethical guidance as they pursue their professional goals and advanced degrees.

Proposal for a National Ethics Congress

We propose that the various mental health professional associations and licensing boards elect representatives to a national ethics congress tasked with developing a mutually acceptable universal standard of ethics. Once the standard is drafted and approved by the congress, each association and licensing board would need to vote to approve the new code. The result would be a unified declaration of all the mental health professions that would be adopted and adhered to by all mental health professionals, whatever their particular discipline or affiliation.

The ethical canons and codes, once consolidated into a single understandable and enforceable form, would be subject to amendment or additions as experience dictates.

The ethical canons and codes, once consolidated into a single understandable and enforceable form, would be subject to amendment or additions as experience dictates. They would always be a work in process, amended annually or semi-annually as circumstances change. When the possibility for unethical acts develop, perhaps due to advancing technology, cyberspace therapy, new theoretical approaches, creative therapists pushing the theoretical envelope or taking a theory further than appropriate or pushing the theory further than the literature indicates or because of the creativity of providers, actions that are not currently specified would be added to the disallowed or proscribed list.

The congress could meet periodically to determine whether modifications or amendments are needed to the national code, which would be subject to the same approval process as the original code.

Faye is a play therapist. Sometimes her children need reinforcement in the form of an occasional hug, a pat, even a squeeze. She has been patting, squeezing, and hugging for years. No parent or child has ever complained. Yet the question arises: Should a counselor hug a child? Would she be vulnerable to a complaint?

Her licensing regulations prohibit sexual physical contact with a client.

The statute does not specifically prohibit hugs.

Because clients sometimes misconstrue a supportive hug, we offer our conservative philosophy: "Don't ever allow yourself to be vulnerable . . . Don't ever touch a client beyond a handshake" to countless groups in seminars. During one question-and-answer period, an experienced, caring, and dedicated, near-retirement school counselor raised her hand. "Mr. Hartsell and Mr. Bernstein," she said, "you lawyers just don't get it. My children need affection, caring, nurturing, and, yes, touching. They don't get enough at home and they will get it here in school and by me as long as I am part of a nurturing and caring school system." "And," she added, "If you think we are going to do away with such an effective supportive method, you're nuts." We backed down, but we are concerned because we know the safe advice is: "No touching."

The best of all possible worlds might be a universally accepted national mental health Ethics Code, taught in every college and university. It would be clearly understood and establish precedents that could be footnoted, clarified, or particularized to accommodate the specific variations of specific disciplines, specialties, or subspecialties. . . . and perhaps, general community attitudes.

Reporting Ethics Violations

In this universal system, names could be included in reporting ethics violations, as is now the case in state and national organizations, or they could be omitted. But wouldn't it be helpful if unethical activities were reported and published on a national level—even without names? Statistical compilations from such data would be helpful to insurance companies for risk analysis and to managed care entities for credentialing purposes. They would also be useful to ethics professors who would know exactly what to emphasize in their classes. If students learned that certain activities are prohibited, perhaps they would act with appropriate restraint when faced with a potentially threatening practice situation or issue. Often the ethical infraction is not an intentional act, but rather a thoughtless or naive act of commission or omission. The therapist may have been unaware of its importance at the time, but after a complaint is filed and client records are scrutinized, the therapist realizes the act was an ethical violation.

Reported ethics infractions should be recorded and clarified, and then precedents established that denote the ethics violation, an explanation, the penalty, and the rationale.

Reported ethics infractions should be recorded and clarified, and then precedents established that denote the ethics violation, an explanation, the penalty, and the rationale. Over the years, these annotated precedents would explain and interpret the written codes and give uniform guidance to professors, students, practitioners, supervisors, authors, and the consuming public.

As greater consideration is given to license portability or reciprocity, a nationwide system or centralized database for sanctions will be just as critical as a uniform ethics code. We are fast becoming a world without geographical boundaries, and when you consider the logistical problems with regulating online therapy, portability and reciprocity makes good sense. Each state and every consumer will need an easy path to determine a professional's eligibility to practice and to record and verify a national complaint history.

Many consumers of mental health services, along with the majority of the general public, are not sophisticated in the area of mental health ethics. Published universal codes with annotations to clarify what might be obscure would be helpful. An informed public with access to compiled information would assist in policing the profession.

Enforcement

A possible solution or approach would be for the state licensing boards to enforce nationally adopted ethical canons. States that do not now provide for complaints to be processed by licensing boards could use the complaint committees of state chapters of the national organizations.

We hesitate to suggest another national governmental bureaucracy to enforce mental health ethics. The possibility of a national mental health policing agency established by the national organizations might be difficult to organize, laborious to augment, and impossible to implement due to turf problems, lack of volunteers and professional staff, and the geographic complexity of our country.

A possible solution or approach would be for the state licensing boards to enforce nationally adopted ethical canons. States that do not now provide for complaints to be processed by licensing boards could use the complaint committees of state chapters of the national organizations. All the legal safeguards, such as procedural due process, would have to be put into place to protect the provider as well as the consuming public.

This solution might not be flawless, but once established, it could be refined by empirical experience and improved over time. This would eliminate the multiple complaint systems a consumer now faces when a therapist has acted unethically. We have represented mental health professionals with two licenses in connection with state licensing board complaint cases in which the two boards reached very different decisions on the same complaint. That is something that can and should be avoided. Considering the same conduct and circumstances, can you imagine a situation when someone—a licensed social worker—is disciplined by the social work board, and the same person—a licensed professional counselor—is not disciplined by the professional counselor board?

Ethical Flash Points

- The ethical canons of all the nonmedical mental health professions are remarkably similar.

- The problem is that they are not identical; therefore, individuals affiliated with different disciplines or who maintain multiple licenses could, and probably do, easily get confused. The consumers of mental health services would, if they were to examine the various codes, get even more confused.

- Enforcement of the ethical canons is divided between national and state organizations and the disciplinary committees of licensing boards. Each has its own rules, processes, and procedures, and the application of these rules changes as personnel changes occur. Thus enforcement, though more than whimsical, is not uniform. Boards change, and member substitutions are common occurrences.

- The consumer of mental health services usually acts instinctively.

- Lawyers, proficient in ethics as it concerns lawyers, and malpractice as it concerns professions, have little training in mental health ethics. Many have no contact at all with the enforcing bodies of the various enforcement agencies.

- Representing clients (therapists of any discipline) before a disciplinary board is not a familiar ritual or procedure for most lawyers.

- Consumers and providers would both benefit from a national system.

Summary

The ethical canons or codes of the nonmedical mental health professions are remarkably similar. The differences are usually semantic, and these semantic differences could be clarified in footnotes, or perhaps in an attachment to a uniform ethical code with a bill of rights to protect such individual differences as exist between the professions, disciplines, specialties, or subspecialties within a discipline.

If this were accomplished in the twenty-first century, the practitioner or the consumer with access to a computer could easily obtain the canons of ethics of the mental health profession, the annotations or the situations which have been decided under the canons, the interpretation of the canons, and the statistical data concerning disciplinary actions. In addition, the necessary procedures for filing a complaint would be readily accessible.

We need to streamline the complaint procedure, make useful information quickly available, and speed up the complaint process from initial alleged ethical infraction to ultimate conclusion. National rules and enforcement procedures would be helpful to both the practitioner and the consuming public. The speed for determination of ethical infractions would also be increased. There is considerable time between the complaint filing and final determination of a case. Anything that results in a speedy resolution of the issues would be helpful to both the provider and the consumer.

Welcome to the twenty-first century!

Appendix A

Mental Health Professional Organizations

The professional associations update their ethical policies and standards regularly. You may obtain the most current version of your organization's ethics code by contacting the national headquarters or by visiting the organization's web site. We have included contact information for several associations here for your convenience.

American Association for Marriage and Family Therapy
1133 15th Street, NW, Suite 300
112 South Alfred Street
Alexandria, VA 22314-3061
(703) 838-9808
(703) 838-9805 (fax)
www.aamft.org

American Counseling Association
5999 Stevenson Avenue
Alexandria, VA 22304
(800) 347-6647
(800) 473-2329 (fax)
(703) 823-6862 (TDD)
www.counseling.org

American Psychological Association
750 First Street, NE
Washington, DC 20002-4242
(800) 374-2721
(202) 336-5500
(202) 336-6123 (TDD/TTY)
www.apa.org

American School Counselor Association
1101 King Street, Suite 625
Alexandria, VA 22314
(703) 683-ASCA
(800) 306-4722
(703) 683-1619 (fax)
www.schoolcounselor.org

National Association of Social Workers
750 First Street, NE, Suite 700
Washington, DC 20002-4241
(202) 408-8600
(800) 638-8799
www.socialworkers.org

Appendix B

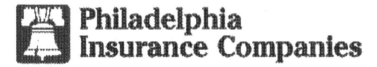

One Bala Plaza, Suite 100, Bala Cynwyd, Pennsylvania 19004

Allied Healthcare Providers Professional and Supplemental Liability Insurance Policy

Source: Philadelphia Insurance Companies—offered through CPH & Associates, Chicago, Illinois.

ALLIED HEALTHCARE PROVIDERS PROFESSIONAL AND SUPPLEMENTAL LIABILITY INSURANCE POLICY

Various provisions in this Policy restrict coverage. Read the entire policy carefully to determine rights, duties, and what is and is not covered.

Throughout this Policy, the words "you" and "your" refer to the Insured shown in the Declarations and any other person or organization qualifying as an Insured under this Policy. The words "we," "us" and "our" refer to the insurance company shown in the Declarations (a stock insurance company, herein called the "Company.")

SECTION I – COVERAGE

A. ALLIED HEALTHCARE PROVIDERS PROFESSIONAL AND SUPPLEMENTAL LIABILITY

1. INSURING AGREEMENT

   a. Coverage A – Professional Liability

   (1) INDIVIDUAL COVERAGE
   The Company will pay on behalf of the **Insured** those sums that the **Insured** becomes legally obligated to pay as **Damages** because of a **Professional Incident** that occurs during the policy period. The **Professional Incident** must result from the practice of the profession shown in the Declarations. This includes services performed by the **Insured** as a member of a credentialing group or utilization review panel, as a case management reviewer or clinical evaluator, or as a member of a board or committee of a hospital or professional society where similar services are performed by the **Insured**.

   (2) ASSOCIATION, PARTNERSHIP OR CORPORATION COVERAGE
   The Company will pay on behalf of the **Insured** those sums that the **Insured** becomes legally obligated to pay as **Damages** because of a **Professional Incident** that occurs during the policy period. The **Professional Incident** must result from the practice of the profession shown in the Declarations.

   b. Coverage B – Supplemental Liability

   (1) BODILY INJURY and PROPERTY DAMAGE COVERAGE
   The Company will pay on behalf of the **Insured** those sums that the **Insured** becomes legally obligated to pay as **Damages**, other than those for which coverage is provided under Coverage A, for Bodily Injury or Property Damage that occurs during the policy period. It must result from a **Professional Incident** that arises out of the profession shown in the Declarations.

   (2) **PERSONAL INJURY** COVERAGE
   The Company will pay on behalf of the **Insured** those sums that the **Insured** becomes legally obligated to pay as **Damages**, other than those for which coverage is provided under Coverage A, for **Personal Injury** that occurs during the policy period and that arises out of the profession shown in the Declarations.

2. EXCLUSIONS

   This insurance does not apply to **Claims** or **Suits** for **Damages**:

   a. arising out of any occupation, business, profession, or personal activity other than the profession specified in the Declarations;

   b. resulting from any actual or alleged breach of contract or agreement. This exclusion does not apply to liability for **Damages** that the **Insured** would have in the absence of the contract or agreement;

   c. you have as a proprietor, owner, superintendent, director, partner, manager, administrator or executive officer of any hospital, nursing home, medical clinic, health maintenance organization, managed care facility, sanitarium, or any other facility with bed and board arrangements;

   d. arising out of the ownership, maintenance, use or entrustment to others of any aircraft, **Auto** or watercraft owned or operated by or rented or loaned to any **Insured**. Use includes operation and **Loading or Unloading**;

   e. arising out of the prescription, utilization, furnishing, or dispensing of drugs or medical, dental or nursing supplies or appliances, except as directed by a physician and in the normal practice as an **Insured**;

   f. arising out of intentional wrongful acts of the **Insured**;

   g. arising out of injury to any **Insured** or any consequential injury to the spouse, child, parent, brother or sister of that **Insured**.

   This exclusion applies:

   (1) whether the **Insured** may be liable as an employer or in any other capacity, and

   (2) to any obligation to share **Damages** with or repay someone else who must pay **Damages** because of the injury;

h. arising out of any obligation of the **Insured** under a workers compensation, disability benefits or unemployment compensation law or any similar law;

i. arising out of any **Claim** made by a person because of any:

(1) refusal to employ that person, or

(2) termination of that person's employment, or

(3) employment-related practices, policies, acts or omissions, such as coercion, demotion, evaluation, reassignment, discipline, defamation, sexual harassment, humiliation or discrimination directed at that person, or

(4) arising out of actual or alleged discrimination.

This exclusion applies:

(1) whether the **Insured** may be liable as an employer or in any other capacity, and

(2) to any obligation to share **Damages** with or repay someone else who must pay **Damages**;

j. arising from **Advertising Injury** or **Personal Injury**.

However, this exclusion does not apply to **Personal Injury** when the offense arises out of a **Professional Incident** and the **Personal Injury** does not arise out of:

(1) oral or written publication of material, if done by or at the direction of the **Insured** with knowledge of its falsity;

(2) oral or written publication of material, whose first publication took place before the beginning of the policy period, or

(3) the willful commission of a criminal act(s);

k. arising out of damage to property:

(1) owned, occupied or used by any **Insured**;

(2) rented to, in the care, custody or control of, or over which physical control is being exercised for any purpose by any **Insured**, or

(3) which is or was in the possession of any **Insured** or any person acting on behalf of any **Insured**, or

(4) that is real property on which you or any contractors or subcontractors working directly or indirectly on your behalf are or were performing operations;

l. arising out of any:

(1) **Pollution Hazard**,

(2) **Nuclear Hazard**,

(3) **Asbestos Hazard**, or

(4) **Lead Hazard**;

m. arising out of unfair competition or violation of any anti-trust laws;

n. arising out of the inability or failure of the **Insured** or others to collect or pay money, including fee disputes and third party reimbursement disagreements;

o. arising out of an **Insured** gaining any personal profit or advantage to which they are not legally entitled;

p. arising out of liability under the Employee Retirement Income Security Act of 1974 (ERISA) and any amendments to that act or any similar federal or state law;

q. arising out of any criminal, dishonest, fraudulent or malicious act or omission. This exclusion does not apply to any **Insured** who did not:

(1) personally participate in committing any such act, or

(2) remain passive after having personal knowledge of any such act or omission;

r. arising out of any **Claim** made or **Suit** brought against an **Insured** by another **Insured**;

s. arising out of sexual therapy, where sexual contact is used as a form of treatment thereof, or where any surrogate sexual therapy related to sexual dysfunction is employed.

t. arising out of any business relationship or venture with any prior or current patient or relative of a prior or current patient of an **Insured**;

u. physical abuse, sexual abuse or licentious, immoral or sexual behavior whether or not intended to lead to, or culminating in any sexual act, whether caused by, or at the instigation of, or at the direction of, or omission by any **Insured**. However, the Company will defend any civil **Suit** against an **Insured** seeking amounts that would be covered if this exclusion did not apply. In such case, the Company will only pay Fees, Costs and Expenses of such defense. Our duty to defend will cease upon admission of guilt by the **Insured**, or if the **Insured** is adjudicated guilty. We will have no obligation to appeal any such judgment or adjudication.

v. any **Claim** arising from professional services that you provide when:

(1) you are not properly licensed or certified by the laws of the state(s) in which you provide such services;

(2) such services are not authorized or permitted by the laws of the state(s) in which your professional services are provided.

B. SUPPLEMENTAL PAYMENTS

We will pay, with respect to any **Claim** or **Suit** we defend:

1. all expenses we incur including defense costs;
2. up to $250 for the cost of bail bonds to release attachments, but only for bond amounts within the applicable limit of insurance. We do not have to furnish these bonds;
3. all reasonable expenses incurred by the **Insured** at our request to assist us in the investigation or defense of the **Claim** or **Suit**, including actual loss of earnings up to $500 a day because of time off from work subject to a maximum of $15,000 for any **Claim** or **Suit**;
4. all costs taxed against the **Insured** in the **Suit**;
5. prejudgment interest awarded against the **Insured** on that part of the judgment we pay. If we make an offer to pay the applicable limit of insurance, we will not pay any prejudgment interest based on that period of time after the offer;
6. all interest on the full amount of any judgment that accrues after entry of the judgment and before we have paid, offered to pay, or deposited in court the part of the judgment that is within the applicable limit of insurance.

These payments will not reduce the limits of insurance.

C. ADDITIONAL POLICY BENEFITS

1. DEPOSITION EXPENSE

We will pay for reasonable legal expenses incurred by an **Insured** for appearance at a deposition, to which the **Insured** is required to submit and that involves the professional occupation shown in the Declarations. No **Insured** will be reimbursed more than $5,000 per **Professional Incident.** This benefit is subject to a limitation of $15,000 per **Insured.**

2. STATE LICENSING BOARD INVESTIGATION EXPENSES

We will pay reasonable expenses that you incur resulting from an investigation or proceeding by a state licensing board or other regulatory body provided that the investigation or proceeding arises out of events which could result in **Claims** covered by this Policy. We will not be responsible for conducting such investigation or providing such defense. The maximum aggregate amount we will pay for this benefit is $25,000.

3. MEDICAL EXPENSES

We will pay, regardless of fault, for necessary medical expenses incurred within a three (3) year period from the date of an accident arising out of professional services rendered by you. The most we will pay for medical expenses is $2,500 per person subject to a $25,000 aggregate in any single policy period. This coverage is provided on the condition that the injured person or someone on their behalf shall give us written proof of a claim for medical expenses, under oath if required. If we request, the injured person shall execute an authorization to enable us to obtain medical reports and copies of all records. The injured person will also submit to physical examinations by physicians selected by us. The examinations will be made when, and as often as, we may reasonably require. Payment by us to an injured person will not imply an admission of liability. Each payment will reduce the total amount payable for such bodily injury if liability is later established.

We will not pay under this extension of coverage for bodily injury:

a. to any person included within the definition of an **Insured.**
b. resulting from selling, serving or giving alcoholic beverages.
c. to any person practicing, instructing, or participating in any physical training, sports, athletic activity or contest whether on a formal or informal basis.
d. arising out of any medical, surgical, dental, X-Ray or other health service or treatment performed by you, including the dispensing of drugs, medical, dental, or surgical supplies, except as directed by a physician and in the normal practice as an Insured.

4. FIRST AID COVERAGE

We will pay up to $2,500 for amounts which you voluntarily pay or incur for first aid rendered to others as a result of bodily injury covered by this policy. The first aid must be provided within a 48 hour period after the bodily injury occurs. This provision does not apply to payments or first aid rendered to any person defined as an **Insured** in this policy. The total amount payable for all first aid coverage shall not exceed $2,500 for all first aid rendered during the policy period.

5. ASSAULT COVERAGE

We will pay for expenses you incur, up to $5,000 for bodily injury to you or property damage to your personal property, other than your mode of transportation, resulting from an assault on you while traveling to and from your place of employment. This coverage is excess over any available insurance specifically written as primary insurance covering such bodily injury or property damage.

These payments are in addition to the applicable limits of liability.

SECTION II – WHO IS AN INSURED

Each of the following is an **Insured** under this Policy to the extent set forth below:

A. if the **Insured** is an individual, the **Insured** so designated in the Declarations;

B. if the **Insured** is a partnership, the partnership so designated in the Declarations and any partner thereof;

C. if the **Insured** is a corporation, the corporation so designated in the Declarations, and any owner, officer, director, trustee, or stockholder thereof, and:

1. any employee of the **Insured** but only for acts within the scope of his/her employment by the **Insured**, and

2. any student in training or volunteer, but solely while such person is acting within the scope of his/her duties for, or on behalf of the **Insured**.

SECTION III – LIMITS OF INSURANCE

A. The Limits of Insurance shown in the Declarations and the provisions below define the most we will pay regardless of the number of:

1. **Insureds**;

2. **Claims** made or **Suits** brought, or

3. persons or organizations making **Claims** or bringing **Suits**.

B. The Aggregate Limit is the most we will pay for all **Damages** to which this insurance applies.

C. Subject to B. above, the Each Incident Limit is the most we will pay for the sum of all **Damages** arising out of the same **Professional Incident** to which this insurance applies. The Limits of Insurance apply separately to each policy period.

D. If both Coverages A and B as shown in the Declarations apply to the same **Claim**, the Company's liability is limited as follows:

1. in no event will the Limits of Liability of Coverages A and B be added together, combined, or stacked to determine the applicable Limit of Liability;

2. the total Limits of Liability under both Coverages A and B will not exceed the highest applicable limit of Coverage A or of Coverage B;

3. the Company, in its sole discretion, will conclusively determine which coverage applies and in what proportion.

SECTION IV – CONDITIONS

A. YOUR AUTHORITY AND DUTIES

You agree to act on behalf of all **Insureds** with respect to cancellation, notice of any **Professional Incident**, **Claim** or **Suit**, payment or return of any premium, or consent to a **Claim** settlement that we recommend. Each **Insured**, by accepting this insurance, agrees to:

1. have you act for them in such matters, and

2. promptly notify you, in writing, of any **Professional Incident** which may result in a **Claim**, or any **Claim** or **Suit** brought against them.

B. DUTIES IN THE EVENT OF A **CLAIM** OR **SUIT**

1. You must promptly notify us in writing of a **Professional Incident** that may result in a **Claim**. To the extent possible, notice should include:

a. all available information concerning the circumstances of the **Professional Incident** including:

(1) how, when, and where it took place, and

(2) the names and addresses of any witnesses and persons seeking **Damages**, and

b. what **Claim** you think may result.

However, even when you notify us of a **Professional Incident**, this does not relieve you of your obligation to also notify us of any resulting **Claim** or **Suit**.

2. If a **Claim** is made or **Suit** is brought against any **Insured**, you must promptly notify us in writing of any **Claim** or **Suit**. **Please submit the requisite information to** the following address:

> Philadelphia Insurance Companies
> 1 Bala Plaza, Suite 100
> Bala Cynwyd, Pennsylvania 19004
> Attention: Claims Department

Such notice shall be effective on the date of receipt by the Company at such address.

3. You and any other involved **Insured** must:

a. immediately send us copies of any demands, notices, summonses, or legal papers received in connection with the **Claim** or **Suit**;

b. authorize us to obtain records and other information;

c. cooperate with us in the investigation, settlement or defense of the **Claim** or **Suit**;

d. assist us, upon our request, in the enforcement of any right against any person or organization which may be liable to the **Insured** because of injury or damage to which this insurance may also apply;

   e. in no way jeopardize our rights after a **Professional Incident**.

C. LEGAL ACTION AGAINST US

No person or organization has a right under this Policy:

1. to join us as a party or otherwise bring us into a **Suit** asking for **Damages** from an **Insured;** or

2. to sue us on this Policy unless all of its terms have been fully complied with.

A person or organization may sue us to recover on an agreed settlement or on a final judgment against an **Insured** obtained after an actual trial; but we will not be liable for **Damages** that are not payable under the terms of this Policy or that are in excess of the applicable limit of insurance. An agreed settlement means a settlement and release of liability signed by us, the **Insured** and the claimant or the claimant's legal representative.

D. OTHER INSURANCE

If all or part of any covered **Claim** or **Suit** is covered by other insurance, whether on a primary, excess, umbrella, contingent, or any other basis, then this Policy:

1. will be excess with respect to Coverage A;

2. will not apply and no coverage will be afforded under this Policy with respect to Coverage B. However, when the limits of this Policy are greater than the limits of all other insurance, then this Policy will provide excess insurance up to an amount sufficient to give the **Insured**, as respects the amount afforded under Coverage B, a total limit of insurance equal to the limit of insurance provided by this Policy.

This will apply even as to fully or partially self-insured programs, and policies in which the **Insured** has a deductible or has retained a self-insured portion of the risk. In no event will this Policy be construed to contribute more than on an excess basis. This provision does not apply to coverage under an excess policy that is specifically written to be excess of this Policy and that specifically refers to this Policy as an underlying policy.

E. REPRESENTATIONS

By accepting this Policy, you agree that:

1. the statements in the application and any supplement are accurate and complete;

2. those statements are based upon representations you made to us, and

3. we have issued this Policy in reliance upon your representations.

F. TRANSFER OF RIGHTS OF RECOVERY AGAINST OTHERS TO US

If the **Insured** has rights to recover all or part of any payment we have made under this Policy, those rights are transferred to us. The **Insured** must do nothing after loss to impair them. At our request, the **Insured** will bring **Suit** or transfer those rights to us and help us enforce them.

G. SETTLEMENT

If you refuse to consent, within a reasonable period of time, to any settlement offer we recommend and elect to contest the **Claim** or continue any legal proceedings in connection with such **Claim** then, subject to provisions of SECTION III – LIMITS OF INSURANCE, our liability for the **Claim** will not exceed the amount for which the **Claim** could have been settled, plus the cost of defense incurred by us up to the date of such refusal.

H. TWO OR MORE COVERAGE PARTS OF POLICIES ISSUED BY US

It is our stated intention that the various coverage parts or policies issued to you by us, or any company affiliated with us, do not provide any duplication or overlap of coverage for the same **Claim** or **Suit**. We have exercised diligence to draft our coverage parts or policies to reflect this intention, but should the circumstances of any **Claim** or **Suit** give rise to such duplication or overlap of coverage then, notwithstanding the other insurance provision, if this Policy and any other coverage part or policy issued to you by us, or any company affiliated with us, apply to the same **Professional Incident**, occurrence, offense, wrongful act, accident or loss, the maximum Limit of Insurance under all such coverage parts or policies combined shall not exceed the highest applicable Limit of Insurance under any one coverage part or policy.

I. LIBERALIZATION

If the Company receives approval to issue a revised version of this form that would broaden the coverage under this Policy during the Coverage Term, the broadened coverage will apply to this Policy on the date of such approval, without additional premium.

J. CANCELLATION/NONRENEWAL/INCREASE IN PREMIUM OR DECREASE IN COVERAGE

1. The **Insured** shown in the Declarations may cancel this Policy by mailing or delivering to us advance written notice of cancellation.

2. If this Policy has been in effect for less than 60 days, we may cancel this Policy by mailing by first class mail or delivering to the **Insured** written notice of cancellation at least:

   a. 10 days before the effective date of cancellation if we cancel for nonpayment of premium, or

   b. 30 days before the effective date of cancellation if we cancel for any other reason.

3. If this Policy has been in effect for 60 days or more, or is a renewal of a policy we issued, we may cancel this Policy by mailing through first-class mail to the **Insured** written notice of cancellation:

   a. including the actual reason, at least 10 days before the effective date of cancellation, if we cancel for nonpayment of premium, or

   b. at least 30 days before the effective date of cancellation if we cancel for any other reason.

4. We may cancel this Policy based on any of the following reasons:

   a. nonpayment of premium;

   b. a false statement knowingly made by the **Insured** on the application for insurance, or

   c. any other legally permissible reason.

5. Notice of cancellation will state the effective date of cancellation. The policy period will end on that date provided proper notice is given.

6. If this Policy is canceled, we will send the **Insured** any premium refund due. If we cancel, the refund will be pro rata. If the **Insured** cancels, the refund will be at least 90% of the pro rata refund.

7. We may decide to not renew this Policy for any legally permissible reason. If we decide not to renew this Policy, we will mail through first-class mail to the **Insured** shown in the Declarations written notice of the nonrenewal at least 30 days before the expiration date.

8. We will not increase the premium unilaterally or decrease the coverage benefits on renewal of this Policy unless we mail through first-class mail written notice of our intention, including the actual reason, to the **Insured's** last mailing address known to us, at least 30 days before the effective date.

9. Any decrease in coverage during the policy term must be based on one or more of the following reasons:

   a. nonpayment of premium;

   b. a false statement knowingly made by the **Insured** on the application for insurance, or

   c. a substantial change in the exposure or risk other than that indicated in the application and underwritten as of the effective date of the policy unless the **Insured** has notified us of the change and we accept such change;

   d. any other legally permissible reason.

10. If any notice is mailed, proof of mailing will be sufficient proof of notice.

SECTION V – DEFINITIONS

A. **Advertising Injury** means injury arising out of one or more of the following offenses committed in the course of advertising your goods, products, or services:

   1. oral or written publication of material that slanders or libels a person or organization or disparages a person's or organization's goods, products, or services;

   2. oral or written publication of material that violates a person's right of privacy;

   3. misappropriation of advertising ideas or style of doing business, or

   4. infringement of copyright, title, or slogan.

B. **Asbestos Hazard** means:

   1. a. inhaling, ingesting, or prolonged physical exposure to asbestos or goods or products containing asbestos;

      b. the use of asbestos in constructing or manufacturing any goods, product, or structure;

      c. the removal of asbestos from any good, product, or structure;

      d. any request, demand, or order for the removal of asbestos from any good, product, or structure, or

      e. the manufacture, sale, transportation, storage of disposal of asbestos or goods or products containing asbestos;

   2. the investigation settlement or defense for any **Claim**, **Suit**, proceeding, **Damages**, loss, cost, or expense excluded by 1. above.

C. **Auto** means a land motor vehicle, trailer, or semitrailer designed for travel on public roads, including any attached machinery or equipment.

D. **Claim** means a demand made upon any **Insured** for **Damages**. All **Claims** arising out of the same act or omission which are logically or causally connected in any way shall be deemed as a single **Claim.**

E. **Coverage Territory** means:

   1. the United States of America (including its territories and possessions), Puerto Rico, and Canada;

   2. all parts of the world if:

   a. the injury or damage arises out of the activities of a person whose home is in the territory described in 1. above but is away temporarily on your business, and

   b. the **Insured's** responsibility to pay **Damages** is determined in a **Suit** on the merits, in the territory described in 1. above or in a settlement we agree to;

  3. if **Suit** is brought within 1. above.

F. **Damages** means a monetary:

  1. judgment,

  2. award, or

  3. settlement,

but does not include fines, sanctions, penalties, punitive or exemplary damages or the multiple portion of any damages.

G. **Insured** means the individual or the association, partnership, or corporation named in the Declarations or qualifying as an **Insured** under the WHO IS AN **INSURED** provision of this form.

H. **Lead Hazard** means:

  1. a. exposure to or existence of lead, paint containing lead, or any other material or substance containing lead, or

    b. manufacture, distribution, sale, resale, rebranding, installation, repair, removal, encapsulation, abatement, replacement, or handling of lead, paint containing lead, or any other material or substance containing lead, whether or not the lead is or was at any time airborne as a particulate, contained in a product ingested, inhaled, transmitted in any fashion, or found in any form whatsoever;

  2. a. any testing for, monitoring, cleaning up, removing, abating, containing, treating or neutralizing lead, paint containing lead, or any other substance or material containing lead or in any way responding to or assessing the effects of lead, or

    b. any request, demand, or order to test for; monitor; clean up; remove; abate; contain; treat or neutralize lead, paint containing lead, or any other substance or material containing lead; or in any way respond to or assess the effects of lead;

  3. the investigation, settlement or defense of any **Claim**, **Suit**, proceeding, **Damages**, loss, cost or expense excluded by 1. and 2. above.

I. **Loading or Unloading** means the handling of property:

  1. after it is moved from its initial place to the place where it is accepted for movement into or onto an aircraft, watercraft, or **Auto**;

  2. while it is in or on an aircraft, watercraft, or **Auto**, or

  3. while it is being moved from an aircraft, watercraft, or **Auto** to the place where it is finally delivered,

but **Loading or Unloading** does not include the movement of property by means of a mechanical device, other than a hand-truck that is not attached to the aircraft, watercraft, or **Auto**.

J. **Nuclear Hazard** means the existence of any nuclear reactor or device, nuclear waste storage or disposal site, or any other nuclear facility, or the transportation of nuclear material, or the hazardous properties of nuclear material which includes but is not limited to, source material, special nuclear material, and by-product material as those terms are defined in the Atomic Energy Act of 1954 and any law amendatory thereof and any similar federal, state or local statutory, civil, or common law.

K. **Personal Injury** means injury, other than bodily injury, arising out of one or more of the following offenses:

  1. false arrest, detention, or imprisonment;

  2. malicious prosecution;

  3. the wrongful eviction from, wrongful entry into, or invasion of the right of private occupancy of a room, dwelling, or premises that a person occupies by or on behalf of its owner, landlord, or lessor;

  4. oral or written publication of material that slanders or libels a person or organization or disparages a person's or organization's goods, products, or services, or

  5. oral or written publication of material that violates a person's right of privacy.

L. **Pollution Hazard** means:

  1. a. any actual, alleged, or threatened emission, discharge, seepage, mitigation, release, or escape of pollutants at any time, or

    b. any clean up of pollutants, or

    c. any request, demand or order for any clean up of pollutants;

  2. the investigation, settlement or defense of any **Claim**, **Suit**, proceeding, **Damages**, loss, cost or expense excluded by 1. above.

Pollutants include any noise, solid, semi-solid, liquid, gaseous, or thermal irritant or contaminant, including smoke vapor, soot, fumes, mists, acids, alkalis, chemical, biological, and etiologic agents or materials, electromagnetic or ionizing radiation and energy, genetically engineered materials, teratogenic, carcinogenic and mutagenic materials, waste and any other irritant or contaminant.

Waste includes any materials to be disposed, recycled, reconditioned, or reclaimed.

Clean up includes monitoring, removal, containment, treatment, detoxification or neutralization of, testing for or response in any way to, or assessment of the effects of pollutants.

M. **Professional Incident** means any actual or alleged negligent:
1. act,
2. error, or
3. omission

in the actual rendering of professional services to others in your capacity as an **Insured** including professional services performed as a member of a credentialing group or utilization review panel, as a case management reviewer or clinical evaluator, or as a member of a board or committee of a hospital or professional society where similar services are performed by the **Insured**.

Any or all **Professional Incidents** arising from interrelated or a series of acts, errors or omissions shall be deemed to be one **Professional Incident** taking place at the time of the earliest **Professional Incident**.

N. **Suit** means a civil proceeding in which **Damages** are sought and to which this insurance applies. **Suit** also includes:
1. an arbitration proceeding in which such **Damages** are sought and to which you must submit or do submit with our consent, or
2. any other alternative dispute resolution proceeding in which such **Damages** are sought and to which you submit with our consent.

IN WITNESS WHEREOF, the Company has caused this Policy to be signed by its President and Secretary, but same shall not be binding upon the Company unless countersigned by an authorized representative of the Company.

President   Secretary

Appendix C

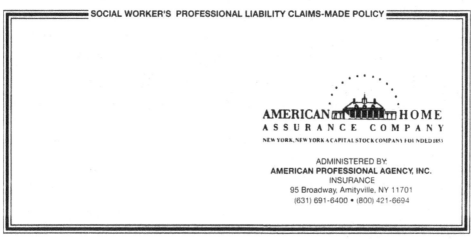

AMERICAN HOME ASSURANCE COMPANY
Executive Offices 70 Pine Street
New York, NY 10270 A Capital Stock Company

NOTICE: THIS IS A CLAIMS-MADE POLICY. COVERAGE IS LIMITED GENERALLY TO LIABILITY FOR CLAIMS FIRST MADE AGAINST YOU AND REPORTED IN WRITING TO US WHILE THE COVERAGE IS IN FORCE.
A LOWER LIMIT OF LIABILITY APPLIES TO JUDGMENTS AND SETTLEMENTS OF ALLEGATIONS OF SEXUAL MISCONDUCT. PLEASE REVIEW THE POLICY CAREFULLY AND DISCUSS POLICY COVERAGE WITH YOUR INSURANCE AGENT OR BROKER.

In consideration of the premium paid and in reliance upon the statements in the Application completed by the **named insured** and upon the Declarations and subject to its terms, conditions, and exclusions, **we** agree to this Policy as a contract with the **named insured**.

I. INSURING AGREEMENTS

A. Wrongful Act

We shall pay those amounts that **you** become legally obligated to pay to compensate others arising out of **your wrongful act**. The **wrongful act** must take place on or after the **retroactive date**, but before the end of the **policy period**, and must arise solely out of **your** performance of professional services as a social worker. A **claim** for a **wrongful act** must be first made against **you** and reported to **us** in writing during the **policy period** or any extended reporting period, if applicable.

B. Premises Liability

We shall pay those amounts that **you** become legally obligated to pay to compensate others for **bodily injury** or **property damage** arising out of an **occurrence** on the premises used principally in the **named insured's** practice as a social worker. The **bodily injury** or **property damage** must take place on or after the **retroactive date**, but before the end of the **policy period**. A claim for **bodily injury** or **property damage** must be first made against **you** and reported to **us** in writing during the **policy period** or any extended reporting period, if applicable.

C. Administrative Hearing

We shall pay reasonable **administrative expenses** arising out of an **administrative hearing**, arising solely out of **your** performance of professional services as a social worker, even if the basis for that **administrative hearing** is groundless or fraudulent. The request or notification for the **administrative hearing** must take place on or after the **retroactive date**, but before the end of the **policy period**.

II. DEFINITIONS

A. **Administrative Expense(s)** means reasonable expenses incurred pursuant to an **administrative hearing** for **attorney's** fees for legal service rendered, pre-hearing discovery and investigation costs and charges for an **attorney's** general services.

B. **Administrative Hearing** means a disciplinary proceeding against **you** and shall be limited to the following:

    1. Proceedings **initiated** by a state licensing board or governmental regulatory body against **you** for unprofessional conduct; or

    2. Proceedings **initiated** by a State Department of Health Services or the Federal Department of Health and Human Services arising out of **your** performance of professional services as a social worker and alleging any violation of guidelines for appropriate utilization of those services.

C. **Attorney** means an individual duly licensed to practice law at the time and place the legal services are rendered.

D. **Automobile** means a land vehicle, whether or not self-propelled, or a trailer or semitrailer, including any machinery or apparatus attached thereto, whether or not designed for use principally on public roads.

E. **Bodily Injury** means physical injury, sickness, disease, sustained by any person, including death resulting therefrom.

Source: American Home Insurance Co. (NASW Insurance Trust)—Administered by Professional Agency, Inc.

F. **Claim(s)** means a demand for money and includes **suit(s)**.

G. **Criminal Prosecution** means any government action for enforcement of criminal laws, including offenses, conviction for which could result in imprisonment.

H. **Defamation** means the publication or utterance of a libel or slander or other defamatory or disparaging material, or a publication or utterance in violation of an individual's right of privacy.

I. **Discrimination** means the violation of any law, whether statutory or common law, including, but not limited to, race, color, religion, national origin, age, sex, marital status, sexual orientation, harassment, handicap, pregnancy, chronic medical condition, or obesity.

J. **Initiated** means the commencement of an **administrative hearing** at the time written notice is received by **you**.

K. **Named Insured** means any organization or individual indicated in Item 1.A. of the Declarations.

L. **Occurrence** means an accident, including continuous or repeated exposure to substantially the same general harmful conditions, which results in **bodily injury** or **property damage** neither expected nor intended from **your** standpoint. **Occurrence** shall not include the rendering of or failure to render any professional service, nor shall it include **defamation**.

M. **Policy Period** means the period commencing on the effective date shown in the Declarations and ending on the effective date of termination, expiration, or cancellation of this Policy.

N. **Pollutants** means any solid, liquid, gaseous, or thermal irritant or contaminant, including: smoke, vapor, soot, fumes, acids, alkalis, chemicals and waste. Waste includes, but is not limited to, material to be recycled, reconditioned or reclaimed, as well as medical waste.

O. **Property Damage** means (1) physical injury to or destruction of tangible property including the loss of use thereof resulting therefrom, or (2) loss of use of tangible property which has not been physically injured or destroyed, provided such loss of use is caused by an **occurrence**.

P. **Retroactive Date** means the date specified as such in the Declarations.

Q. **Suit** means a civil proceeding seeking money damages, and includes an arbitration, mediation or any other alternative dispute resolution procedure seeking such damages, to which **you** shall submit or may submit with **our** consent. **Suit** shall not include an **administrative hearing**.

R. **You** and **Your** means any Insured as set forth in Section III. Who Is An Insured.

S. **We**, **Our** and **Us** means the Company providing this insurance.

T. **Wrongful Act** means any actual or alleged negligent act, error, or omission, or any actual or alleged **defamation**.

III. WHO IS AN INSURED

The following is an Insured and is referred to as **you** or **your**:

A. The individual, partner or corporation designated as **named insured** in Item 1.A. of the Declarations, including any partner, executive officer, director or stockholder thereof, and the individual(s) designated as Additional Named Insured in Item 1.B. of the Declarations; and

B. Any present or former employee, partner, executive officer, director or stockholder of the **named insured** designated in Item 1.A. of the Declarations, but only while acting in the capacity as such; and

C. Any individual, partnership or corporation designated in Item 2 of the Declarations, but only as to matters for which a **named insured** may be liable under this policy.

IV. DEFENSE COSTS, CHARGES AND EXPENSES

The following shall apply only to Insuring Agreements A and B:

We shall pay the costs related to the following which are in addition to the Limits of Liability:

A. **We** have the right and duty to defend and appoint counsel, at **our** expense for any **suit** brought against **you** for a covered **wrongful act**, **bodily injury**, or **property damage** even if the **suit** is groundless or fraudulent. **Our** duty to defend **suit** ends after the applicable Limit of Liability has been exhausted by payment of judgments, awards, and interest accruing thereon prior to entry of judgment or issuance of an award and settlements.

B. **We** have the right to investigate any **claim** or **suit** and, with the **named insured's** written consent, settle any **claim** or **suit** that **we** believe is proper. **Our** duty to defend any **suit** ends if the **named insured** refuses to consent to a settlement **we** recommend and the claimant shall accept. The **named insured** shall then defend the **suit** at the **named insured's** own expense and negotiate any settlement. **Our** liability for any settlement or judgment shall not be more than the amount for which **we** could have settled had the **named insured** consented.

C. 1. **We** shall pay all reasonable costs, other than loss of earnings, **we** ask **you** to incur while defending a **suit**.

    2. **We** shall pay premiums for appeal bonds, or bonds to release property used to secure legal obligation, if required in a **suit** **we** defend. **We** shall only pay, however, for bonds valued up to **our** applicable Limit of Liability. **We** have no obligation to appeal or to obtain these bonds.

    3. Up to two hundred fifty dollars ($250) per day with a maximum amount payable of five thousand dollars ($5,000) per **suit** as lost earnings when **your** practice as a social worker was suspended due to attendance at hearings or trials at **our** request.

D. **We** shall pay all interest and all costs taxed on that amount of any judgment up to **our** Limit of Liability:

    1. Which accrues after entry of judgment; and

    2. Before **we** pay, offer to pay, or deposit in court that part of the judgment within **our** applicable Limit of Liability.

The following shall only apply to Insuring Agreement C:

A. **We** shall defend **you** and pay **administrative expenses** at an **administrative hearing** arising solely out of **your** profession as a social worker up to **our** Limit of Liability stated in the Declarations.

B. Duties in the event of an **administrative hearing:**
   1. **You** shall notify **us** as soon as practicable of any **administrative hearing.**
   2. **You** shall notify **us** whether **you** have legal services available or require **us** to select an **attorney** for **you.**
   3. a. Send to **us,** as soon as practicable, copies of any notices, summons, or legal papers received in connection with t **administrative hearing.**
      b. Furnish **us,** upon request, with records and other information and submit to an interview by **us** or **our** representat concerning the full extent of his/her knowledge of the events leading to the **administrative hearing. We** shall also entitled to immediately receive upon request copies of any agency or departmental correspondence **you** receive relat to the **administrative hearing,** including specifically any correspondence which may have predated the date of applicat for coverage under this Policy.
      c. Cooperate and assist **us** with all reasonable requests in the handling of an **administrative hearing** including, but (limited to:
         i. Attending depositions and hearings;
         ii. Securing and giving evidence; and
         iii. Obtaining the attendance of witnesses.
C. All **administrative expenses** incurred with respect to appeals and proceedings, or a series of continuous or interrelat appeals and proceedings arising out of an **administrative hearing** shall be considered as part of the original **administrat hearing.**
D. 1. **We** shall pay **administrative expenses** in excess of any other insurance or coverage **you** maintain, no matter how the coverages are described, if:
      a. **You** have legal services other than those provided in this Policy which have the right and duty to defend **you** at **administrative hearing;** and
      b. **You** have paid directly or indirectly for those legal services before the **administrative hearing** was **initiated.**
   If **you** do not have these other legal services:
   2. **We** shall have the right to freely select any **attorney** to represent **you** in the defense of an **administrative hearing.**

V. LIMITS OF LIABILITY

A. The limits shown in the Declarations to the Policy and the information contained in this section indicate the most **we** shall p regardless of the number of:
   1. Persons or organizations covered by this Policy; or
   2. **Claims** made or **suits** brought.
B. Each **wrongful act, bodily injury,** or **property damage** limit is the most **we** shall pay for all loss that results from a sin **wrongful act, bodily injury,** or **property damage.**
C. Aggregate Limit is the most **we** shall pay for all losses covered under this Policy.
D. All **claims** arising from continuous, repeated, or related **wrongful acts** or **occurrences** shall be treated as one **claim.** Such wrong **acts** or **occurrences** shall be considered to have taken place when the earliest **wrongful act** or **occurrence** takes place.
E. Coverage for an **administrative hearing** shall cease when the **Administrative Hearing** Limit is exhausted. For each individ named in Item 1.A. or 1.B. of the Declarations, a separate **Administrative Hearing** Limit shall apply.
F. For each individual named in Item 1.A. or 1.B. of the Declarations a separate Limit of Liability shall apply for each **wrongful a**

VI. EXCLUSIONS FOR ALL INSURING AGREEMENTS

We shall not defend or pay any **claims** against **you** under Insuring Agreements A, B, and C:
A. For any dishonest, criminal, fraudulent or malicious act, error, or omission;
B. For any liability as a proprietor or owner of any clinic with bed and board facilities, hospital, sanitarium, nursing home laboratory or to acts, errors or omissions arising out of or in the course of any trade, business, employment or profession oth than that of a social worker;
C. For any medical, surgical, dental, x-ray or nursing service or treatment, the furnishing of food or beverages in connect therewith or the furnishing or dispensing of drugs or medical, dental or surgical supplies or appliances. The term medi service or treatment used in this exclusion shall not be construed to mean such service performed by **you** at the direction c physician, or the furnishing or use of biofeedback equipment as is usual in **your** practice as a social worker;
D. For matters involving overbilling, miscoding, reimbursement requests, and other fee related matters or inquiries, unless ' action involves an actual disciplinary proceeding where **your** license or ability to practice is threatened;
E. For any **discrimination** on any basis;
F. For any **wrongful act** of a managerial or administrative nature. This exclusion shall not apply to **your** activities as a membe a formal accreditation or professional review board of a hospital or professional society, or professional licensing board;
G. Brought by any Insured, as set forth in Section III. Who Is An Insured, against any other Insured, as set forth in Section III. W Is An Insured;
H. For any **bodily injury** or **property damage** arising out of the ownership, maintenance, operation, use, loading or unloadinç any **automobile,** aircraft or watercraft;
I. For any **bodily injury** or **property damage** to any employee of **yours** or independent contractor working for **you,** or to ; obligation of **you** to indemnify another because of damages arising out of any **bodily injury** or **property damage;**
J. For any actual or alleged infringement of copyright;
K. For any liability arising out of any obligation under a workers' compensation, disability benefits, unemployment compensat law, or any similar law;
L. For **property damage** to:
   1. Property owned or occupied by or rented to **you;**
   2. Property used by **you;**
   3. Property in **your** care, custody or control, or property of which **you** are exercising physical control for any purpose; or

4. Premises sold, given away or abandoned by **you**, if the **property damage** arises out of any part of those premises;

M. For any **wrongful act** committed with knowledge by **you** that it was a **wrongful act**;

N. Any **occurrence** or **wrongful act** of which any **named insured** was aware, prior to the effective date of this Policy, which any **named insured** could have reasonably believed would result in an **administrative hearing**;

O. For:
   1. The actual, alleged or threatened discharge, dispersal, release or escape of **pollutants**; or
   2. Any direction or request to test for, monitor, clean up, remove, contain, treat, detoxify or neutralize **pollutants**;

P. For any of **your** employment activities including, but not limited to, application for employment, refusal to employ, termination of employment, coercion, demotion, evaluation, re-assignment, discipline, **defamation**, harassment including sexual harassment, humiliation, or violation of civil rights;

Q. Arising out of any **wrongful act** committed while **you** did not have a license required by law or while **your** license was suspended;

R. Arising out of any **wrongful act** while **you** were under the influence of an illegal substance or drug or while intoxicated; or

S. Arising out of any business relationship or venture with any prior or current client of **yours**.

VII. EXCLUSIONS FOR INSURING AGREEMENT C, ADMINISTRATIVE HEARING

In addition to the Exclusions for all Insuring Agreements A, B, and C, **we** shall not pay for any **administrative expenses** against **you** under Insuring Agreement C for:

A. Any defense of **criminal prosecution**;

B. Any legal or disciplinary matter other than an **administrative hearing**;

C. Any application for initial placement on a staff as a professional social worker;

D. Any legal action including, but not limited to, **administrative hearing**, commenced by **you**.

VIII. SEXUAL MISCONDUCT PROVISION

A. **Our** Limit of Liability shall not exceed $25,000 in the aggregate for all damages with respect to the total of all **claims** and **suits** against **you** involving any actual or alleged erotic physical contact, or attempt thereat or proposal thereof:
   1. By **you** or by any other person for whom **you** may be legally liable; and
   2. With or to any former or current client of **yours**, or with or to any relative or member of the same household as any said client, or with or to any person with whom said client or relative has an affectionate personal relationship.

B. In the event that any of the foregoing are alleged at any time, either in a complaint, during discovery, at trial or otherwise, any and all causes of action alleged and arising out of the same or related courses of professional treatment and/or relationships shall be subject to the aforesaid $25,000 aggregate Limit of Liability and shall be part of, and not in addition to, the Limits of Liability otherwise afforded by this Policy.

C. **We** shall not be obligated to undertake nor continue to defend any **suit** or proceeding subject to the $25,000 aggregate Limit of Liability after the $25,000 aggregate Limit of Liability has been exhausted by payment of judgments, settlements and/or other items included within the Limits of Liability.

IX. PUNITIVE DAMAGES PROVISION

We shall not pay for fines or penalties or punitive, exemplary or multiplied damages; wherever permitted by law **we** shall pay up to $25,000 in the aggregate for all damages with respect to the total of all **claims** and **suits** against **you** involving punitive, exemplary or multiplied damages as part of and not in addition to the applicable Limits of Liability of this Policy.

X. CONDITIONS

A. WHERE COVERAGE APPLIES

We cover **wrongful acts, bodily injury, property damage** or **administrative hearings** anywhere in the world, but only if a **claim** is made, a **suit** is brought or **administrative hearing initiated** for such **wrongful act, bodily injury, property damage** or **administrative hearing** in the United States of America, its territories and possessions, Puerto Rico, or Canada.

B. **YOUR** ASSISTANCE AND COOPERATION
   1. **You** agree to cooperate with and help **us**:
      a. Make settlements;
      b. Enforce any legal rights **you** or **we** may have against anyone who may be liable to **you**;
      c. Attend depositions, hearings and trials; and
      d. Secure and give evidence, and obtain the attendance of witnesses.

   You shall not admit any liability, assume any financial obligation, or pay out any money without **our** prior consent. If **you** do, it shall be at **your** own expense.

C. LAWSUITS AGAINST **US**
   1. No one can sue **us** to recover under this Policy unless all of the terms have been honored.
   2. A person or organization may sue **us** to recover up to the Limits of Liability under this Policy only after **your** liability has been decided by:
      a. Trial, after which a final judgment has been entered; or
      b. A written settlement agreement signed by **you, us**, and the party making the **claim**.

D. BANKRUPTCY

You or **your** estate's bankruptcy or insolvency shall not relieve **us** of **our** obligations under this Policy.

E. CHANGES

The **named insured** shown in the Declarations is authorized to make changes in the terms of this Policy with **our** written consent. This Policy's terms can be amended or waived only by endorsement issued by **us** and made a part of this Policy.

F. TITLES OF PARAGRAPHS

Titles of paragraphs are inserted solely for convenience of reference and shall not be deemed to limit, expand or otherwise affect the provisions to which they relate.

TRANSFER OF **YOUR** RIGHTS AND DUTIES UNDER THIS POLICY

Your rights and duties under this Policy may not be transferred without **our** written consent. If **you** are declared lega incompetent, **your** rights and duties shall be transferred to **your** legal representative but only while acting within the scope his duties as **your** legal representative.

CONFORMANCE TO STATUTE

To the extent a term of this Policy conflicts with a statute of the State within which this Policy is issued, the term shall deemed amended so as to conform to minimum requirements of the statute.

DUTIES IN THE EVENT OF AN INCIDENT, **CLAIM** OR **SUIT**

1. If, during the **policy period**, incidents or events occur which **you** reasonably believe may give rise to a **claim** or **suit** which coverage may be provided, **you** shall, during the **policy period**, give written notice to **us**. Such written notice sh contain:

    a. The identity of the person(s) alleging the **bodily injury, property damage,** or **wrongful act**:

    b. The identity of the person(s) who allegedly were involved in the incidents or events; and

    c. The date the alleged incidents or events took place.

    And, if **you** submit written notice containing Items a. through c. above, then any **claim** or **suit** that may subsequently made against **you** arising out of such incidents or events shall be deemed, for the purpose of this insurance, to have be first made during the **policy period** in effect at the time such written notice was submitted to **us**.

2. If a **claim** is made or **suit** is brought against **you, you** shall:

    a. Immediately record the specifics of the **claim** and the date received; and

    b. Notify **us** as soon as practicable.

    You shall see to it that **we** receive written notice of this **claim** as soon as practicable.

3. **You** shall:

    a. Immediately send **us** copies of any demands, notices, summonses or legal papers received in connection with a **claim** or **suit**;

    b. Authorize **us** to obtain records and other information;

    c. Cooperate with **us** in the investigation, settlement, or defense of the **claim** or **suit**; and

    d. Assist **us**, upon **our** request, in the enforcement of any right against any person or organization which may be liable **you** because of injury or damage to which this insurance may also apply.

OTHER INSURANCE

If there is other insurance which applies to the loss resulting from **bodily injury, property damage,** or **wrongful act** the oth insurance shall pay first. This Policy applies to the amount of loss which is more than:

a. The Limits of Liability of the other insurance; and

b. The total of all deductibles and self-insured amounts under all such other insurance.

We shall not pay more than **our** Limits of Liability.

MULTIPLE POLICIES

1. Two or more policies may be issued by **us** or other member companies of American International Group, Inc. These polici may provide coverage for:

    a. **Claims** or **suits** arising from the same or related **wrongful act** or **occurrence**; or

    b. Persons or organizations covered in those policies that are jointly and severally liable.

2. In such a case, **we** shall not be liable under this Policy for an amount greater than the proportion of the loss that this Policy applicable Limit of Liability bears to the total applicable Limits of Liability under all such policies.

In addition, the total amount payable under all such policies is the highest applicable Limit of Liability among all such policie

REPRESENTATIONS

1. By accepting this Policy, the **named insured** agrees that the statements in the Application and Declarations are true, ar that they are the **named insured's** agreements and representations.

2. The **named insured** agrees that this Policy is issued in reliance upon the truth of those representations.

3. Any and all relevant provisions may be voided by **us** in any case of fraud, intentional concealment, or misrepresentation material fact by **you**.

TRANSFER OF RIGHTS OF RECOVERY AGAINST OTHERS TO **US**

If **you** have rights to recover all or part of any payment **we** have made under this Policy, those rights are transferred to **us**. Yo shall do nothing to impair them. At **our** request, **you** shall bring **suit** or transfer those rights to **us** and help **us** enforce them

ARBITRATION

1. Any controversy arising out of or relating to this Policy or its breach shall be settled by arbitration in accordance with th rules of the American Arbitration Association. The arbitration panel shall consist of three (3) arbitrators. One of the arbitrato shall be chosen by the **named insured** and one arbitrator shall be chosen by **us**. Those two arbitrators shall then choo the third arbitrator. Unless the parties otherwise agree, the arbitration shall be held in New York, New York.

2. Unless the parties otherwise agree, within thirty (30) days of the parties submitting their case and related documentatio the arbitration panel shall issue a written decision resolving the controversy and stating the facts reviewed, conclusior reached, and the reasons for reaching those conclusions. The arbitration panel may make an award of compensato damages, but shall not award punitive or exemplary damages. The findings of the arbitration panel, however, shall b binding upon **you** or **us**.

3. The **named insured** shall bear the expense of the arbitrator chosen by the **named insured**. **We** shall bear the expense the arbitrator chosen by **us**. The **named insured** and **we** shall share equally the expense of the other arbitrator. Th arbitration panel shall allocate any remaining costs of the arbitration preceding.

AUTOMATIC LIMITED REPORTING PERIOD

1. The **named insured** shall have an automatic limited reporting period of ninety (90) days, starting with the end of the polic **period**, during which **claims** arising out of **wrongful acts, bodily injury** or **property damage** which take place on or aft the **retroactive date** but before the end of the **policy period** may be first made or brought.

2. This automatic limited reporting period shall not extend the **policy period** or change the scope of coverage provided. **We** shall consider any **claim** first made or **suit** brought during the automatic limited reporting period to have been made on the last date on which this Policy is in effect.

3. The automatic limited reporting period shall apply only if this insurance is canceled or not renewed for any reason. Coverage under the automatic limited reporting period cannot be canceled.

4. The automatic limited reporting period, however, shall not apply to **claims** if other insurance **you** buy covers them or would cover them if its Limits of Liability had not been exhausted.

5. The Limits of Liability that apply at the end of the **policy period** are not renewed or increased for **claims** first made or **suits** first brought during the automatic limited reporting period.

P. OPTIONAL REPORTING ENDORSEMENT

1. If the **named insured** or **we** cancel or do not renew this Policy, the **named insured** has the right to buy an Optional Reporting Endorsement. The **named insured** shall not have this right if **we** cancel for non-payment of premium.

2. The endorsement applies only to covered **claims** arising solely out of a **wrongful act, bodily injury**, or **property damage** on or after the **retroactive date** but before the end of the **policy period**. The **claim** shall first be made against you and reported to **us** in writing during the Optional Reporting Period immediately after the **policy period**.

3. To obtain this Optional Reporting Endorsement the **named insured** shall request this endorsement in writing within ninety (90) days after the **policy period** ends and pay the premium when due. If the **named insured** does so, **we** cannot cancel the endorsement. If **we** do not receive the written request and payment as required, the **named insured** may not exercise this right at a later date. If the **named insured** cancels the endorsement, **we** shall not pay any return premium.
   If **you**:
   a. die, or
   b. become permanently disabled so **you** cannot continue as a social worker, or
   c. permanently retire as a social worker;
   We will not charge **you** a premium for the reporting endorsement. **You** will still have to request the reporting endorsement from **us** in writing within 90 days after the **policy period** ends. **You** will have to give **us** reasonable proof of death, permanent disability or permanent retirement. **You** will also have to give **us** written confirmation that during the past 5 years, there have been no **claims** against **you** for sexual misconduct, as described in the "Sexual Misconduct" section of the Policy.

4. Any change in premium or terms from this Policy shall not be considered a refusal to renew.

5. The provision of an Optional Reporting Endorsement shall not increase the Aggregate Limit of Liability described in the Limits of Liability section of this Policy.

XI. CANCELLATION/NONRENEWAL

A. The **named insured** shown in the Declarations may cancel this Policy by mailing or **delivering to us** advance written notice of cancellation.

B. **We** may cancel this Policy by mailing or **delivering to the named insured** written notice of cancellation at least:
   1. Ten (10) days before the effective date of cancellation if **we** cancel for non-payment of premium; or
   2. Sixty (60) days before the effective date of cancellation if **we** cancel for any other reason.

C. **We** shall mail or deliver **our** notice to the **named insured's** address shown in the Declarations.

D. Notice of cancellation shall state the **effective date of cancellation. The policy period** shall end on that date.

E. If this Policy is canceled, **we** shall send the **named insured** any premium refund due. If **we** cancel, the refund shall be pro rata. If the **named insured** cancels, the refund may be less than pro rata. The cancellation shall be effective even if **we** have not made or offered a refund.

F. If notice is mailed, proof of mailing shall be sufficient proof of notice.

G. The Policy cannot be canceled by either party after the premium for an Optional Reporting Period is paid.

H. If **we** decide not to renew this Policy, **we** shall mail or deliver to the first **named insured** shown in the Declarations written notice of the nonrenewal not less than sixty (60) days before the expiration date.
   If notice is mailed, proof of mailing shall be sufficient proof of notice.

IN WITNESS WHEREOF, we have caused this Policy to be signed by **our** President and Secretary and countersigned where required by law on the Declarations page by **our** duly authorized representative.

_____
Secretary

_____
President

ENDORSEMENT

This endorsement, effective   12:01   A.M.,
forms a part of

Policy Number: issued to :

By: American Home Assurance Company

In consideration of the premium charged, it is hereby understood and agreed that
Section II, **Definitions (B), Administrative Hearings,** is deleted in its entirety
and replaced with the following:

Administrative Hearing means a disciplinary proceeding against **you** and shall
be limited to the following:

1. Proceedings initiated by a state licensing board or governmental regulatory
    body against **you** for unprofessional conduct; or

2. Proceedings initiated by a State Department of Health Services or the
    Federal Department of Health and Human Services arising out of **your**
    performance of professional services as a social worker and alleging any
    violation of guidelines for appropriate utilization of those services; or

3. Civil proceedings in which **you** are not a defendant but have been ordered to
    offer deposition testimony regarding treatment rendered to a patient or client;
    or

4. Civil proceedings in which **you** are not a party but have received a subpoena
    for record production.

All other terms, conditions and exclusions shall remain unchanged.

Authorized Representative

83191 (10/03)

Appendix D

Sample Jurisprudence
Exam Questions

Jurisprudence exam questions are often included in initial licensing examinations or constitute a separate examination for license renewal in many states. The following list of questions can be used to prepare for these kinds of examinations. Each question should be answered by applying the laws and rules of the mental health professional's discipline and license.

1. How long can you practice after the expiration of your license?
2. What amount is acceptable remuneration for referral of a client to another licensee?
3. What obligations do you have if a client provides credible information of a sexual relationship with a former therapist?
4. An improper dual relationship occurs when you treat two members of the same family?
5. What are five circumstances when it is permissible for you to violate a client's confidentiality?
6. What is the minimum client record retention period for an adult client?
7. What is the minimum client record retention period for a minor client?
8. Can you have an independent practice, though supervised, with a provisional license or intern status?
9. What is the number of supervised hours an applicant needs for licensure?
10. Who can provide supervision to an applicant for licensure?
11. If you are introduced as Dr. _____ to an audience to whom you are about to deliver a speech and you do not have a PhD or MD, what should you do?

12. Before initiating services what should you inform your clients of in writing?

13. Are you prohibited from raising fees and making the new fees applicable to a client who has not achieved the therapeutic goals and with whom therapy is continuing?

14. Under what circumstances can you refuse to provide a client with a copy of the client's therapy records?

15. If a client moves to another state and wants to continue counseling can you provide distance therapy (i.e., phone or Internet therapy)?

16. A child's divorced mother initially presents the child for therapy and brings the child to 14 therapy sessions. Six months after therapy is concluded, the child contacts you seeking access to all of his or her therapy records. What should you do?

17. What should you do if you observe another licensee snorting cocaine during a Christmas party?

18. Is it permissible for you to include on your business card and in your promotional material that you offer "superior therapeutic services"?

19. A client confesses to you during a therapy session that just after he and his wife moved into the state 10 years ago, he "accidentally" killed his wife during an argument. He then buried her body in a swamp. He has never reported her missing to authorities and since the wife had no close family members no one has asked about her. What should you do?

20. You are served with a subpoena requesting production of a client's therapy records including psychotherapy notes. What should you do?

21. Can you administer a projective assessment instrument?

22. Is an applicant with a felony conviction ineligible for licensing?

23. What is the consequence to you if you choose *not* to submit a licensing renewal application while a complaint filed against you is being investigated by your licensing board?

24. When seeking representation in a divorce, you are assigned a lawyer by the law firm you retained who turns out to be the spouse of one of your clients. What should you do?

25. A client who has lost his job and insurance asks if he can exchange yard maintenance work for therapy. What should you do?

26. Under what circumstance can a dual relationship with a client be acceptable?

27. What information are you required to disseminate to clients regarding your license and the licensing board?

28. A client reveals to you during a therapy session that she strongly believes her husband is sexually touching their 11-year-old daughter. What should you do?

29. A client presents you with a $50.00 gift certificate for a health spa in appreciation for the services you have provided to this client. What should you do?

30. A prospective new client shows up for her first appointment and on an intake form indicates she is currently seeing another therapist. What should you do?

31. What items should be included in each client's file?

32. What should you do if a client expresses suicidal ideation?

33. What should you do if a client expresses homicidal ideation? Does your answer change if the client identifies a potential victim?

34. Is it permissible to charge a client for skipping an appointment without contacting you before the scheduled appointment?

35. Is it permissible to charge a client for skipping an appointment even if the client contacts you in advance of the scheduled session?

36. What are you required to do with respect to the possibility of your death or incapacity in the future?

37. What must you advise a client with respect to confidentiality?

38. What kinds of services and therapies does your license allow you to offer to clients?

39. Once licensed, what are the continuing education requirements required by your licensing board?

40. What do you do if a client, who is still in therapy with you, files a complaint against you with your licensing board?

References and Reading Material

Sources of Current Information

FMS (False Memory) Foundation
3401 Market Street, Suite 130
Philadelphia, PA 19104-3318
(215) 387-1865

Mental Health Law Reporter
Bonnie Becker (Editor)
951 Pershing Drive
Silver Springs, MD 20910-4464
(301) 587-6300

Practice Strategies: A Business Guide for Behavioral Health Care Providers
442½ East Main Street, Suite 2
Clayton, NC 27520
(919) 553-0637

Psychotherapy Finance: Managing Your Practice and Your Money
P.O. Box 8979
Jupiter, FL 33468
(800) 869-8450

References

American Counseling Association. 2007. *2007 mental health professions statistics.* www.counseling.org/Counselors/LicensureAndCert.aspx? (accessed December 24, 2007).

American Psychiatric Association. 1994. *Diagnostic and statistical manual of mental disorders.* 4th ed. Washington, DC: Author.

Bernstein, B., and T. Hartsell. 2004. *The portable lawyer for mental health professionals: An A–Z guide for protecting your clients, your practice, and yourself.* 2nd ed. Hoboken, NJ: John Wiley & Sons.

Bernstein, B., and T. Hartsell. 2005. *The portable guide to testifying in court: An A–Z guide to being an effective witness.* Hoboken, NJ: John Wiley & Sons.

Corey, G., M. S. Corey, and P. Callanan. 1998. *Issues and ethics in the helping professions.* 5th ed. Belmont, CA: Brooks/Cole.

Davis, K. C. 1993. *Administrative law.* New York: Aspen Publishers.

Lawless, L. L. 1999. *How to build and market your mental health practice.* Hoboken, NJ: John Wiley & Sons.

Psychotherapy Finances. 1995. *Managed care handbook: The practitioner's guide to behavioral managed care.* Ridgewood, NJ: Ridgewood Financial Institute.

Roach, W. H., Jr., R. G. Hoban, B. M. Broccolo, A. B. Roth, and T. P. Blanchard. 2006. *Medical records and the law.* 4th ed. New York: Aspen Publishers.

Simon, R. I. 1992. *Clinical psychiatry and the law.* 2nd ed. Arlington, VA: American Psychiatric Press.

Special report: You should be concerned about repressed memory lawsuits. 1998. *Psychotherapy Finances* 24, no. 2 (286), 7.

Stout, C. E., G. A. Theis, and J. Oher. 1996. *The complete guide to managed behavioral healthcare.* Hoboken, NJ: John Wiley & Sons.

U.S. Department of Labor, Bureau of Labor Statistics. (n.d.). Occupational employment statistics: May 2006. www.bls.gov/oes/ (accessed December 24, 2007).

Wiger, D. E. 2005. *The clinical documentation sourcebook: A comprehensive collection of mental health practice forms, handouts, and records.* 2nd ed. Hoboken, NJ: John Wiley & Sons.

Organizations with Periodic Publications on Law and Mental Health

American Association for Marriage and Family Therapists (AAMFT)

American Association of Pastoral Counselors (AAPC)

American Bar Association (ABA; especially mental health or hospital law sections)

American Counseling Association (ACA)

American Medical Association (AMA)

American Mental Health Counselors Association (AMHCA)

American Psychiatric Association

American Psychological Association (APA)

National Association of Social Workers (NASW)

Note: All state licensing boards publish lists of licensed practitioners who have been disciplined by the boards. Usually, the names of the individuals who have been disciplined are given, together with the rule allegedly violated.

Library List for Background

Applebaum, P. *Clinical Handbook of Psychiatry and Law*. Baltimore: Lippincott Williams & Wilkins, 2006.

Banton, R. *The Politics of Mental Health*. London: Macmillan, 1985.

Corey, G., M. Corey, and P. Callanan, *Issues and Ethics in the Helping Professions*, 6th ed. San Francisco, CA: Thomson Learning/Brooks Cole, 2006.

Dutton, M. A. *Empowering and Healing the Battered Woman*. New York: Springer Publishing, 2000.

Hunter, E., and D. Hunter. *Professional Ethics and Law in the Health Sciences*. Melbourne, FL: Krieger Publishing, 1990.

Pederson, P. *Handbook of Cross-Cultural Counseling and Therapy*. Westport, CT: Greenwood Publishing Group, 1987.

Rosner, R., ed. *Ethical Practice in Psychiatry and the Law*. Berlin: Kluwer, 1990.

Shuman, D. W. *Law and Mental Health Professionals*, 3rd ed., Washington, DC: American Psychological Association Press, 2004.

Steiner, H., ed. *Handbook of Mental Health Interventions in Children and Adolescents: An Integrated Developmental Approach.* San Francisco: Jossey-Bass, 2004.

Web Sites

American Association for Marriage and Family Therapists
www.aamft.org

American Counseling Association
www.counseling.org

American Psychological Association
www.apa.org

National Association of Social Workers
www.naswdc.org

American School Counselor Association
www.schoolcounselor.org

Art Therapy Credentials Board
www.atcb.org

Index